NEUROSCIENCE RESEARCH PROGRESS

SYNAPTIC FUNDAMENTALS OF MEMORY PERFORMANCE

NEUROSCIENCE RESEARCH PROGRESS

Additional books in this series can be found on Nova's website under the Series tab.

Additional e-books in this series can be found on Nova's website under the e-book tab.

NEUROSCIENCE RESEARCH PROGRESS

SYNAPTIC FUNDAMENTALS OF MEMORY PERFORMANCE

IGNACIO GONZÁLEZ-BURGOS
EDITOR

nova publishers
New York

Library of Congress Cataloging-in-Publication Data

ISBN: 978-1-63483-279-3
Library of Congress Control Number: 2015943819

Published by Nova Science Publishers, Inc. † New York

CONTENTS

PREFACE

Synaptic activity is how neurons communicate, transmitting chemical information between one another. Synaptic activity is regulated by many factors, including neurotransmitters, hormones and glial cells. Through very dynamic bioelectric signals, synaptic activity provokes the transmission of information that becomes integrated into the post-synaptic element of the synaptic complex. These interactions can provoke the plastic changes in neuronal cytoarchitecture that are subsequently translated into a wide range of responses, which when integrated into functional circuits reflect the organization of various psychoneural processes that underlie behavior. One group of such processes is known generically as cognitive processes, including learning and memory. Both these processes stand out as an essential link between the individual and his environment, by virtue of which both favor adaptation that joins the present with the past and future, whether in the short- or long-term. Memory performance may be normal or atypical, the latter expressing some unusual features, such as those that constitute part of illnesses that course with cognitive impairment.

Synaptic Fundamentals of Memory Performance aims to describe some of the microenvironmental factors that modulate synaptic activity and how this relates to the cerebral organization of learning and memory under certain conditions, be they normal or atypical. Among the microenvironmental factors addressed in this book are several subcellular elements and events as genes, synapse-associated molecules and signaling pathways, coupled to hormonal actions to favor plastic changes underlying cerebral organization of learning and memory. Furthermore, long-term spatial memory and some of its time course-related determinants, the impact of music-induced emotions in short- or long-term memory encoding, some genetics-associated mental illness, and memory impairments in neuroinflammation and in Alzheimer's disease, are also addressed in the light of synaptic activity.

Dr. Ignacio González-Burgos, PhD
Centro de Investigación Biomédica de Occidente
Instituto Mexicano del Seguro Social
Sierra Mojada #800 Col. Independencia
C.P. 44340 Guadalajara, Jalisco, México
Email: igonbur@hotmail.com

In: Synaptic Fundamentals of Memory Performance
Editor: Ignacio González-Burgos
ISBN: 978-1-63483-279-3

Chapter 1

SYNAPTOGENES, SIGNALING PATHWAYS AND INTELLECTUAL DISABILITY SYNDROMES

Patricio Barros Núñez[1,*], Mónica Alejandra Rosales Reynoso[2] and Berenice Ochoa Hernández[1]

[1]División de Genética, Centro de Investigación Biomédica de Occidente, Instituto Mexicano del Seguro Social. Guadalajara, Jalisco, México
[2]División de Medicina Molecular, Centro de Investigación Biomédica de Occidente, Instituto Mexicano del Seguro Social, Guadalajara, Jalisco, México

ABSTRACT

The proteome of synapse includes a very large number of proteins involved in several highly complex metabolic signaling pathways, which are frequently disturbed by a number of gene mutations and causing over 100 brain diseases; among them, intellectual disability syndromes represent a major health problem.

The discovery of the genetic causes of intellectual disabilities and disorders associated with autism spectrum has improved our understanding of the molecular pathways critical for normal synaptic function. Intellectual disability disorders have been found associated with numerous mutated genes that code for proteins involved in the synapse construction, the dendritic spine morphology, the regulation of the synaptic cytoskeleton or the synthesis and degradation of specific synapse proteins. Most studies have strongly demonstrated that even mild alterations in synapse morphology and function give rise to mild or severe alteration in intellectual abilities. Analyzes of the underlying mechanisms using gain and loss of function approaches have revealed alterations of spine morphology, density or plasticity, raising the possibility that these disorders result from synaptopathies. Although a multiplicity of genes and proteins has been involved, data points to specific signaling pathways as implicated in the pathogenesis of many synaptopathies, among which small guanine tri phosphatases (GTPases), the cytoskeletal regulatory signaling proteins, the cell adhesion molecules (CAMs), and the calcium and cyclic nucleotide signaling, appear to play a central role.

* Corresponding author: Dr. Patricio Barros Núñez. División de Genética, Centro de Investigación Biomédica de Occidente. Instituto Mexicano del Seguro Social. Sierra Mojada 800. Colonia Independencia, CP: 44340. Guadalajara, Jalisco, México. E-mail: pbarros_gdl@yahoo.com.mx.

1. INTRODUCTION

During embryonic neuronal development, axons migrate in the brain and body towards specific target regions to establish functional synaptic connections. Synapses are specialized neural structures that communicate a presynaptic neuron with a postsynaptic cell.

For the majority of neurons, an action potential in the presynaptic axon stimulates the release of chemical neurotransmitters that activate a specific receptor on the postsynaptic membranes, opening ion channels and activating signaling cascades. There are numerous types of synapses which can be identified by the type of neurotransmitter released from the presynaptic terminal and the specific involved cells. Synaptogenesis (formation of new synapses) involves some functional and structural cell changes that are initiated through ligand-receptor interactions, intracellular signaling, and remodeling of actin filamentous. Complex intracellular processes contribute actively to the formation of synaptic components long before the dendrite or axon arrives at the synaptic sites. Together, other mechanisms inhibit the formation of abnormal synapses (Shen and Cowan, 2009). The detailed molecular processes that control synaptogenesis are still poorly understood. Advances in microscopy and modern molecular and genetic research have allowed identify key steps in the synapse formation. An important portion of this knowledge was obtained from analysis of either the neuromuscular junction or the axodendritic synapse between two neurons.

Obviously, substantial differences exist between both processes as also between the molecules involved in these two types of synapses. Furthermore, each subtype of the synapse (excitatory, inhibitory or neuromodulatory), has distinct mechanisms controlling its formation and plasticity. On the other hand, functionally mature synapses are not inert; instead modify their strength and number in response to an activity to facilitate complex behavioral plasticity (Shen and Cowan, 2009). By what means a neuron (axon or dendrite) choose among numerous available neurons to build a functional and durable synapse? Rarely synapses are made at their first encounter. Instead, the long marriage of the pre- and postsynaptic partners is a consequence of a lengthy process that involves a series of meetings, dancing and touching. Only the correct partners eventually merge. The cellular and molecular mechanisms underlying the formation of specific synaptic connections are intricate and even not completely known. Regardless of its complexity, synaptogenesis involves two sequential processes. First, the presynaptic axon and postsynaptic dendrites need to have the right "physical chemistry". Second, after initial molecular interactions that ensure the parties have the right matches, an activity-dependent process occurs. The synaptic meeting between two cells does not occur in a one-by-one mode; instead, often there are competitions. The synapse gets refined and strengthened if the pre- and postsynaptic partners negotiate in synchrony; those partners who cannot speak harmoniously (asynchronously) are eliminated (Lu et al., 2009). In this chapter, the most recent progress in identifying synaptogenic and anti-synaptogenic factors that strengthen the appropriate connections will be highlighted.

An actualized review of new studies show how the early axon-dendritic interactions help to find the correct synaptic partners; how these process are controlled by signaling cascades and genetic pathways, and how the neuronal activity controls the expression of genes that shape and coordinate the formation and stability of neuronal circuits, and finally, which pathologies affecting the neuronal development are related to specific genes or genetic signaling pathways.

2. SYNAPTOGENESIS

2.1. Preselecting of Synaptic Partners

Dendritic filopodia, the precursor of dendritic spines, seem to know which axonal targets are suitable for a long-term relationship after initial contacts (Figure 1). In cultures of hippocampal CA3 pyramidal cells, Lohmann and Bonhoeffer (2008) observed that filopodia grow, retract, and search for appropriate sites along the axons to make contacts. The lifetimes for the majority of the contacts are very short (one minute), and only a few contacts eventually become stable synapses on glutamatergic axons. Remarkably, although dendritic filopodia frequently contacted GABAergic axons, such contacts never form stable synapses (Lohmann and Bonhoeffer, 2008). On the contrary, protrusions from GABAergic axons also make transient contacts with the dendritic shaft, but they are never transformed into stable contacts. Unlike glutamatergic synapses, new GABAergic synapses were formed exclusively by new boutons at pre-existing axon-dendrite crossings without the involvement of any dendritic or axonal protrusions (Wierenga et al., 2008).

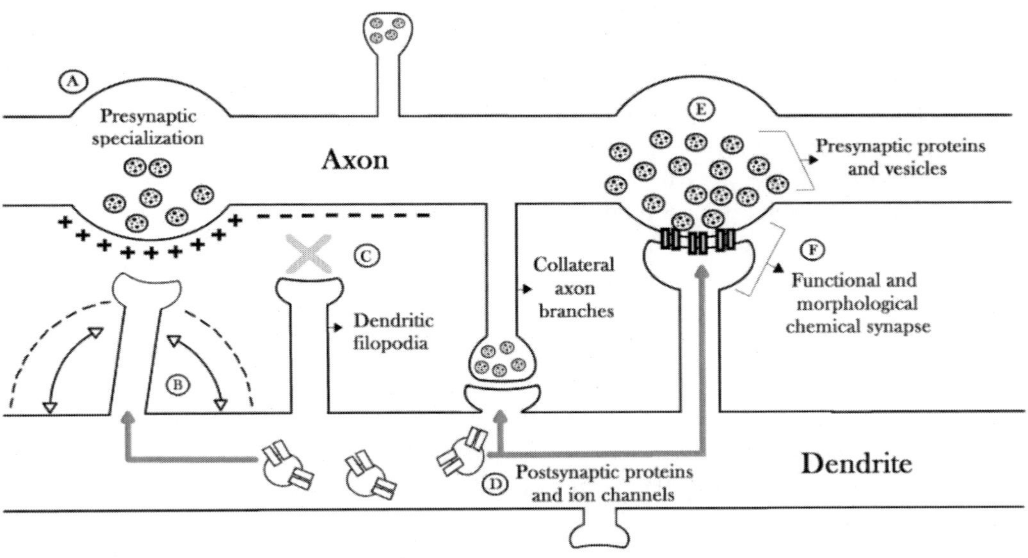

Modified from Shen and Cowan, 2009.

Figure 1. The basic mechanism of axo-dendritic synaptogenesis. The diagram illustrates the time-line of synaptogenesis showing key steps involved in forming a passant type of synapses. (A) Axon and nearby dendrite interact via cell–cell contacts mediated by collateral axon branches and filopodial dendritic extensions. (B) Pre-established presynaptic specializations mark the location of future synapses (+++), whereas (C) inappropriate axonal regions impede synapse formation (- - -). Frequently, random interactions between axon and dendrite filopodia form transient cell–cell adhesions. If the contacts are stable, presynaptic and postsynaptic proteins, vesicles, and ion channels are recruited to the contact site (D). Stable contacts are then matured into functional and morphological chemical synapses (F).

While specific molecules that inhibit the bonding between GABAergic axons and dendritic spines remain to be identified, there exist evidence that local Ca^{2+} in dendritic filopodia play a critical role: 1) Ca^{2+} transients increases after filopodia-axon contacts are made; 2) the increase in local Ca^{2+} is more pronounced at stable contacts than at transitory contacts; 3) the Ca^{2+} change is not observed in filopodia contacting GABAergic axons (Lohmann and Bonhoeffer, 2008).

Since this Ca^{2+} transient was independent of glutamatergic transmission, non-synaptic signaling initiated by contact, perhaps through cell adhesion molecules (CAMs), might contribute to the initial selection of appropriate synaptic partners (Lohmann and Bonhoeffer, 2008). The appropriate targeting of axons is a crucial process for proper neural circuit formation, and the axon is an obligate partner of the functional synapse (Figure 1). The axon guidance involves the interaction of receptor proteins on the surface of navigating growth cones with secreted or cell surface-bound ligands found in the target field.

Binding of ligand to receptor often stimulates intracellular signaling that coordinate complex cell morphological changes in the axon growth cone to move toward (attraction) or away from (repulsion) the guidance cue source. At seems, the interaction between an axon and a postsynaptic cell appears to trigger signaling events necessary for synapse formation, and in some cases, involves complex morphological changes that are mediated by assembly and disassembly of the F-actin cytoskeleton. The main process controlling the morphological changes in both navigating growth cones and dendritic spines is the regulation of F-actin. Spines are on 90% of excitatory glutamatergic synapses in the mature brain, and, although the detailed role of dendritic spines is still incomplete, probably they are crucial in proper synaptic transmission (Shen and Cowan, 2009).

In the navigating axon, guidance cues trigger localized changes in the growth cone morphology that promote axon outgrowth or turning (attraction or repulsion). In a similar mode, the dendritic spines provide an anatomic compartment to dendrite that may restrict synaptic activity by signaling events to the activated synapse (Goldberg et al., 2003; Soler-Llavina and Sabatini 2006). In an axon growth cone, rapidly extending and retracting filopodial structures are thought to search the local environment for guidance cues. Similarly, highly dynamic, dendritic filopodia extend from the dendritic shaft during the robust periods of synaptogenesis, and appear to search the proximal space for a potential presynaptic axon in the vicinity. This process likely increases the probability of making axodendritic contacts and forming functional synapses.

However, the physical interaction between dendritic filopodium and axon is not sufficient to induce a synapse as many contacts are transient. Cell-surface proteins and intracellular signaling pathways likely determine whether an axodendritic interaction proceeds to form a synapse or whether the contact is "repelled" (Shen and Cowan, 2009).

2.2. Synaptogenic and Anti-Synaptogenic Factors

After initial contacts, development of synapse depends basically on the right molecular chemistry. Probably, neuroligins and neurexins are the best known trans-synaptic CAMs connecting pre- and postsynaptic cells. Analyzes *in vitro* demonstrated that neuroligins and neurexins can initiate pre- and postsynaptic specializations, suggesting that these molecules participate to build bidirectional synaptogenesis (Sudhof, 2008).

Analyzes *in vivo* suggest however that neuroligins are not required for initial establishment of synapses, but play critical roles in the regulation of the functional maturation of synapses. Neuroligin 1 (NLGN1) is preferentially localized at excitatory synapses whereas neuroligin 2 (NLGN2) at inhibitory synapses (Song et al., 1999; Varoqueaux et al., 2004). Overexpression of *Nlgn-1* or *Nlgn-2* in neuronal cultures increases excitatory or inhibitory synaptic responses, respectively (Chubykin et al., 2007).

Meanwhile a point mutation of *Nlgn-3* increases inhibitory synaptic transmission, possibly due to a gain-of-function effect (Tabuchi et al., 2007). Together, these results demonstrate that the balance between NLGN1, 2 and 3 signaling perhaps regulate the excitatory/inhibitory ratio and the proper maturation of synaptic junctions.

Eph/ephrin is another known synaptic receptor-ligand pair, which mediates trans-bidirectional synaptic signaling. Studies on EphB1-3 knockout mice showed that the binding of presynaptic ephrins to, and the activation of postsynaptic Eph receptors, is required for spine morphogenesis (Klein, 2009). EphrinBs are also present in the dendrites of hippocampal neurons, and its reverse signaling can trigger spine and synapse formation in postsynaptic neurons (Segura et al., 2007).

Also to synaptogenic factors, anti-synaptogenic factors have also been studied in synapse formation. For example, Wnt4 could act as an anti-synaptogenic signal, preventing the development of the neuromuscular synapse in *Drosophila* (Inaki et al., 2007). Wnt/Lin-44 and Unc-6/Netrin are expressed in different tissues and act in concert to restrict synapse formation in specific domains of the axon where both molecules are absent.

These results indicate that the spatial specificity of synapses is regulated not only by attraction from the target but also by exclusion from neighboring cells or local environments (Klassen and Shen, 2007).

Some anti-synaptogenic factors can also control timing of synaptogenesis. As an example, Slit1a, through the Robo2 receptor, inhibits arborization and synaptogenesis of retinal ganglion cells in zebrafish. When Slit-Robo signaling is absent, arbors form earlier, suggesting that Slit-Robo prevents premature synapse formation. Similarly, polysialic acid (PSA), which is attached to NCAM, prevents precocious maturation of GABAergic synapses in the visual cortex of mammals (Campbell et al., 2007; Di Cristo et al., 2007).

2.3. Activity-Regulated Gene Expression

Certainly, genetically established molecular recognition mechanisms should be important in joining specific synaptic partners; however, neural activity-regulated gene expression appear to orchestrate the assembly of neural circuits, which contain synaptic connections among diverse types of neurons. Genome-wide gene expression analyzes have revealed several hundreds of genes regulated by membrane depolarization or neural transmitter release. In a general mode, these genes encode both transcription factors and downstream effectors and regulators of synaptogenesis. Recent studies have showed the importance of several activity-regulated transcription factors in controlling synapse development. They can regulate the concentration of glutamatergic or GABAergic synapses, and affect this balance through activity-dependent positive or negative feedback loops in individual cells or across neuronal circuits (Flavell and Greenberg, 2008). MeCP2, a transcriptional regulator that binds to methylated DNA, promote the number and strength of excitatory synaptic connections. Loss of MeCP2 in mice cause decreased excitatory synaptic responses and reduced excitatory synapse numbers, although inhibitory synaptic responses are normal. Conversely, increased MeCP2 expression enhances the excitatory synaptic responses and synapse formation (Dani et al., 2005). Neuronal activity produces the phosphorylation of MeCP2, which is necessary for induction of target genes and modulation of dendritic growth and spine maturation; MeCP2 participate in an activity-dependent positive feedback to promote excitatory synaptogenesis. In contrast, the activity-dependent transcription factor MEF2 restricts the number of excitatory synapses (Zhou et al., 2006).

Disrupted *MEF2* function *in vitro* or *in vivo* results in an increase, whereas overexpression of MEF2 results in a decrease of excitatory synapses. Since increased neuronal activity dephosphorylates MEF2, activates MEF2 mediated transcription of target genes, and suppresses excitatory synapse numbers (Flavell et al., 2006; Barbosa et al., 2008).

Another group of activity-regulated genes encodes molecules that are effectors or regulators of synapses such as Arc, Homer, Cpg15, MHC Class I (Chowdhury et al., 2006; Wang et al., 2006; Goddard et al., 2007). Of particular interest is the activity-dependent transcription of BDNF through promoter IV. Disruption of *Bdnf*-promoter IV function appears to affect selectively the development of cortical inhibition (Hong et al., 2008).

3. Signaling Mechanisms Regulating Synapse Formation and Function

Major progress has been carried out in the last two decades in the identification of genetic alterations associated with intellectual disability (ID) and autism spectrum disorders (ASD). In many instances, these defects concern genes coding for synaptic proteins or proteins involved in the regulation of synaptic properties. Research of causal mechanisms using gain and loss of function approaches have revealed alterations of spine morphology, density or plasticity, raising the possibility that these disorders result from synaptopathies. There are some genes and proteins involved in specific signaling pathways like GTPases, which seem to play a central role in this type of genetic alterations. Recent studies in some molecular pathways that regulate axon guidance and synaptogenesis in early brain development demonstrate mutations in genes involved in synapse formation and increase the risk of developing autism and neurodevelopment disorders.

3.1. GTPases Signaling Pathway

Among the genes currently related to ID or ASD, there exist several groups implicated in the postsynaptic signaling. Evidently, a significant fraction of these genes codes for synaptic proteins associated with signaling by GTPases and functioning as regulators or effectors (Figure 2). The GTPases represent a large family of proteins characterized by their capacity to bind and hydrolyze GTP. They act as molecular switches affecting various biological activities regulating growth and migration of many cell types. Their mechanism of action is, therefore, not restricted to neurons and synapses, and some of these non-synaptic roles could be important for their pathophysiological implication in ID.

The complexity of their action is in great part related to the variety of these modulators and the different molecular partners or protein complexes with which they interact, affecting in this way multiple systems.

The principal modulators include guanine-nucleotide exchange factors (GEFs) and inhibitors such as GTPase activating proteins (GAPs) and guanine nucleotide dissociation inhibitors or GDIs (Chen et al., 2009).

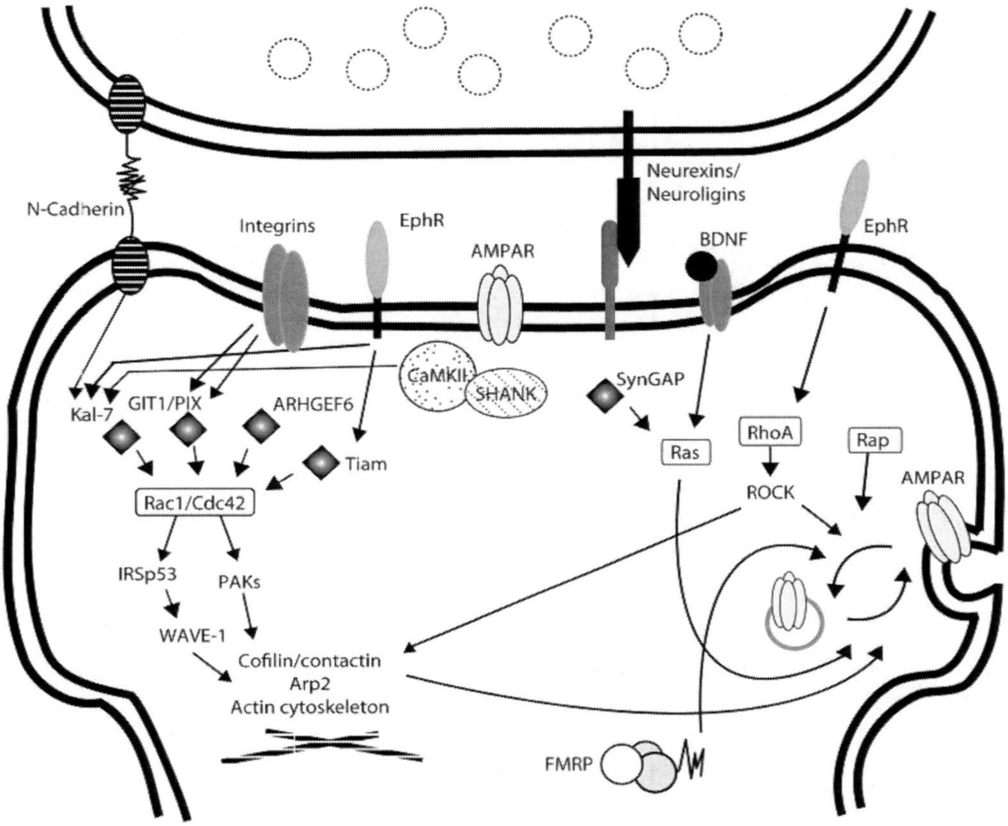

Modified from Boda et al., 2010.

Figure 2. Diagram illustrating the signaling pathways related with small GTPases at synapses. These signaling pathways converge directly on the regulation of receptor trafficking, and indirectly through the control of the actin cytoskeleton. Not all the signaling interactions are illustrated.

3.1.1. Ras and Rho GTPases

Ras and Rho-GTPase signaling pathways represent two distinct molecular networks that have opposing functions in developing axons (Figure 2). Classically, Ras GTPases promote axon outgrowth by regulating the stability of microtubules in the axon. Ras activation inactivates glycogen synthase kinase 3β (GSK-3β) a microtubule destabilizing protein, through the activation of the PI3-kinase/Akt signaling pathway (Govek et al., 2004; Khelfaoui et al., 2007; Nadif et al., 2008; Nadif et al., 2009; Khelfaoui et al., 2009).

Normally, when an axon growth cone encounters a repulsive cue (Figure 1), Ras signaling is decreased while Rho-GTPase signaling is increased to reorganize the F-actin cytoskeleton (Nakano-Kobayashi et al., 2009).

Although the role of Ras signaling is crucial in coordinating guidance and outgrowth, its precise regulation and function in repulsive axon guidance is poorly understood. Several studies on the Sema4D/PlexinB1 receptor revealed coordinated regulation of the Rho and Ras signaling pathways in repulsive axon guidance (Ito et al., 2006). Plexins possess intracellular Ras-GAP functional domains. PlexinB1 activation results in a decrease in R-Ras activity and destabilization of microtubules in the axon (Govek et al., 2004; Fu et al., 2007). Similar and coordinated Rho/Ras signaling has been reported for the Eph Receptors, such that activated EphB receptors recruit p120-Ras-GAP, which in turn facilitates the inhibition of R-Ras signaling by accelerating its GTP hydrolysis.

The interplay of the Rho/Ras GTPases in axon guidance is obviously complex, but it highlights the importance of these signaling factors for axon guidance (Bernstein and Bamburg, 2010; Rex et al., 2009).

3.1.2. Ras/Rap GTPases Family

Ras and Rap are closely related GTPases that function in different but interconnected signaling networks (Figure 2). Their specificity is given by their different upstream regulatory proteins and downstream effectors (Meng et al., 2002). Their implication in MR is currently linked to two regulatory proteins: SynGAP, a Ras/Rap GTPase-activating protein, recently described to be mutated in patients with MR (Boda et al., 2004) and Epac2 or Rap-GEF4, for which variants have been detected in autism (Node-Langlois et al., 2006). SynGAP was demonstrated to play an important role in the regulation of AMPA receptors (AMPAR) (Meng et al., 2005). Carlisle et al., in 2008 showed that heterozygous deletion of SynGAP also affected spine morphology, promoting an increase in mushroom spines, which was associated with increased levels of Ras and Rac-GTP, and increased phosphorylation of cofilin. The authors suggested that SynGAP could have acted through Rac signaling and the cytoskeleton. Other evidence however directly implicates Ras and Rap signaling in the control of receptor trafficking. Activation of this pathway in mice expressing constitutively active Rap2 resulted in fewer and shorter dendritic spines in CA1 neurons, defects in spatial learning and extinction of contextual fear (Haditsch et al., 2009). Hu et al., reported a selective deficit in the synaptic delivery of GluR1 containing AMPARs resulting in a loss of GluR1-dependent LTP in these mice. This effect was associated with a defect in the signaling between Ras, phosphoinositide3-kinase (PI3K) and protein kinase B (PKB) consistent with an inefficient signaling. All together these studies support the hypothesis that Ras and Rap have opposing effects in the regulation of AMPAR delivery to synapses and that this mechanism could represent a primary cause for the alterations of spine morphology (Hu et al., 2008).

3.1.3. Ras and Rho-GTPases Signaling

Ras and Rho-GTPase molecules are two of the most commonly employed signaling molecules in the developing axon growth cone, and both molecules fall into the Ras GTPase superfamily of nearly 200 proteins. Interestingly, this protein superfamily participates in a broad range of cellular and developmental processes. Small GTPases, like other G proteins, are active when bound to guanosine triphosphate (GTP), and are inactivated following hydrolysis of bound GTP to guanosine diphosphate (GDP). This molecular switch is regulated by guanine nucleotide exchange factors (GEFs), which promote the release of bound GDP and allow for binding to GTP. In contrast, inactivation of the GTPases is regulated by GTPase activating proteins (GAPs), which bind to and accelerate GTP hydrolysis (Xie et al., 2007; Sawallisch et al., 2009).

Rho-family GTPases are key regulators of the F-actin cytoskeleton, and function by promoting the formation, branching, or disassembly of F-actin scaffolds (Figure 2). These F-actin scaffolds support the cells shape, and they provide dynamic control over cell membrane protrusion, retraction, or key internalization mechanisms of cell migration. Rho-GTPases, of which there are over 20 different genes, play important roles in the dynamics, forward movement, and retraction of the F-actin cytoskeleton in a navigating axon growth cone (Penzes et al., 2003; Tolias et al., 2007). Rho-family is divided into three major subgroups: Rho, Rac, and Cdc42.

In general, Rac-GTP promotes the formation of highly branched F-actin structures called lamellipodia while Cdc42-GTP promotes the formation of unbranched F-actin structures called filopodia. Finally, RhoA-GTP is reported to regulate F-actin severing and contractility via regulation of F-actin and type-II myosin structures (Xie et al., 2008).

Netrin1 is an axon guidance protein that binds to the Deleted Colorectal Cancer (DCC) receptor in growth cones and induces attraction and axon growth cone extension during the development of various mammalian white matter tracts, including commissural axons in the spinal cord (Webb et al., 2007) and the cerebral cortex (Wu et al., 2008). Netrin binding to the DCC receptor promotes the generation of active Rac1-GTP and Cdc42-GTP while RhoA and its downstream effector Rho-kinase (ROCK), are switched off (Raaijmakers et al., 2009). The coordinated increase in Rac/Cdc42 and the decrease in RhoA activity promote axon outgrowth (Hamdan et al., 2009).

For axon growth cone repulsion, many ligand-activated guidance receptors activate or at least require, RhoA-GTP to initiate F-actin disassembly and retraction (Rumbaugh et al., 2006; Carlisle, 2008). Thus, RhoA-mediated growth cone remodeling is a common downstream signaling cascade resulting in growth cone repulsion or collapse.

More evidence related to RhoA signaling in MR comes from studies of the synaptic function of Oligophrenin1, a Rho-GAP for which several mutations or deletions have been identified in patients suffering from MR (Zhu et al., 2005). Upon knockdown of Oligophrenin1 in pyramidal neurons, several important defects have been reported. The first one was a decrease in spine length. Constitutively active RhoA could mimic this effect and rescued by an inhibitor of the RhoA effector, suggesting a regulation by RhoA of the spine actin skeleton (Ryu et al., 2008).

Further studies of Oligophrenin1 deficient mice also revealed behavioral deficits in spatial memory and social recognition, as well as alterations of presynaptic facilitation (Kielland et al., 2009). In another study, Nadif-Kasri et al., (2009), using an acute down-expression or over-expression approach in slice cultures, showed that Oligophrenin1 suppression decrease in AMPA and NMDA receptor-mediated currents, while over-expression selectively increased AMPA currents; moreover, suppression of Oligophrenin1 was associated with impairment of LTP and structural plasticity. Consistent with this, Oligophrenin1 is driven by NMDA activity in dendritic spines, where it co-localizes with AMPAR and co-precipitates with them. This suggested, therefore, that Oligophrenin1 could promote AMPAR stabilization at synapses, thus enhancing transmission and favoring spine maturation and maintenance. Interestingly, the defects in Oligophrenin 1 null mice could be rescued by ROCK inhibitors, opening new avenues for the development of therapeutic strategies.

These new data demonstrate a critical role played by RhoA/ROCK signaling in regulating AMPAR endocytosis at excitatory synapses and provide a new understanding of the mechanisms through which Oligophrenin1 could contribute to cognitive deficits. Another interesting issue is to understand how this RhoA/ROCK pathway is activated at synapses. The work of Nadif-Kasri et al., (2009), indicates that this activity certainly plays a major role by promoting the translocation of Oligophrenin1 in dendritic spines. Another mechanism could involve the MR gene *MAGI2*, coding for a scaffolding molecule (S-SCAM) that has multiple functions at the synapse. One of them could be to activate RhoA in response to NMDA receptor stimulation. The RhoA/ROCK pathway might be regulated by other molecules among which are Ephrin receptors.

Specifically, Fu et al., (2007) showed that Eph4A may regulate the activation of RhoA at synapses through activation of Cdk5 and the RhoA guanosine exchange factor ephexin1. Activation of this pathway resulted in dendritic spine retraction.

3.2. Rac1/Cdc42/PAKs Signaling

The Rac/Cdc42/PAK signaling pathway has been associated in multiple ways with ID. Some proteins linked to this pathway have been found mutated in ID patients. These include not only upstream regulators of Rac/Cdc42 such as ARHGEF6, SrGAP3, and FGD1, but also downstream effectors such as PAK3 and LIMK. These effectors are important regulators of the actin cytoskeleton and, in particular, their activation leads to the phosphorylation of cofilin, one of the central functional players in the regulation of actin dynamics (Figure 2). Cofilin can be phosphorylated through two GTPase cascades: Rac/Cdc42/PAK or RhoA/ROCK, both of them through LIMK (Rex et al., 2009; Bernstein and Bamburg, 2010).

In these mechanisms, Rac/Cdc42/PAK signaling is believed to transfer information from transmembrane proteins to the actin cytoskeleton and thus control a great variety of biological functions including not only cell motility, but also receptor delivery to the cell surface. ARHGEF6, PAK3, and LIMK have shown to be expressed at synapses and result in alterations of spine morphology or function upon knockdown or over-expression (Boda et al., 2004). Expression of mutant variants of ARHGEF6 and PAK3 was found to result in morphological alterations of spines with an increase in spines with small immature heads and a decrease in classical mushroom type spines.

In cells expressing PAK3 mutants, this effect was associated with a decrease in the ratio of AMPA/NMDA receptors, and an impairment of LTP. PAK3 deficient mice also showed impaired LTP and deficiencies in learning and memory (Meng et al., 2005). Moreover, the defects observed in cells expressing mutant AHRGEF6 could be rescued by PAK3 activation, confirming that the two molecules are involved in the same signaling pathway (Node-Langlois et al., 2006). Some evidence also suggests that Cdc42 might play a more important role than Rac1 in these synaptic mechanisms (Kreis et al., 2007).

More recent works revealed that phosphorylation of PAK and cofilin is a critical step in the mechanisms of long-term potentiation (Chen et al., 2007; Fedulov et al., 2007). Evidence from *in vivo* experiments in which Rac1 was selectively suppressed in forebrain excitatory neurons showed that this affects spine morphology, impairs synaptic plasticity and interferes with spatial learning (Haditsch et al., 2009). In a recent and very elegant *in vitro* study, Rex et al., showed that RhoA/ROCK signaling, and the Rac/Cdc42/PAK cascade both regulate in different ways synaptic plasticity. While RhoA/ROCK was required to induce stable LTP, inhibition of Rac or PAK leads to a prolonged vulnerability of LTP to reversal, indicating that this signaling pathway is critical for the stabilization of the increase in synaptic efficacy. This finding thus suggests that actin might shift from a dynamic to a stable state following the induction of LTP and thus eventually account for the consolidation of LTP (Rex et al., 2009).

Regulation of the Rac/Cdc42/PAK signaling cascade probably be quite complex and implicate several potential partners. For example, the Rho GAP SrGAP3, which has associated with the scaffolding protein WAVE-1 and inhibits Rac function (Endris et al., 2002). Suppression of WAVE-1 was found to affect growth cone dynamics and spine density and to result in altered synaptic plasticity and learning deficits (Soderling et al., 2007).

More recent evidence has also implicated IRSp53 (insulin receptor substrate of 53 kDa) in this signaling. IRSp53 is an adapter protein that binds Rac and Cdc42 and acts downstream of Rac/Cdc42. It interacts with Shank and various actin regulatory proteins to control actin polymerization and filopodia formation. Two recent studies that analyzed IRSp53 deficient mice show that the suppression of IRSp53 is associated with a reduced AMPA/NMDA ratio, an increased long-term potentiation, but learning deficits (Kim et al., 2009; Sawallisch et al., 2009). Another interesting question regarding Rac1/Cdc42/PAK signaling concerns the mechanisms that activate the cascade. Theta burst activity is certainly capable of triggering the signaling in the hippocampus since it is associated with a marked increase in phosphorylated PAK in individual spines (Chen et al., 2007). One mechanism that could account for this activity-dependency involves the phosphorylation of kalirin-7 a Rho-GEF present at synapses and shown to regulate the size of dendritic spines through activation of Rac1 and PAKs (Xie et al., 2007).

There are however several adhesion systems that could also participate in this activation. EphrinB receptors have been proposed to act through activation of kalirin-7 (Penzes et al., 2003). They could also participate together with NMDA receptors to the activation of another Rac1 specific GEF, Tiam, and thus regulate spine morphogenesis (Tolias et al., 2007). There is also evidence that N-cadherin could signal to the cytoskeleton via activation of Rac/Cdc42/PAK. Studies of Xie et al., (2008) showed that N-cadherin adhesion modulates the morphology of spines through an interaction with the scaffolding protein AF-6/afadin that forms a multi-molecular complex containing kalirin-7, thus leading to Rac1 and PAK activation and an enlargement of the spine head. Finally, integrins have also been linked to Rac1 signaling through the adaptor protein GIT1 (Webb et al., 2007).

Altogether these results suggest that the Rac/Cdc42/PAK signaling cascade integrates activity and trans-synaptic signals to fine-tune the spine actin cytoskeleton, controlling in this way the growth, size, and morphology of spines, but possibly also exocytotic mechanisms and receptor trafficking. Cdc42, for example, has been directly implicated in the control of exocytosis and the trafficking of membrane proteins in the synaptic terminals (Wu et al., 2008).

3.3. Cytoskeletal Regulatory Signaling

While Rho-GTPases are a common signaling component of axon guidance signaling, some receptors regulate the F-actin cytoskeleton through association with actin-modifying proteins. F-actin cytoskeletal changes occur largely in the outer peripheral zone of the axon growth cone, where F-actin polymers are structured in bundles and interweaving meshworks. Actin-modifying proteins generate and protect pointed, or "barbed," F-actin ends that are required for polymer elongation and axonal extension. Other accessory proteins server or depolymerize F-actin filaments to break down the F-actin cytoskeleton.

While this F-actin severing process is most commonly associated with growth cone repulsion, the severing of actin filaments also creates new sites for actin filament polymerization and membrane protrusion that is an important part of axonal growth cone extension (Dent et al., 2011). It is interesting to note that the presumed axon guidance functions of many of the actin-modifying or associating proteins are based, at least in part, on their roles in non-neuronal cell morphology and cell migration.

Over a dozen actin-regulating proteins have been identified in growth cones, but their precise roles and regulation in axon growth cones are less well understood (Dent et al., 2011).

Ena/VASP is an important actin-regulatory protein that functions during axon guidance by binding barbed F-actin polymers and promoting the polymerization during axon outgrowth or by coordinating F-actin remodeling during axon repulsion (Drees and Gertler, 2008). Thus, the same F-actin regulatory protein can be essential for either axonal attraction/outgrowth or repulsion, depending on the guidance receptor and developmental context. F-actin severing and depolymerizing proteins promote the disassembly of F-actin polymers into G-actin monomers, a process thought to be critical for axon guidance. Cofilin and gelsolin are also two well-studied F-actin severing proteins that play critical roles in axon guidance (Lu et al., 1997; Aizawa et al., 2001).

3.4. CAMs and Co-Receptors Signaling

Cell adhesion molecules or CAMs, are transmembrane proteins that adhere to substrates in the extracellular matrix, including other CAMs. CAM mediated adhesion is necessary for proper axonal outgrowth in many different neuronal cell types (Raper and Mason, 2010). The CAMs are tethered to the underlying intracellular actin cytoskeleton within a growth cone, and they cooperate with guidance receptors to recruit and activate signaling proteins during axon guidance. L1-CAM is a surface protein that contains extracellular immunoglobulin-like and fibronectin type domains that form a cis-association with Neuropilin-1 (Nrp1), a guidance receptor that binds Sema3A (Raper, 2000; Maness and Schachner, 2007). This L1-CAM/Nrp1 co-receptor interaction is required for Sema3A binding and growth cone repulsion in spinal cord axons. Interestingly, L1-CAM can also bind to Nrp1 in trans, and this stable co-receptor complex binds Sema3A and promotes growth cone attraction rather than repulsion (Castellani et al., 2002). Similarly, another CAM protein, Nr-CAM, associates in cis with Neuropilin-2 (Nrp2) to convert the axonal response from Sema3B and Sema3F from repulsion to the attraction (Falk et al., 2005). Indeed, CAMs are thought to attract initially commissural axons to the ventral midline of the forebrain but then switch to promote repulsion after the axons cross the midline region (Falk et al., 2005). PlexinA receptors form co-receptor complexes with Nrp1 and Nrp2 and the tyrosine kinase-like transmembrane protein, Off-track (OTK). These co-receptor complexes are necessary for growth cone repulsion in response to class 3 semaphorins in different developing neuronal cell types (Tran et al., 2007). As with CAM complexes, PlexinA co-receptor complexes likely function as docking stations that recruit additional and specific signaling proteins to orchestrate axonal repulsion through F-actin remodeling. For example, FARP2 is a Rac-GEF that binds to the PlexinA1/Nrp1 co-receptor complex, but not PlexinA1 alone (Toyofuku et al., 2005). Also, Sema3A binding to the

PlexinA1/Nrp1 complex triggers recruitment of Rnd1, a Rho-family GTPase that regulates PlexinA Ras-GAP activity (Toyofuku et al., 2005).

3.5. Morphogenic Signaling

In addition to "traditional" axon guidance molecules, a class of proteins called morphogens including Hedgehog (Hh) and Wnt (short for Wingless Integration), regulate axon guidance through a unique set of morphogenic receptors. The membrane-bound Hh protein interacts with the Patched (Ptc) receptor to manipulate the axon growth cone through cAMP and SFK-dependent local signaling pathways (Trousse et al., 2001; Tenzen et al., 2006; Charron and Tessier-Lavigne, 2007; Yam et al., 2009). Wnt proteins are secreted factors and they bind to either the Frizzled family of G-protein-coupled receptors or to Ryk receptor tyrosine kinases, which are both capable of initiating an array of signaling pathways (Salinas and Zou, 2008; Mulligan and Cheyette, 2012).

Wnt4 is expressed at the ventral midline of the developing spinal cord and plays a critical role in directing the anterior growth of spinal cord axons after they cross the midline. In the crossed axons, Wnt4 binds to the Frizzled receptor and initiates a heterotrimeric G-protein signaling cascade that ultimately activates the atypical protein kinase C (aPKC) to promote anterior growth of crossed axons (Wolf et al., 2008). Interestingly, Wnt5A can promote either axon outgrowth or axonal repulsion in developing cortical axons, depending on the manner in which the Wnt is presented (Li et al., 2009). The addition of a uniform concentration of Wnt5A stimulates axonal outgrowth through binding and activating the Ryk receptor, which in turn activates phosphoinositide signaling and release of intracellular Ca^{2+} stores. Thus, the specific mechanisms by which Wnt5A trigger a cytoplasmic Ca^{2+} rise determines whether the ligand-receptor binding promotes attractive or repulsive axonal responses. This Wnt5A-mediated switch between attraction and repulsion appears to be critical for midline crossing of axons forming the corpus callosum, a major inter hemispheric cortical fiber tract in the mammalian brain (Hutchins et al., 2011).

3.6. Calcium and Cyclic Nucleotide Signaling

Another way of signaling related to axonal regulation is a calcium pathway. A rise in intracellular Ca^{2+} concentration regulates axon guidance processes. In general, moderate Ca^{2+} levels signal attractive growth cone responses, whereas very high or very low Ca^{2+} levels promote axonal repulsion (Gomez and Zheng, 2006). In addition, the spatiotemporal rise in Ca^{2+} instructs directional growth cone turning, such that stimulation of a calcium rise on one side of the growth cone is sufficient to induce axon outgrowth toward the stimulated side (Zheng, 2000). Calcium triggers growth cone remodeling in large part by binding and activating calcium-binding proteins such as the calcium calmodulin kinase II (CaMKII) or the calcium-activated protein phosphatases, calcineurin (CaN), and protein phosphatase-1 (PP1). Activation of CaMKII often promotes axon outgrowth, whereas activation of CaN and PP1 often promotes axonal repulsion (Wen et al., 2004; To et al., 2007).

It is thought that most of the calcium-activated signaling pathways ultimately control the activity of the Rho-GTPases to regulate the F-actin cytoskeleton. For example, the artificial release of intracellular Ca^{2+} in cerebellar granule cells induces axonal outgrowth through activation of Rac and Cdc42 GTPases, and the inhibition of RhoA GTPases. Similar Rho-family GTPase mechanisms have been proposed for attractive axon guidance cues, netrin-1 or brain-derived neurotrophic factor (BDNF) (Jin et al., 2005). Netrin binding to the DCC receptor triggers a calcium influx as a result of TRP-C channel activation, which in turn depolarizes the growth cone membrane and activates voltage-dependent calcium channels (VDCCs).

The activated VDCCs promote the influx of extracellular Ca^{2+}, which in turn facilitates the turning of the growth cone toward the source of netrin (Hong et al., 2000; Wang and Poo, 2005). The cyclic molecules, cAMP, and cGMP also regulate growth cone guidance. A change in cAMP/cGMP levels is sufficient to define a growth cone response. Increased cAMP levels induce attractive growth cone turning while elevated cGMP levels induce repulsive growth cone turning (Song et al., 1998). Netrin-1 signaling through the DCC receptor increases cAMP levels in the growth cone, which in turn stimulates PKA activity (Corset et al., 2000). Netrin-1 binding to DCC increases the activity of a soluble form of adenylyl cyclase (sAC), the enzyme that produces cAMP (Wu et al., 2006).

Also to PKA, netrin stimulation of embryonic DRGs triggers the cAMP-dependent activation of the Rap-GEF, Epac, to promote attractive axon guidance (Murray et al., 2009). In comparison, Sema1A binding to PlexinA receptors in fly motor neurons stimulates the recruitment of Gyc7GC, a receptor guanylyl cyclase, to increase cGMP levels and promote axonal repulsion (Ayoob et al., 2004). Together, these and other studies illustrate how regulation of cAMP and cGMP levels in growth cones controls axon guidance during early neural development.

4. Genes Involved in Abnormal Synaptogenesis and Resultant Pathologies

In recent years, many neuropsychiatric disorders, including autism, schizophrenia, epilepsy and intellectual disability (ID), have been linked to inherited mutations and dysfunction of a number of proteins implicated in synaptogenesis, synaptic growth, development, and stability; hence, the understanding of the basic biology of synaptogenesis is critical to unraveling the pathogenesis of neuropsychiatric disorders (Mitchell, 2010; Melom and Mittleton, 2011). Autism genetics is highly complex, involving many genes and different genetic alterations, such as deletions, translocations, single nucleotide polymorphisms (SNP) and copy number variations (CNV) (Ye, 2010). In this literature review, the main genes and proteins participating in abnormal synaptogenesis processes occurring in patients with intellectual disability, autism, and other neurodevelopmental disorder are described.

4.1. Autism and Features

Autism is a severe neurodevelopmental disorder usually beginning in the first 30 months of life, a crucial moment in the maturation of neural circuits. It is characterized by impaired social interactions, communication deficient, restricted interests and stereotypic and repetitive activities (García-Peñas et al., 2012; Lu et al., 2014). Autism spectrum disorders (ASDs) refer to a broad definition of autism, including classical and atypical autism, Asperger syndrome and pervasive developmental disorder not otherwise specified (Sousa, 2010). Autism is a heritable neurodevelopmental disorder, and although the major inheritance pattern is not known (Zhiling et al., 2008), in the last 10 years, there has been a progressive advance regard the genetic basis of autism.

It has been associated with an increasing number of genes related to a variety of neurobiological functions. Among them, especially important is the presence of anomalies in synaptogenesis and an imbalance between excitatory and inhibitory circuits in the brain development (García-Peñas, 2012).

4.1.1. Genetic Alterations in Synaptogenesis and Autism

There is strong evidence that altered homeostasis mechanisms of Central Nervous System (CNS) synapses play a major role in the genesis of ASD. Recent genetic and genomic studies have identified a great number of candidate genes for autism, including but not limited to semaphorins, SynCAM1, contactins, cadherins, neurexins, SHANK3, and CNTNAP2, which has been related to synaptogenesis, maturation, and/or modification after maturation (Abrahams et al., 2008; García-Peñas et al., 2012).

4.1.2. Alterations in Semaphoring

Autism spectrum disorders are consistent with primary defects in cell migration, axon guidance and synaptogenesis in many brain areas. From this perspective, genes in the semaphorin (Sema) families emerge as promising candidates. Semaphorins provide a tight spatiotemporal control of sensory and motor axon growth and guidance; plexins and neuropilins serve as coreceptors for semaphorins (Mann et al., 2007).

The transmembrane semaphorin, semaphorin-6A (Sema6A), interacts with the transmembrane proteins plexin-A2 and plexin-A4 and, together with Sema6B controls the axon guidance, laminar connectivity, neuronal migration, and dendrite development.

The mutation of Sema6A results in widespread but subtle derangements of cytoarchitecture and neuronal connectivity in different parts of the brain (Rünker et al., 2011).

Semaphorins act through a functional interaction with the Wnt system, mainly in the cerebellum and limbic system, inhibiting the formation of inappropriate synapses. Abnormalities of lamination, cortical neuronal organization and synaptic connections have been described in mouse models carrying mutations of sema6A and showing psychotic features and impaired reciprocal social interaction and working memory (Ye et al., 2010; Melom and Litleton., 2011; Rünker et al., 2011; García-Peñas et al., 2012).

Similarly, histochemical studies of brains in autistic subjects have shown anomalies in the plexin-A4 protein, mostly in the primary motor cortex and the anterior cingulate cortex; Furthermore, alterations in expression levels of multiple semaphorins, plexins or semaphorin signalling proteins have been observed in the cortex of post-mortem brains of patients with schizophrenia or autism (Suda et al., 2011).

4.1.3. Alterations in SynCAM1

SynCAM1 (CADM1), a member of the immunoglobulin superfamily (IgSF), is another synaptic adhesion molecule sufficiently important for promoting the formation of presynaptic terminals and to induce the functional synapse (García-Peñas et al., 2012).

Zhiling et al., examined the relationship between mutations in the CADM1 gene and ASDs. They found two missense mutations, C739A (H246N) and A755C (Y251S), in the *CADM1* gene of Caucasian male patients with ASD and their relatives. The mutated CADM1 exhibited reduced amount of high molecular weight oligosaccharides, defective trafficking to the cell surface and increased susceptibility to cleavage and or degradation.

These findings provide key support for the unified idea that impaired synaptogenesis underlies the pathogenesis of autism (Zhiling et al., 2008). A Cadm1-knockout (KO) mice showed increased anxiety-related behavior in open-field and abnormal light-dark transition tests. Social behavior of Cadm1-KO mice was impaired in social interaction, resident-intruder, and social memory/recognition tests.

Furthermore, motor coordination and gait were impaired in rotarod and footprint tests. This finding demonstrates that CADM1 plays roles in regulating emotional behaviors, social behaviors, and motor performances and that CADM1 has an important role in the origin of autism (Takayanagi et al., 2010).

4.1.4. Alterations in Synaptic Adhesion Proteins

One of the earliest steps in synaptogenesis is the induction and adhesion of precisely opposed presynaptic and postsynaptic domains. Multiple trans-synaptic cell adhesion complexes operate in parallel to ensure proper synaptic alignment. Mutation of synaptic adhesion proteins has been linked to various neuropsychiatric disorders, indicating that abnormal formation or maintenance of synaptic contacts may cause several neurological diseases. Various anomalies in cell adhesion molecules (CAM), mainly contactins and similar molecules involved in the early stages of synaptogenesis are known (Giagtzoglou et al., 2009).

4.1.5. Contactin (CNTN)

Contactins are a family of Ig-type CAMs involved in synaptogenesis, axonal growth, and synaptic plasticity. This family harbors at least four members that have genetically been implicated in autism: CNTN3, CNTN4, CNTN5, and CNTN6. Deletions of CNTN3 (3p12.3) and CNTN4 (3p26.3), and duplications of CNTN4 have been described in autistic children with and without intellectual disability (Melom and Litleton, 2011; Zuko et al., 2013).

Contactin associated protein-like 2 (CNTNAP2), a protein structurally similar to contactin, is a neurexin family member involved in local axonal differentiation and synaptic adhesiveness. Single nucleotide polymorphisms (SNPs) in this gene (rs2710102) are related with language development in general population and children with autism (Jonsson et al., 2014). Interestingly, carboxyl-terminal truncation of CNTNAP2 is associated with severe autism, seizures, language regression and low IQ (Strauss et al., 2006).

L1-type adhesion molecules (L1CAM) are transmembrane proteins with an evolutionary well-conserved domain structure of usually six immunoglobulins and five fibronectin type III domains. This glycoprotein cell adhesion is involved in synaptogenesis, neuronal migration and deployment of dendritic spines. Mutations have been reported in L1CAM in syndromic autism patients (Hortsch et al., 2014).

4.1.6. Alterations in Cadherins Y Protocadherins

Cadherins (CDH) are a superfamily of cell adhesion molecules, also involved in the adhesion between pre and postsynaptic cells; specifically N-cadherin (CDH2) acts as a basic adhesion molecule for the development of excitatory and inhibitory synapses. Moreover, the protocadherins (PCDH) appear also to be essential in the development of synaptic specificity (Crepel et al., 2014).

SNPs polymorphisms in CDH9 and CDH10 have been associated both with autism and social interaction impairment (Pourcain et al., 2010). Partial deletion of CDH11 and the presence of rare variants in this gene, confirm the involvement of CDH11 in autism, which is consistent with the association of other CDHs as CDH15 and CDH18 showing mutations in patients with autism (Crepel et al., 2014).

4.1.7. Alterations in Neurexins and Neuroligins

The Neurexin (Nrx) and Neuroligin (Nlg) proteins play a major role in synapse formation and function (Giagtzoglou et al., 2009). Mutations in neurexins and neuroligins have been identified in several families with heritable neurological disorders, including autism (Zhiling et al., 2008; Melom and Litleton, 2011).

The neurexins family are type-1 transmembrane proteins containing epidermal growth factor-like repeats (EGF-like) and laminin G domains in their extracellular region. There are three neurexins (NRXN1, NRXN2, NRXN3) and five contactin-associated proteins (CNTNAP1–5) in this family (Ye et al., 2010). Each of the three neurexin genes reported has two promoters that enable expression of two distinct protein isoforms, a long α- and a short β-isoform (Giagtzoglou et al., 2009).

NRXN1 has been associated with autism in several studies. In an independent study, two missense structural variants in the neurexin 1β signal peptide region were identified in 4 autism patients (Feng, 2006). Translocations and intragenic rearrangements within or near *NRXN1* gene have also been identified in patients with autism (Wisniowiecka-Kowalnik et al., 2010). Beta-neurexins also interact with neuroligins and as such are compelling candidates for involvement in the ASDs. Identification of *de novo* deletions overlapping with *NRXN1* in affected sisters, along with rare missense mutations in other cases, provides strong support for the involvement of this molecule in the ASDs (Abrahams et al., 2008).

Neuroligins are postsynaptic proteins that bind to presynaptic neurexins; correct assembly between them is basic in synaptogenesis and the correct function of synapses (Scheiffele et al., 2000; Dean et al., 2003).

There are five neuroligins in the human genome, *NLGN1*, *NLGN2*, *NLGN3*, *NLGN4X* and *NLGN4Y*. Neuroligins share similar domain structures: an esterase domain, a single transmembrane domain followed by a short cytoplasmic domain (Jamain et al., 2003).

Different mutations have been described in NLGN1, NLGN3, NLGN4 and NLGN4Y in autistic patients. The implication of NLGN3 and NLGN4X in the imbalance between inhibition and excitation in different neural circuits has been proposed as one of the key pathogenetic mechanisms of autism, mainly in the forms associated with epilepsy (Melom and Litleton, 2011).

Autism has been associated with the X chromosome-linked *NLGN3* and *NLGN4X* also to *NLGN1*. Jamain et al., (2003) reported the first mutations in *NLGN4X* and *NLGN3* genes from patients with autism and Asperger syndrome.

The R451C mutation in *NLGN3* causes deficits both in neuroligin 3 trafficking from the endoplasmic reticulum (ER) to the cell surface and in its binding to neurexin (Comoletti et al., 2004); moreover, it has been described that type R87W mutation in NLGN4 alter normal glycosylation of this neuroligin and cause its retention in the endoplasmic reticulum of neurons and glia, such that block the final transport to the cell surface and alter the synaptic assembly (Zhang et al., 2009).

4.1.8. Alterations in SHANK

SHANK is a family of genes encoding for large synaptic scaffold proteins whence these proteins play a crucial role in the formation and stabilization of synapses. Deletions, duplications and coding mutations in the SHANK genes have been recurrently reported in patients with autism (Grabrucker et al., 2011).

There are three SHANK proteins, SHANK1–3. SHANKs are crucial components of the postsynaptic density (PSD) that link ionotropic and metabotropic glutamate receptor complexes to the cytoskeleton; SHANK also binds to neuroligins directly or indirectly in the PSD (Boeckers et al., 2002). The human *SHANK3* gene is located on chromosome 22q13, a region deleted or amplified in some autistic patients. Two mutations in *SHANK3* gene, one at an intronic donor splice site and one missense in the coding region, have been identified in ASD patients (Ye et al., 2010), also de novo or truncating mutations in SHANK3 have also been observed in this patients (Boccuto et al., 2012). SHANK3 haploinsufficiency has been identified in more than 900 patients affected with chromosome 22q13 deletion syndrome, known as Phelan–McDermid syndrome; the majority of these patients have moderate to severe intellectual disability (ID), absent to severely delayed speech and more than 80% of the cases, autism or autistic-like behavior is present (Phelan and McDermid, 2012; Betancur and Buxbaum, 2013).

Few studies have explored SHANK1 and SHANK2 in ASD, but all have led to the conclusion that deleterious mutations in these genes contribute to the disorder (Leblond et al., 2012; Sato et al., 2012). A recent meta-analysis by Leblond et al., (2014) found that mutations in SHANK1 are rare (0.04%) and present in males with normal IQ and autism; mutations in SHANK2 were present in 0.17% of patients with ASD and mild intellectual disability; mutations in SHANK3 were present in 0.69% of patients with ASD and up to 2.12% of the cases with moderate to profound intellectual disability.

4.2. Synaptogenes in Other Neurodevelopmental Disorders

In addition to Autism, diverse disorders such as schizophrenia, epilepsy, and intellectual disability have been associated with mutations, deletions, translocations, SNP polymorphisms, CNV and dysfunction of a number of proteins implicated in synaptogenesis.

Mutations in SHANK2 and SHANK3 have been identified in patients with ID and schizophrenia (Berkel et al., 2010; Gauthier et al., 2010; Boccuto et al., 2012). Mutations in neurexins and neuroligins have been identified in several families with heritable neurological disorders, including schizophrenia and ID (Sudhof, 2008). Further neurexin 1α-deficient mice displayed abnormal behaviors, such as a decrease in prepulse inhibition, an increase in grooming behaviors and impairment in nest building activity. The deficit in prepulse inhibition is a hallmark of schizophrenia. Therefore, some of the behavior changes in the neurexin 1α-deficient mice correlate, at least in part, with impairments observed in schizophrenic patients (Ye et al., 2010). Similar to neurexins and neuroligins, mutations in synaptic adhesion molecules have been associated with schizophrenia and are thought to promote synapse formation. The netrin-G ligand (NGL) proteins form a subfamily of synaptic adhesion molecules implicated in the etiology of schizophrenia and bipolar disorders (Ko et al., 2009; Woo et al., 2009; Sousa et al., 2010).

On the other hand, it is well known the presence of mutations in protocadherin PCDH19 in women with refractory epilepsy and ID (Depienne et al., 2009). Contactin-associated protein-2 (CNTNAP2) is a single-pass transmembrane protein distantly related to neurexins that have been associated with schizophrenia, ID, and epilepsy by genome-wide linkage analysis (Burbach and van der Zwaag, 2009).

A recessive frameshift mutation was also identified in *CNTNAP2*, in Amish individuals presenting with cortical dysplasia-focal epilepsy syndrome, a congenital disorder characterized by seizures and language regression (Strauss et al., 2006).

Recently have been reported a Q555X mutation in synapsin 1 (*SYN1*), an X-linked gene encoding for a neuron-specific phosphoprotein implicated in the regulation of neurotransmitter release and synaptogenesis. This nonsense mutation was found in all affected individuals from a large French-Canadian family segregating epilepsy and ASDs. Additional mutations in SYN1 (A51G, A550T, and T567A) were found in 1.0 and 3.5% of French-Canadian individuals with autism and epilepsy, respectively (Fassio et al., 2011).

Several Wnt pathway components have been implicated in the pathogenesis of schizophrenia and Alzheimer disease, raising the question of how anomalies in this pathway alter the synapse (Freyberg et al., 2010). Single nucleotide polymorphisms in GSK-3b, a crucial protein in Wnt-β-catenin pathway, are associated with schizophrenia; besides, GSK-3b was found to interact with *DISC1*, a major schizophrenia susceptibility gene (Mao et al., 2009). Certain cases of schizophrenia may be caused by an imbalance in the development and/or activity of excitatory and inhibitory synapses; moreover, de novo CNV analyses indicate an enrichment of genes of the PSD95 complex in schizophrenia, and rare exonic deletions implicate Gephyrin as a risk factor for seizures and schizophrenia (Lionel et al., 2013).

GRIN2B, located on 12p13.1, encodes the NMDA receptor subunit NR2B, which is required for neuronal pattern formation and synaptic plasticity (Cull-Candy et al., 2001; Akashi et al., 2009). Mutations and disruptions of *GRIN2B* have recently been described in patients with intellectual disability (Dimassi et al., 2013) and autism spectrum disorders (O'Roak et al., 2012).

4.3. Genes Involved in Synaptogenesis in Fragile X Syndrome

Fragile X syndrome (FXS), caused by the transcriptional silencing of fragile X mental retardation protein (FMRP), has been proposed to result in an excessive signaling of synaptic metabotropic glutamate receptors, leading to alterations of synapse maturation and plasticity, as well as impaired dendrite maturation. Lack of FMRP leads to dysregulation of synaptic protein synthesis and impairments of intellect, cognition, and behavior; a disorder that currently has no effective therapeutics (Cheng et al., 2013; Boda et al., 2014; Sun et al., 2014). Nimchinsky et al., (2001) reported that patients and adult *FMR1* knock-out mice have abnormally long dendritic spines of increased density suggesting that the disorder might involve abnormal spine development. In a recently study, Wang et al., (2014) used variance-mean analysis and peak-scaled non-stationary variance analysis to examine changes in both presynaptic and postsynaptic parameters during repetitive activity at excitatory CA3-CA1 hippocampal synapses in a mouse model of FXS; the results indicate that FMRP regulates neurotransmission at excitatory hippocampal synapses specifically during repetitive activity via modulation of release probability in a presynaptic manner, suggesting that FMRP function in regulating neurotransmitter release is an activity-dependent phenomenon that may contribute to the pathophysiology of FXS.

The *Drosophila* FXS model has been shown to functionally conserve the roles of human FMRP in synaptogenesis, and has been centrally important in generating mechanistic understanding of the FXS disease state (Doll et al., 2014). In an interesting study, screening for upregulated neural proteins in *Drosophila fmr1* (*dfmr1*) null mutants, suggest that FMRP negatively regulates heparan sulfate proteoglycans co-receptors controlling trans-synaptic signaling during synaptogenesis, and that loss of this regulation causes synaptic structure and function defects characterizing the FXS disease state (Friedman et al., 2013).

Synaptic Rac1 GTPase activity was shown to be regulated by FMRP and DISC1, raising the possibility that both Fragile X and Schizophrenia may have impaired BMP mediated activity-dependent synaptic growth (Chen et al., 2010; Hayashi-Takagi et al., 2010).

Conclusion

In summary, synaptogenesis includes a quite large amount of genes and proteins involved in highly complex metabolic signaling pathways, frequently disturbed by a number of gene mutations and causing intellectual disability syndromes and more than 100 brain diseases.

Intellectual disability disorders are associated with numerous abnormal proteins involved in synapse formation, dendritic spine morphology, synaptic cytoskeleton regulation or synthesis and degradation of specific synapse proteins.

Different GTPases families appear to form an intricate network of signaling pathways, integrating information through transmembrane proteins and from the neuronal activity to precisely regulate the size of synaptic structures and the trafficking of receptors. Interestingly, the GTPases signaling cascade integrates activity and trans-synaptic signals to fine-tune the spine actin cytoskeleton, controlling in this way the growth, size and morphology of spines, but also the exocytotic mechanisms and receptor trafficking.

Most genetic defects associated with MR appear to perturb somehow this signaling and interfere with the regulation of surface expression of receptors. This trafficking is crucial for synapse function, plasticity, and dynamics and represents a common primary alteration that leads to cognitive dysfunctions.

ACKNOWLEDGMENTS

To Myrna González Ramírez and Pablo Barros Medina for their excellent artwork support.

REFERENCES

Abrahams, B. S. and Geschwind, D. H. (2008) Advances in autism genetics: on the threshold of a new neurobiology. *Nat. Rev. Genet.*, 9, 341–355.

Aizawa, H., Wakatsuki, S., Ishii, A., Moriyama, K., Sasaki, Y., Ohashi, K., Sekine-Aizawa, Y., Sehara-Fujisawa, A., Mizuno, K., Goshima, Y., and Yahara, I. (2001) Phosphorylation of cofilin by LIM-kinase is necessary for semaphorin 3A-induced growth cone collapse. *Nat. Neurosci.*, 4, 367–373.

Akashi, K., Kakizaki, T., Kamiya, H., Fukaya, M., Yamasaki, M., Abe, M., Natsume R., Watanabe, M., and Sakimura, K. (2009) NMDA receptor GluN2B (GluR épsilon 2/ NR2B) subunit is crucial for channel function, postsynaptic macromolecular organization, and actin cytoskeleton at hippocampal CA3 synapses. *J. Neurosci.*, 29: 10869–10882.

Ayoob, J. C., Yu, H. H., Terman, J. R., and Kolodkin, A. L. (2004) The Drosophila receptor guanylyl cyclase Gyc76C is required for semaphorin-1a-plexin A-mediated axonal repulsion. *J. Neurosci.*, 24, 6639–6649.

Barbosa, A. C., Kim, M. S., Ertunc, M., Adachi, M., Nelson, E. D., McAnally, J., Richardson, J. A., Kavalali, E. T., Monteggia, L. M., Bassel-Duby, R., and Olson, E. N. (2008) MEF2C, a transcription factor that facilitates learning and memory by negative regulation of synapse numbers and function. *Proc. Natl. Acad. Sci. US*, 105, 9391–9396.

Berkel, S., Marshall, C. R., Weiss, B., Howe, J., Roeth, R., Moog, U., Endris V., Roberts, W., Szatmari, P., Pinto, D., Bonin, M., Riess, A., Engels, H., Sprengel, R., Scherer, S. W., and Rappold, G. A. (2010) Mutations in the SHANK2 synaptic scaffolding gene in autism spectrum disorder and mental retardation. *Nat. Genet.*, 42, 489-491.

Bernstein, B. W. and Bamburg, J. R. (2010) ADF/Cofilin: a functional node in cell biology. *Trends Cell Biol.*, 20, 187-195.

Betancur, C. and Buxbaum, J. D. (2013) SHANK3 haploinsufficiency: a “common” but underdiagnosed highly penetrant monogenic cause of autism spectrum disorders. *Mol. Autism*, 4, 17.

Boccuto, L., Lauri, M., Sarasua, S. M., Skinner, C. D., Buccella, D., Dwivedi, A., Orteschi, D., Collins, J. S., Zollino, M., Visconti, P., Dupont, B., Tiziano, D., Schroer, R. J., Neri, G., Stevenson, R. E., Gurrieri, F., and Schwartz, C. E. (2012) Prevalence of SHANK3 variants in patients with different subtypes of autism spectrum disorders. *Eur. J. Hum. Genet.*, 3, 310–316.

Boda, B., Alberi, S., Nikonenko, I., Node-Langlois, R., Jourdain, P., Moosmayer, M., Parisi-Jourdain, L., and Muller, D. (2004) The mental retardation protein PAK3 contributes to synapse formation and plasticity in hippocampus, *J. Neurosci.*, 24, 10816-10825.

Boda, B., Mendez, P., Boury-Jamot, B., Magara, F., and Muller, D. (2014) Reversal of activity-mediated spine dynamics and learning impairment in a mouse model of Fragile X syndrome. *Eur. J. Neurosci.*, 39, 1130-1137.

Boeckers, T. M., Bockmann, J., Kreutz, M. R., and Gundelfinger, E. D. (2002) ProSAP/Shank proteins a family of higher order organizing molecules of the postsynaptic density with an emerging role in human neurological disease. *J. Neurochem.*, 81, 903–910.

Burbach, J. P. and van der Zwaag, B. (2009) Contact in the genetics of autism and schizophrenia. *TINS*, 32, 69-72.

Campbell, D. S., Stringham, S. A., Timm, A., Xiao, T., Law, M. Y., Baier, H., Nonet, M. L., and Chien, C. B. (2007) Slit1a inhibits retinal ganglion cell arborization and synaptogenesis via Robo2-dependent and –independent pathways. *Neuron*, 55, 231–245.

Carlisle, H. J., Manzerra, P., Marcora, E., and Kennedy, M. B. (2008) SynGAP regulates steady-state and activity-dependent phosphorylation of cofilin. *J. Neurosci.*, 28, 13673-13683.

Castellani, V., De Angelis, E., Kenwrick, S., and Rougon, G. (2002) Cis and trans interactions of L1 with neuropilin-1 control axonal responses to semaphorin 3A. *EMBO J.*, 21, 6348–6357.

Charron, F. and Tessier-Lavigne, M. (2007) The Hedgehog, TGF-beta/BMP and Wnt families of morphogens in axon guidance. *Adv. Exp. Med. Biol.*, 621, 116-133.

Chen, L., Melendez, J., Campbell, K., Kuan, C. Y., and Zheng, Y. (2009) Rac1 deficiency in the forebrain results in neural progenitor reduction and microcephaly. *Dev. Biol.*, 325, 162-170.

Chen, L. Y., Rex, C. S., Babayan, A. H., Kramar, E. A., Lynch, G., Gall, C. M., and Lauterborn, J. C. (2010) Physiological activation of synaptic Rac > PAK (p-21 activated kinase) signaling is defective in a mouse model of fragile X syndrome. *J. Neurosci.*, 30, 10977-10984.

Chen, L. Y., Rex, C. S., Casale, M. S., Gall, C. M., and Lynch, G. (2007) Changes in synaptic morphology accompany actin signaling during LTP. *J. Neurosci.*, 27, 5363-5372.

Cheng, Y., Corbin, J. G. and Levy, R. J. (2013) Programmed cell death is impaired in the developing brain of FMR1 mutants. *Dev. Neurosci.*, 35, 347-358.

Chowdhury, S., Shepherd, J. D., Okuno, H., Lyford, G., Petralia, R. S., Plath, N., Kuhl, D., Huganir, R. L., and Worley, P. F. (2006) Arc/Arg3.1 interacts with the endocytic machinery to regulate AMPA receptor trafficking. *Neuron*, 52, 445–459.

Chubykin, A. A., Atasoy, D., Etherton, M. R., Brose, N., Kavalali, E. T., Gibson, J. R., and Sudhof, T. C. (2007) Activity dependent validation of excitatory versus inhibitory synapses by neuroligin-1 versus neuroligin-2. *Neuron*, 54, 919–931.

Comoletti, D., De Jaco, A., Jennings, L. L., Flynn, R. E., Gaietta, G., Tsigelny, I., Ellisman, M. H., and Taylor, P. (2004) The Arg451Cys-neuroligin-3 mutation associated with autism reveals a defect in protein processing. *J. Neurosci.*, 24, 4889–4893.

Corset, V., Nguyen-Ba-Charvet, K. T., Forcet, C., Moyse, E., Chedotal, A., and Mehlen, P. (2000) Netrin-1-mediated axon outgrowth and cAMP production requires interaction with adenosine A2b receptor. *Nature*, 407, 747–750.

Crepel, A., De Wolf, V., Brison, N., Ceulemans, B., Walleghem, D., Peuteman, G., Lambrechts, D., Steyaert, J., Noens, I., Devriendt, K., and Peeters, H. (2014) Association of CDH11 with non-syndromic ASD. *Am. J. Med. Genet. B. Neuropsychiatr. Genet.*, 165 B, 391-398.

Cull-Candy, S., Brickley, S. and Farrant, M. (2001) NMDA receptor subunits: Diversity, development and disease. *Curr. Opin. Neurobiol.*, 11, 327–335.

Dani, V. S., Chang, Q., Maffei, A., Turrigiano, G. G., Jaenisch, R., and Nelson, S. B. (2005) Reduced cortical activity due to a shift in the balance between excitation and inhibition in a mouse model of Rett syndrome. *Proc. Natl. Acad. Sci. US*, 102, 12560–12565.

Dean, C., Scholl, F. G., Choih, J., DeMaria, S., Berger, J., Isacoff, E., and Scheiffele, P. (2003) Neurexin mediates the assembly of presynaptic terminals. *Nat. Neurosci.*, 6, 708–716.

Dent, E. W., Gupton, S. L. and Gertler, F. B. (2011) The growth cone cytoskeleton in axon outgrowth and guidance, *Cold Spring Harb. Perspect. Biol.*, 3, a001800.

Depienne, C., Bouteiller, D., Keren, B., Cheuret, E., Poirier, K., Trouillard, O., Benyahia, B., Quelin, C., Carpentier, W., Julia, S., Afenjar, A., Gautier, A., Rivier, F., Meyer, S., Berquin, P., Hélias, M., Py, I., Rivera, S., Bahi-Buisson, N., Gourfinkel-An, I., Cazeneuve, C., Ruberg, M., Brice, A., Nabbout, R., and Leguern, E. (2009) Sporadic infantile epileptic encephalopathy caused by mutations in PCDH19 resembles Dravet syndrome but mainly affects females. *PLoS Genet.*, 5, e1000381.

Di Cristo, G., Chattopadhyaya, B., Kuhlman, S. J., Fu, Y., Belanger, M. C., and Wu, C. Z. (2007) Rutishauser U, Maffei L, Huang ZJ. Activity-dependent PSA expression regulates inhibitory maturation and onset of critical period plasticity. *Nat. Neurosci.*, 10, 1569–1577.

Dimassi, S., Andrieux, J., Labalme, A., Lesca, G., Cordier, M. P., Boute, O., Neut, D., Edery, P., Sanlaville, D., and Schluth-Bolard, C. (2013) Interstitial 12p13.1 deletion involving GRIN2B in three patients with intelectual disability. *Am. J Med. Genet. Part A.*, 116A, 2564–2569.

Doll, C. A. and Broadie, K. (2014) Impaired activity dependent neural circuit assembly and refinement in autism spectrum disorder genetic models. *Front. Cell. Neurosci.*, 8, 30.

Drees, F. and Gertler, F. B. (2008) Ena/VASP: proteins at the tip of the nervous system. *Curr. Opin. Neurobiol.*, 18, 53-59.

Endris, V., Wogatzky, B., Leimer, U., Bartsch, D., Zatyka, M., Latif, F., Maher, E. R., Tariverdian, G., Kirsch, S., Karch, D., and Rappold, G. A. (2002) The novel Rho-GTPase activating gene MEGAP/srGAP3 has a putative role in severe mental retardation. *Proc. Natl. Acad. Sci. US*, 99, 11754-11759.

Falk, J., Bechara, A., Fiore, R., Nawabi, H., Zhou, H., Hoyo-Becerra, C., Bozon, M., Rougon, G., Grumet, M., Puschel, A. W., Sanes, J. R., and Castellani, V. (2005) Dual functional activity of semaphorin 3B is required for positioning the anterior commissure. *Neuron*, 48, 63-75.

Fassio, A., Patry, L., Congia, S., Onofri, F., Piton, A., Gauthier, J., Pozzi, D., Messa, M., Defranchi, E., Fadda, M., Corradi, A., Baldelli, P., Lapointe, L., St-Onge, J., Meloche, C., Mottron, L., Valtorta, F., Khoa, Nguyen, D., Rouleau, G. A., Benfenati, F., and Cossette, P. (2011) *SYN1 loss-of-function mutations in autism and partial epilepsy cause impaired synaptic function*. 20, 2297-2307.

Fedulov, V., Rex, C. S., Simmons, D. A., Palmer, L., Gall, C. M., and Lynch, G. (2007) Evidence that long-term potentiation occurs within individual hippocampal synapses during learning. *J. Neurosci.*, 27, 8031-8039.

Flavell, S. W., Cowan, C. W., Kim, T. K., Greer, P. L., Lin, Y., Paradis, S., Griffith, E. C., Hu, L. S., Chen, C., and Greenberg, M. E. (2006) Activity-dependent regulation of MEF2 transcription factors suppresses excitatory synapse number, *Science*, 311, 1008–1011.

Flavell, S. W. and Greenberg, M. E. (2008) Signaling mechanisms linking neuronal activity to gene expression and plasticity of the nervous system. *Annu. Rev. Neurosci.*, 31, 563–590.

Freyberg, Z., Ferrando, S. J. and Javitch, J. A. (2010) Roles of the Akt/GSK-3 and Wnt signaling pathways in schizophrenia and antipsychotic drug action. *Am. J. Psych.*, 167, 388-396.

Friedman, S. H., Dani, N., Rushton, E., Kendal, T., and Broadie, K. (2013) Fragile X mental retardation protein regulates trans-synaptic signaling in Drosophila. *Dis. Mod. Mech.*, 6, 1400-1413.

Fu, W. Y., Chen, Y., Sahin, M., Zhao, X. S., Shi, L., Bikoff, J. B., Lai, K. O., Yung, W. H., Fu, A. K., Greenberg, M. E., and Ip, N. Y. (2007) Cdk5 regulates EphA4-mediated dendritic spine retraction through an ephexin1-dependent mechanism. *Nat. Neurosci.*, 10, 67-76.

García-Peñas, J. J., Domínguez-Carral, J. and Pereira-Bezanilla, E. (2012) Alteraciones de la sinaptogénesis en el autismo. Implicaciones etiopatogénicas y terapéuticas. *Rev. Neurol.*, 54S, 41-50.

Gauthier, J., Champagne, N., Lafreniere, R. G., Xiong, L., Spiegelman, D., Brustein, E., Lapointe, M., Peng, H., Côté, M., Noreau, A., Hamdan, F. F., Addington, A. M., Rapoport, J. L., Delisi, L. E., Krebs, M. O., Joober, R., Fathalli, F., Mouaffak, F., Haghighi, A. P., Néri, C., Dubé, M. P., Samuels, M. E., Marineau, C., Stone, E. A., Awadalla, P., Barker, P. A., Carbonetto, S., Drapeau, P., and Rouleau, G. A. (2010) De novo mutations in the gene encoding the synaptic scaffolding protein SHANK3 in patients ascertained for schizophrenia. *Proc. Natl. Acad. Sci. US*, 107, 7863-7868.

Giagtzoglou, N., Ly, C. V. and Bellen, H. J. (2009) Cell adhesion, the backbone of the synapse: 'vertebrate' and 'invertebrate' perspectives. *Cold Spring Harb. Perspect. Biol.*, 1, a003079.

Goddard, C. A., Butts, D. A. and Shatz, C. J. (2007) Regulation of CNS synapses by neuronal MHC class I. *Proc. Natl. Acad. Sci. US*, 104, 6828–6833.

Goldberg, J. H., Tamas, G., Aronov, D., and Yuste, R. (2003) Calcium microdomains in aspiny dendrites. *Neuron*, 40, 807–821.

Gomez, T. M. and Zheng, J. Q. (2006) The molecular basis for calcium-dependent axon pathfinding. *Nat. Rev. Neurosci.*, 7, 115-125.

Govek, E. E., Newey, S. E., Akerman, C. J., Cross, J. R., Van der Veken, L., and Van Aelst, L. (2004) The X-linked mental retardation protein oligophrenin-1 is required for dendritic spine morphogenesis. *Nat. Neurosci.*, 7, 364-372.

Grabrucker, A. M., Schmeisser, M. J., Schoen, M., and Boeckers, T. M. (2011) Postsynaptic ProSAP/Shank scaffolds in the cross-hair of synaptopathies. *Trends Cell Biol.* 21, 594–603.

Haditsch, U., Leone, D. P., Farinelli, M., Chrostek-Grashoff, A., Brakebusch, C., Mansuy, I. M., McConnell, S. K., and Palmer, T. D. (2009) A central role for the small GTPase Rac1 in hippocampal plasticity and spatial learning and memory. *Mol. Cell. Neurosci.*, 41, 409-419.

Hamdan, F. F., Gauthier, J., Spiegelman, D., Noreau, A., Yang, Y., Pellerin, S., Dobrzeniecka, S., Cote, M., Perreau-Linck, E., Carmant, L., D'Anjou, G., Fombonne, E., Addington, A. M., Rapoport, J. L., Delisi, L. E., Krebs, M. O., Mouaffak, F., Joober, R., Mottron, L., Drapeau, P., Marineau, C., Lafrenière, R. G., Lacaille, J. C., Rouleau, G. A., and Michaud, J. L. (2009) Mutations in SYNGAP1 in autosomal nonsyndromic mental retardation. *N. Engl. J. Med.*, 360, 599-605.

Hayashi-Takagi, A., Takaki, M., Graziane, N., Seshadri, S., Murdoch, H., Dunlop, A. J., Makino, Y., Seshadri, A. J., Ishizuka, K., Srivastava, D. P., Xie, Z., Baraban, J. M., Houslay, M. D., Tomoda, T., Brandon, N. J., Kamiya, A., Yan, Z., Penzes, P., and Sawa, A. (2010) Disrupted-in-Schizophrenia 1 (DISC1) regulates spines of the glutamate synapse via Rac1. *Nat. Neurosci.*, 13, 327-332.

Hong, E. J., McCord, A. E. and Greenberg, M. E. (2008) A biological function for the neuronal activity-dependent component of Bdnf transcription in the development of cortical inhibition. *Neuron*, 60, 610–624.

Hong, K., Nishiyama, M., Henley, J., Tessier-Lavigne, M., and Poo, M. (2000) Calcium signaling in the guidance of nerve growth by netrin-1. *Nature*, 403, 93-98.

Hortsch, M., Nagaraj, K. and Mualla, R. (2014) The L1 family of cell adhesion molecules: a sickening number of mutations and protein functions. *Adv. Neurobiol.* 8, 195-229.

Hu, H., Qin, Y., Bochorishvili, G., Zhu, Y., Van Aelst, L., and Zhu, J. J. (2008) Ras signaling mechanisms underlying impaired GluR1-dependent plasticity associated with fragile X syndrome. *J. Neurosci.*, 28, 7847-7862.

Hutchins, B. I., Li, L. and Kalil, K. (2011) Wnt/calcium signaling mediates axon growth and guidance in the developing corpus callosum. *Dev. Neurobiol.*, 71, 269-283.

Inaki, M., Yoshikawa, S., Thomas, J. B., Aburatani, H., and Nose, A. (2007) Wnt4 is a local repulsive cue that determines synaptic target specificity. *Curr. Biol.*, 17, 1574–1579.

Ito, Y., Oinuma, I., Katoh, H., Kaibuchi, K. and Negishi, M. (2006) Sema4D/ plexin-B1 activates GSK-3beta through R-Ras GAP activity, inducing growth cone collapse. *EMBO Rep.*, 7, 704–709.

Jamain, S., Quach, H., Betancur, C., Rastam, M., Colineaux, C., Gillberg, I. C., and Bourgeron, T. (2003) Mutations of the X-linked genes encoding neuroligins NLGN3 and NLGN4 are associated with autism. *Nat. Genet.*, 34, 27–29.

Jin, M., Guan, C. B., Jiang, Y. A., Chen, G., Zhao, C. T., Cui, K., Song, Y. Q., Wu, C. P., Poo, M. M., and Yuan, X. B. (2005) Ca^{2+}-dependent regulation of rho GTPases triggers turning of nerve growth cones. *J. Neurosci.*, 25, 2338-2347.

Jonsson, L., Zettergren, A., Pettersson, E., Hovey, D., Anckarsäter, H., Westberg, L., Lichtenstein, P., Lundström, S., and Melke, J. (2014) Association study between autistic-like traits and polymorphisms in the autism candidate regions RELN, CNTNAP2, SHANK3, and CDH9/10. *Mol. Autism*, 5, 55.

Khelfaoui, M., Denis, C., van Galen, E., de Bock, F., Schmitt, A., Houbron, C., Morice, E., Giros, B., Ramakers, G., Fagni, L., Chelly, J., Nosten-Bertrand, M., and Billuart, P. (2007) Loss of X-linked mental retardation gene oligophrenin1 in mice impairs spatial memory and leads to ventricular enlargement and dendritic spine immaturity. *J. Neurosci.*, 27, 9439-9450.

Khelfaoui, M., Pavlowsky, A., Powell, A. D., Valnegri, P., Cheong, K. W., Blandin, Y., Passafaro, M., Jefferys, J. G., Chelly, J., and Billuart, P. (2009) Inhibition of RhoA pathway rescues the endocytosis defects in Oligophrenin1 mouse model of mental retardation. *Hum. Mol. Genet.*, 18, 2575-2583.

Kielland, A., Bochorishvili, G., Corson, J., Zhang, L., Rosin, D. L., Heggelund, P., and Zhu, J. J. (2009) Activity patterns govern synapse-specific AMPA-receptor trafficking between deliverable and synaptic pools. *Neuron*, 62, 84-101.

Kim, M. H., Choi, J., Yang, J., Chung, W., Kim, J. H., Paik, S. K., Kim, K., Han, S., Won, H., Bae, Y. S., Cho, S. H., Seo, J., Bae, Y. C., Choi, S. Y., and Kim, E. (2009) Enhanced NMDA receptor-mediated synaptic transmission, enhanced long-term potentiation, and impaired learning and memory in mice lacking IRSp53. *J. Neurosci.*, 29, 1586-1595.

Klassen, M. P. and Shen, K. (2007) Wnt signaling positions neuromuscular connectivity by inhibiting synapse formation in C. Elegans. *Cell*, 130, 704–716.

Klein, R. (2009) Bidirectional modulation of synaptic functions by Eph/ephrin signaling. *Nat. Neurosci.*, 12, 15–20.

Ko, J., Fuccillo, M. V., Malenka, R. C., and Sudhof, T. C. (2009) LRRTM2 functions as a neurexin ligand in promoting excitatory synapse formation. *Neuron*, 64, 791-798.

Leblond, C. S., Heinrich, J., Delorme, R., Proepper, C., Betancur, C., Huguet, G., Konyukh, M., Chaste, P., Ey, E., Rastam, M., Anckarsäter, H., Nygren, G., Gillberg, I. C., Melke, J., Toro, R., Regnault, B., Fauchereau, F., Mercati, O., Lemière, N., Skuse, D., Poot, M., Holt, R., Monaco, A. P., Järvelä, I., Kantojärvi, K., Vanhala, R., Curran, S., Collier, D. A., Bolton, P., Chiocchetti, A., Klauck, S. M., Poustka, F., Freitag, C. M., Waltes, R., Kopp, M., Duketis, E., Bacchelli, E., Minopoli, F., Ruta, L., Battaglia, A., Mazzone, L., Maestrini, E., Sequeira, A. F., Oliveira, B., Vicente, A., Oliveira, G., Pinto, D., Scherer, S. W., Zelenika, D., Delepine, M., Lathrop, M., Bonneau, D., Guinchat, V., Devillard, F., Assouline, B., Mouren, M. C., Leboyer, M., Gillberg, C., Boeckers, T. M., and Bourgeron, T. (2012) Genetic and functional analyses of SHANK2 mutations suggest a multiple hit model of autism spectrum disorders. *PLoS Genet.*, 8, e1002521.

Li, L., Hutchins, B. I. and Kalil, K. (2009) Wnt5a induces simultaneous cortical axon outgrowth and repulsive axon guidance through distinct signaling mechanisms. *J. Neurosci.*, 29, 5873–5883.

Lionel, A. C., Vaags, A. K., Sato, D., Gazzellone, M. J., Mitchell, E. B., Chen, H. Y., Costain, G., Walker, S., Egger, G., Thiruvahindrapuram, B., Merico, D., Prasad, A., Anagnostou, E., Fombonne, E., Zwaigenbaum, L., Roberts, W., Szatmari, P., Fernandez, B. A., Georgieva, L., Brzustowicz, L. M., Roetzer, K., Kaschnitz, W., Vincent, J. B., Windpassinger, C., Marshall, C. R., Trifiletti, R. R., Kirmani, S., Kirov, G., Petek, E., Hodge, J. C., Bassett, A. S., and Scherer, S. W. (2013) Rare exonic deletions implicate the synaptic organizer Gephyrin (GPHN) in risk for autism, schizophrenia and seizures. *Hum. Mol. Gen.*, 22, 2055–2066.

Lohmann, C. and Bonhoeffer, T. (2008) A role for local calcium signaling in rapid synaptic partner selection by dendritic filopodia. *Neuron*, 59, 253-260.

Lu, B., Wang, K. H. and Nose, A. (2009) Molecular mechanisms underlying neural circuit formation. *Curr. Opin. Neurobiol.*, 19, 162–167.

Lu, M., Witke, W., Kwiatkowski, D. J., and Kosik, K. S. (1997) Delayed retraction of filopodia in gelsolin null mice. *J. Cell Biol.*, 138, 1279-1287.

Lu, L., Guo, H., Peng, Y., Xun, G., Liu, Y., Xiong, Z., Tian, D., Liu, Y., Li, W., Xu, X., Zhao, J., Hu, Z., and Xia, K. (2014) Common and rare variants of the THBS1 gene associated with the risk for autism. *Psychiatr. Genet.*, 24, 235-240.

Maness, P. F. and Schachner, M. (2007) Neural recognition molecules of the immunoglobulin superfamily: signaling transducers of axon guidance and neuronal migration. *Nat. Neurosci.*, 10, 19-26.

Mann, F., Chauvet, S. and Rougon, G. (2007) Semaphorins in development and adult brain: Implication for neurological diseases. *Prog. Neurobiol.*, 82, 57–79.

Mao, Y., Ge, X., Frank, C. L., Madison, J. M., Koehler, A. N., Doud, M. K., Tassa, C., Berry, E. M., Soda, T., Singh, K. K., Biechele, T., Petryshen, T. L., Moon, R. T., Haggarty, S. J., and Tsai, L. H. (2009) Disrupted in schizophrenia 1 regulates neuronal progenitor proliferation via modulation of GSK3beta/beta-catenin signaling. *Cell*, 136, 1017-1031.

Melom, J. E. and Littleton, J. T. (2011) Synapse development in health and disease. *Curr. Opin. Genet. Dev.*, 21, 256-261.

Meng, J., Meng, Y., Hanna, A., Janus, C., and Jia, Z. (2005) Abnormal long-lasting synaptic plasticity and cognition in mice lacking the mental retardation gene Pak3. *J. Neurosci.*, 25, 6641-6650.

Meng, Y., Zhang, Y., Tregoubov, V., Janus, C., Cruz, L., Jackson, M., Lu, W. Y., MacDonald, J. F., Wang, J. Y., Falls, D. L., and Jia, Z. (2002) Abnormal spine morphology and enhanced LTP in LIMK-1 knockout mice. *Neuron*, 35, 121-133.

Mitchell, K. J. (2010) The genetics of neurodevelopmental disease. *Curr. Opin. Neurobiol.*, 21, 197-203.

Mulligan, K. A. and Cheyette, B. N. (2012) Wnt signaling in vertebrate neural development and function. *J. Neuroimm. Pharmacol.*, 7, 774-787.

Murray, A. J., Tucker, S. J. and Shewan, D. A. (2009) cAMP-dependent axon guidance is distinctly regulated by Epac and protein kinase A. *J. Neurosci.*, 29, 15434-15444.

Nadif-Kasri, N., Nakano-Kobayashi, A., Malinow, R., Li, B., and Van Aelst, L. (2009) The Rho-linked mental retardation protein oligophrenin-1 controls synapse maturation and plasticity by stabilizing AMPA receptors. *Genes Dev.*, 23, 1289-1302.

Nadif-Kasri, N. and Van Aelst, L. (2008) Rho-linked genes and neurological disorders. *Pflugers Arch.*, 455, 787-797.

Nakano-Kobayashi, A., Kasri, N. N., Newey, S. E., and Van Aelst, L. (2009) The Rho-linked mental retardation protein OPHN1 controls synaptic vesicle endocytosis via endophilin A1. *Curr. Biol.*, 19, 1133-1139.

Nimchinsky, E. A., Oberlander, A. M. and Svoboda, K. (2001) Abnormal Development of Dendritic Spines in FMR1 Knock-Out Mice. *J. Neurosci.*, 21, 5139–5146.

Node-Langlois, R., Muller, D. and Boda, B. (2006) Sequential implication of the mental retardation proteins ARHGEF6 and PAK3 in spine morphogenesis. *J. Cell. Sci.*, 119, 4986-4993.

O'Roak, B. J., Vives, L., Girirajan, S., Karakoc, E., Krumm, N., Coe, B. P., Levy, R., Ko, A., Lee, C., Smith, J. D., Turner, E. H., Stanaway, I. B., Vernot, B., Malig, M., Baker, C., Reilly, B., Akey, J. M., Borenstein, E., Rieder, M. J., Nickerson, D. A., Bernier, R., Shendure, J., and Eichler, E. E. (2012) Sporadic autism exomes reveal a highly interconnected protein network of de novo mutations. *Nature*, 485, 246–250.

Penzes, P., Beeser, A., Chernoff, J., Schiller, M. R., Eipper, B. A., Mains, R. E., and Huganir, R. L. (2003) Rapid induction of dendritic spine morphogenesis by trans-synaptic ephrinB-EphB receptor activation of the Rho-GEF kalirin. *Neuron*, 37, 263-274.

Phelan, K. and McDermid, H. E. (2012) The 22q13.3 Deletion Syndrome (Phelan-McDermid Syndrome). *Mol. Syndromol.*, 2, 186–201.

Pourcain, B. S., Wang, K., Glessner, J. T., Golding, J., Steer, C., Ring, S. M., Skuse, D. H., Grant, S. F., Hakonarson, H., and Davey Smith, G. (2010) Association between a high-risk autism locus on 5p14 and social communication spectrum phenotypes in the general population. *Am. J. Psychiat.*, 167, 1364–1372.

Raaijmakers, J. H. and Bos, J. L. (2009) Specificity in Ras and Rap signaling. *J. Biol. Chem.*, 284, 10995-10999.

Raper, J. and Mason, C. (2010) Cellular strategies of axonal pathfinding. *Cold Spring Harb. Perspect. Biol.*, 2, a001933.

Raper, J. A. (2000) Semaphorins and their receptors in vertebrates and invertebrates. *Curr. Opin. Neurobiol.*, 10, 88-94.

Rex, C. S., Chen, L. Y., Sharma, A., Liu, J., Babayan, A. H., Gall, C. M., and Lynch, G. (2009) Different Rho GTPase-dependent signaling pathways initiate sequential steps in the consolidation of long-term potentiation. *J. Cell Biol.*, 186, 85-97.

Rumbaugh, G., Adams, J. P., Kim, J. H., and Huganir, R. L. (2006) SynGAP regulates synaptic strength and mitogen-activated protein kinases in cultured neurons. *Proc. Natl. Acad. Sci. US*, 103, 4344-4351.

Rünker, A. E., O´Tuathaigh, C., Dunleavy, M., Morris, D. W., Little, G. E., Corvin, A. P., Gill, M., Henshall, D. C., Waddington, J. L., and Mitchell, K. J. (2011) Mutation of semaphorin-6a disrupts limbic and cortical connectivity and models. neurodevelopmental psychopathology. *PLoS ONE*, 6, e26488.

Ryu, J., Futai, K., Feliu, M., Weinberg, R., and Sheng, M. (2008) Constitutively active Rap2 transgenic mice display fewer dendritic spines, reduced extracellular signal-regulated kinase signaling, enhanced long-term depression, and impaired spatial learning and fear extinction. *J. Neurosci.*, 28, 8178-8188.

Salinas, P. C. and Zou, Y. (2008) Wnt signaling in neural circuit assembly. *Annu. Rev. Neurosci.*, 31, 339-358.

Sato, D., Lionel, A. C., Leblond, C. S., Prasad, A., Pinto, D., Walker, S., O'Connor, I., Russell, C., Drmic, I. E., Hamdan, F. F., Michaud, J. L., Endris, V., Roeth, R., Delorme, R., Huguet, G., Leboyer, M., Rastam, M., Gillberg, C., Lathrop, M., Stavropoulos, D. J., Anagnostou, E., Weksberg, R., Fombonne, E., Zwaigenbaum, L., Fernandez, B. A., Roberts, W., Rappold, G. A., Marshall, C. R., Bourgeron, T., Szatmari, P., and Scherer, S. W. (2012) SHANK1 Deletions in males with autism spectrum disorder. *Am. J. Hum. Genet.*, 90, 879–887.

Sawallisch, C., Berhorster, K., Disanza, A., Mantoani, S., Kintscher, M., Stoenica, L., Dityatev, A., Sieber, S., Kindler, S., Morellini, F., Schweizer, M., Boeckers, T. M., Korte, M., Scita, G., Kreienkamp, H. J. (2009) The insulin receptor substrate of 53 kDa (IRSp53) limits hippocampal synaptic plasticity. *J. Biol. Chem.*, 284, 9225-9236.

Scheiffele, P., Fan, J., Choih, J., Fetter, R., and Serafini, T. (2000) Neuroligin expressed in nonneuronal cells triggers presynaptic development in contacting axons. *Cell*, 101, 657–669.

Segura, I., Essmann, C. L., Weinges, S., and Acker-Palmer, A. (2007) Grb4 and GIT1 transduce ephrinB reverse signals modulating spine morphogenesis and synapse formation. *Nat. Neurosci.*, 10, 301–310.

Shen, K. and Cowan, C. W. (2009) Guidance molecules in synapse formation and plasticity. *Cold Spring Harb. Perspect. Biol.*, 2, a001842.

Soderling, S. H., Guire, E. S., Kaech, S., White, J., Zhang, F., Schutz, K., Langeberg, L. K., Banker, G., Raber, J., and Scott, J. D. (2007) A WAVE-1 and WRP signaling complex regulates spine density, synaptic plasticity, and memory. *J. Neurosci*., 27, 355-365.

Soler-Llavina, G. J. and Sabatini, B. L. (2006) Synapse-specific plasticity and compartmentalized signaling in cerebellar stellate cells. *Nat. Neurosci*., 9, 798–806.

Song, H., Ming, G., He, Z., Lehmann, M., McKerracher, L., Tessier-Lavigne, M., and Poo, M. (1998) Conversion of neuronal growth cone responses from repulsion to attraction by cyclic nucleotides. *Science*, 281, 1515-1518.

Song, J. Y., Ichtchenko, K., Sudhof, T. C., and Brose, N. (1999) Neuroligin 1 is a postsynaptic cell-adhesion molecule of excitatory synapses. *Proc. Natl. Acad. Sci. US*, 96, 1100–1105.

Sousa, I., Clark, T. G., Holt, R., Pagnamenta, A. T., Mulder, E. J., and Minderaa, R. B. (2010) Polymorphisms in leucine-rich repeat genes are associated with autism spectrum disorder susceptibility in populations of European ancestry. *Mol. Autism*, 1, 7.

Strauss, K. A., Puffenberger, E. G., Huentelman, M. J., Gottlieb, S., Dobrin, S. E., Parod, J. M., Stephan, D. A., and Morton, D. H. (2006) Recessive symptomatic focal epilepsy and mutant contactin-associated protein-like 2. *N. Engl. J. Med*., 354, 1370–1377.

Suda, S., Iwata, K., Shimmura, C., Kameno, Y., Anitha, A., Thanseem, I., Nakamura, K., Matsuzaki, H., Tsuchiya, K. J., Sugihara, G., Iwata, Y., Suzuki, K., Koizumi, K., Higashida, H., Takei, N., and Mori, N. (2011) Decreased expression of axon-guidance receptors in the anterior cingulate cortex in autism. *Mol. Autism*., 2, 14.

Sudhof, T. C. (2008) Neuroligins and neurexins link synaptic function to cognitive disease. *Nature*, 455, 903-911.

Sun, M. K., Hongpaisan, J., Lim, C. S., and Alkon, D. L. (2014) Bryostatin-1 restores hippocampal synapses and spatial learning and memory in adult fragile x mice. *J. Pharmacol. Exp. Ther*., 349, 393-401.

Tabuchi, K., Blundell, J., Etherton, M. R., Hammer, R. E., Liu, X., Powell, C. M., and Sudhof, T. C. (2007) A neuroligin-3 mutation implicated in autism increases inhibitory synaptic transmission in mice. *Science*, 318, 71–76.

Takayanagi, Y., Fujita, E., Yu, Z., Yamagata, T., Momoi, M. Y., Momoi, T., and Onaka, T. (2010) Impairment of social and emotional behaviors in Cadm1-knockout mice. *Biochem. Biophys. Res. Commun*., 396, 703-708.

Tenzen, T., Allen, B. L., Cole, F., Kang, J. S., Krauss, R. S., and McMahon, A. P. (2006) The cell surface membrane proteins Cdo and Boc are components and targets of the Hedgehog signaling pathway and feedback network in mice. *Dev. Cell*, 10, 647-656.

Tolias, K. F., Bikoff, J. B., Kane, C. G., Tolias, C. S., Hu, L., and Greenberg, M. E. (2007) The Rac1 guanine nucleotide exchange factor Tiam1 mediates EphB receptor-dependent dendritic spine development. *Proc. Natl. Acad. Sci. US*, 104, 7265-7270.

Toyofuku, T., Yoshida, J., Sugimoto, T., Zhang, H., Kumanogoh, A., Hori, M., and Kikutani, H. (2005) FARP2 triggers signals for Sema3A-mediated axonal repulsion. *Nat. Neurosci*., 8, 1712-1719.

Tran, T. S., Kolodkin, A. L. and Bharadwaj, R. (2007) Semaphorin regulation of cellular morphology. *Annu. Rev. Cell Dev. Biol*., 23, 263-292.

Trousse, F., Marti, E., Gruss, P., Torres, M., and Bovolenta, P. (2001) Control of retinal ganglion cell axon growth: a new role for Sonic hedgehog. *Development*, 128, 3927-3936.

Varoqueaux, F., Jamain, S. and Brose, N. (2004) Neuroligin 2 is exclusively localized to inhibitory synapses. *Eur. J. Cell Biol.*, 83, 449–456.

Wang, G. X. and Poo, M. M. (2005) Requirement of TRPC channels in netrin-1-induced chemotropic turning of nerve growth cones. *Nature*, 434, 898-904.

Wang, K. H., Majewska, A., Schummers, J., Farley, B., Hu, C., Sur, M., and Tonegawa, S. (2006) In vivo two-photon imaging reveals a role of arc in enhancing orientation specificity in visual cortex. *Cell*, 126, 389–402.

Wang, X. S., Peng, C. Z., Cai, W. J., Xia, J., Jin, D., Dai, Y., Luo, X. G., Klyachko, V. A., and Deng, P. Y. (2014) Activity-dependent regulation of release probability at excitatory hippocampal synapses: a crucial role of fragile X mental retardation protein in neurotransmission. *Eur. J. Neurosci.*, 39, 1602-12.

Webb, D. J., Zhang, H., Majumdar, D., and Horwitz, A. F. (2007) alpha5 integrin signaling regulates the formation of spines and synapses in hippocampal neurons. *J. Biol. Chem.*, 282, 6929-6935.

Wen, Z., Guirland, C., Ming, G. L., and Zheng, J. Q. (2004) A CaMKII/calcineurin switch controls the direction of $Ca(^{2+})$-dependent growth cone guidance. *Neuron*, 43, 835-846.

Wierenga, C. J., Becker, N. and Bonhoeffer, T. (2008) GABAergic synapses are formed without the involvement of dendritic protrusions. *Nat. Neurosci.*, 11, 1044-1052.

Wisniowiecka-Kowalnik, B., Nesteruk, M., Peters, S. U., Xia, Z., Cooper, M. L., Savage, S., Amato, R. S., Bader, P., Browning, M. F., Haun, C. L., Duda, A. W., Cheung, S. W., and Stankiewicz, P. (2010) Intragenic rearrangements in NRXN1 in three families with autism spectrum disorder, developmental delay, and speech delay. *Am. J. Med. Genet. B Neuropsychiatr. Genet.*, 153B, 983–993.

Wolf, A. M., Lyuksyutova, A. I., Fenstermaker, A. G., Shafer, B., Lo, C. G., and Zou, Y. (2008) Phosphatidylinositol-3-kinase-atypical protein kinase C signaling is required for Wnt attraction and anterior-posterior axon guidance. *J. Neurosci.*, 28, 3456-3467.

Woo, J., Kwon, S. K. and Kim, E. (2009) The NGL family of Leucine-rich repeat-containing synaptic adhesion molecules. *Mol. Cell Neurosci.*, 42, 1-10.

Wu, H., Rossi, G. and Brennwald, P. (2008) The ghost in the machine: small GTPases as spatial regulators of exocytosis. *Trends Cell Biol.*, 18, 397-404.

Wu, K. Y., Zippin, J. H., Huron, D. R., Kamenetsky, M., Hengst, U., Buck, J., Levin, L. R., and Jaffrey, S. R. (2006) Soluble adenylyl cyclase is required for netrin-1 signaling in nerve growth cones. *Nat. Neurosci.*, 9, 1257-1264.

Xie, Z., Srivastava, D. P., Photowala, H., Kai, L., Cahill, M. E., Woolfrey, K. M., Shum, C. Y., Surmeier, D. J., and Penzes, P. (2007) Kalirin-7 controls activity-dependent structural and functional plasticity of dendritic spines. *Neuron*, 56, 640-656.

Yam, P. T., Langlois, S. D., Morin, S., and Charron, F. (2009) Sonic hedgehog guides axons through a noncanonical, Src-family-kinase-dependent signaling pathway. *Neuron*, 62, 349-362.

Zhang, C., Milunsky, J. M., Newton, S., Ko, J., Zhao, G., Maher, T. A., Tager-Flusberg, H., Bolliger, M. F., Carter, A. S., Boucard, A. A., Powell, C. M., and Südhof, T. C. (2009) A neuroligin-4 missense mutation associated with autism impairs neuroligin-4 folding and endoplasmic reticulum export. *J. Neurosci.*, 29, 10843–10854.

Zheng, J. Q. (2000) Turning of nerve growth cones induced by localized increases in intracellular calcium ions. *Nature*, 403, 89-93.

Zhiling, Y., Fujita, E., Tanabe, Y., Yamagata, T., Momoi, T., and Momoi, M. Y. (2008) Mutations in the gene encoding CADM1 are associated with autism spectrum disorder. *Biochem. Biophys. Res. Commun.*, 377, 926–929.

Zhou, Z., Hong, E. J., Cohen, S., Zhao, W. N., Ho, H. Y., Schmidt, L., Chen, W. G., Lin, Y., Savner, E., Griffith, E.C., Hu, L., Steen, J. A., Weitz, C. J., and Greenberg, M. E. (2006) Brain-specific phosphorylation of MeCP2 regulates activity-dependent Bdnf transcription, dendritic growth, and spine maturation. *Neuron*, 52, 255–269.

Zhu, Y., Pak, D., Qin, Y., McCormack, S. G., Kim, M. J., Baumgart, J. P., Velamoor, V., Auberson, Y. P., Osten, P., van Aelst, L., Sheng, M., and Zhu, J. J. (2005) Rap2-JNK removes synaptic AMPA receptors during depotentiation. *Neuron*, 46, 905-916.

Zuko, A., Kleijer, K. T., Oguro-Ando, A., Kas, M. J., van Daalen, E., van der Zwaag, B., and Burbach, J. P. (2013) Contactins in the neurobiology of autism. *Eur. J. Pharmacol.*, 719, 63-74.

In: Synaptic Fundamentals of Memory Performance
Editor: Ignacio González-Burgos
ISBN: 978-1-63483-279-3

Chapter 2

The Cellular and Molecular Mechanisms Driving the Estrogenic Modulation of Synaptic Activity in Mnemonic Information Processing

Oscar González-Flores[1,*], Raymundo Domínguez-Ordóñez[1,2] and Ignacio González-Burgos[3]

[1]Centro de Investigación en Reproducción Animal, UAT-CINVESTAV, IPN. Panotla, Tlaxcala, México
[2]Centro Tlaxcala de Biología de la Conducta-Universidad Autónoma de Tlaxcala. Panotla, Tlaxcala, México
[3]Laboratorio de Psicobiología, División de Neurociencias, Centro de Investigación Biomédica de Occidente, IMSS. Guadalajara, Jalisco, México

Abstract

Estrogen receptors (ER) can be activated by their natural ligand estradiol (E_2), although several cytoplasmic and nuclear ERs have been identified that may be activated in a different manner, such as ER-α66 and ER-β. The cloning of human ER-α66 led to the identification of variants of this receptor, including the ER-α46 splice variant and more recently, the novel ERα-36 variant. On the other hand, five splice variants of ER-β have also been identified named Erb1, Erb2, Erb1d3, Erb2d3 and Erb1d4, possibly with distinct biological activities. Both ER-α and ER-β receptors are expressed extensively in the brain, and even in the spinal cord. Furthermore, ER-α/ER-β receptor expression overlaps in several brain regions, although often to a different extent, and the functional role of such an overlapping distribution is still unclear. While ER-α plays a key role in

* Send correspondence to: Oscar González-Flores, PhD, Centro de Investigación en Reproducción Animal, Universidad Autónoma de Tlaxcala-CINVESTAV, Instituto Politécnico Nacional. Panotla, Tlaxcala. México. Email: oglezflo@gmail.com.

the regulation of reproductive behavior and neuroendocrine activity, ER-β is more strongly involved in non-reproductive psychoneural processes of a cognitive nature, such as learning and memory.

In fact, ER-β expression predominates over ERα in several cognition-related brain regions, such as the hippocampus and prefrontal cortex. Nevertheless, both ER-α and ER-β are thought to modulate the excitatory synaptic activity underlying the transmission of cognitive information at dendritic spines, both in the hippocampus and prefrontal cortex. In this sense they favor and protect the integrity of learning- and mnemonic-associated information to yield adequate behavioral patterns, although the precise role of the α and β ERs in these events has yet to be elucidated. In addition, ER activation could have a distinct cognitive significance depending on the origin of E_2 synthesis (i.e., gonadal or locally in the brain).

1. Introduction

Estrogens are steroid hormones synthesized from cholesterol molecules in different organs, such as the ovaries, uterus, mammary and adrenal glands, placenta, skin and brain among others. These hormones are involved in a wide range of physiological processes including reproduction, development, cardiovascular protection and brain function. However, the cellular mechanism by which estrogens exert their effects has not been well established. Nevertheless, it is known that estradiol (E_2) is the most potent estrogen given its higher affinity for both intracellular and membrane receptors.

The classic estrogen receptors (ER) belong to a nuclear receptor superfamily that includes the androgen receptor, vitamin D receptor and thyroid hormone receptor. Most of the biological effects of estrogens are mediated by the ERs, ER-α and ER-β, which up- or downregulate the expression of their target genes by binding to site-specific DNA sequences (estrogen response elements -EREs) and/or specific co-regulatory proteins, including co-activators and co-repressors. In addition, non-genomic activity of ERs and rapid effects initiated at the membrane have been described in the brain, which influence a wide range of brain functions, including learning and memory.

Both ER subtypes are expressed in different regions of the human forebrain, although they show distinct distributions. ER-α mRNA is expressed predominantly in the hypothalamus and amygdala, indicating that the α-subtype might modulate neuronal cell populations involved mainly in autonomic and reproductive neuroendocrine functions, or in emotional interpretation and processing. By contrast, ER-β is predominantly found in the hippocampal formation, cortex and thalamus, suggesting a key role for ER-β in cognition.

It is also well documented that E_2 can also provoke many fast 'non-genomic' effects and that these may be mediated by extranuclear ERs or by non-classic membrane bound receptors. In fact, both genomic and non-genomic effects of ERs are involved in cognition as they modulate plastic changes occurring in the dendritic spines that form synaptic contacts. Thus, E_2, whether synthesized in the gonads (neuroactive steroids) or locally in the brain (neurosteroids), can influence synaptic transmission in brain regions involved in cognitive information processing, such as the hippocampus and prefrontal cortex.

2. Estrogen Synthesis

2.1. E_2 Synthesis in Peripheral Organs

As indicated above, estrogens are produced from cholesterol, primarily in the ovaries, corpus luteum and placenta. However, other organs such as the liver, heart, skin and brain also produce small but significant amounts of estrogens (Cui et al., 2013). The biosynthesis of estrogens (Figure 1) begins when pregnenolone is converted to progesterone by 3β-hydroxysteroid dehydrogenase (3β-HSD) in both thecal and granulosa cells.

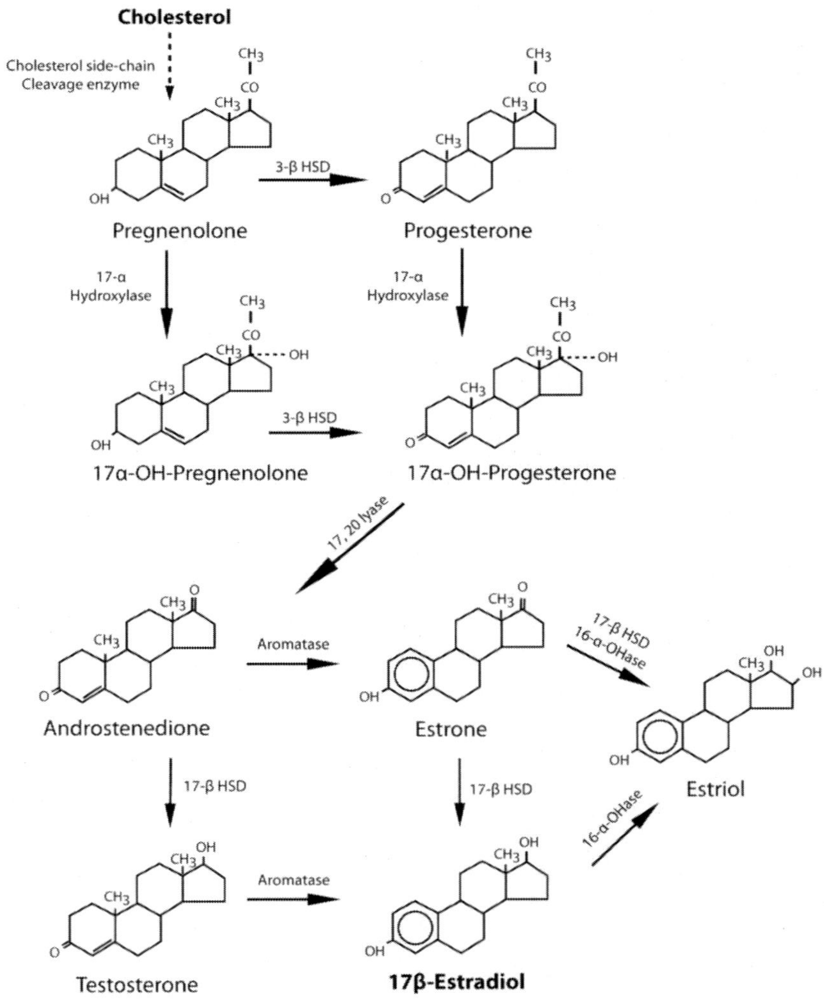

Figure 1. Estradiol synthesis starts with the conversion of cholesterol to pregnenolone through cytochrome P450 side-chain cleavage enzyme (P450scc). Pregnenolone is then converted to progesterone by 3β-hydroxysteroid dehydrogenase (3β HSD), which is converted to androgens by cytochrome P450 17 β-hydroxylase and 17β-hydroxysteroid dehydrogenase (17β-HSD). Finally aromatase (P450Arom) catalyzes the synthesis of E_2 from androgens.

Progesterone can be converted to androgens via cytochrome P450 17α-hydroxylase (P45017α) and 17β-hydroxysteroid dehydrogenase (17β-HSD) in the thecal cells during the follicular phase.

The conversion of androgens to estrogens is then catalyzed by aromatase (P450Arom) in granulosa cells (Hillier et al., 1994; Cui et al., 2013). In female mammals, three major forms of physiological estrogens are synthesized: estrone (E_1), estradiol (E_2, or 17β-estradiol), and estriol (E_3). E_2 is synthesized from E_1 by 16α-hydroxylation and it is the most potent estrogen, as well as being the main product of the entire biosynthesis pathway during the reproductive cycle. E_2 is largely synthesized in the placenta, which is strongly associated with its crucial role during pregnancy (Cui et al., 2013).

2.2. E_2 Synthesis in the Brain

Aromatase (P450scc) is the sole enzyme that mediates the conversion of cholesterol to pregnenolone, and it has been identified in the hippocampus, hypothalamus, caudate nucleus, thalamus, cerebral cortex, cerebellum and limbic areas like the amygdala. Aromatase expression has also been discovered in non-primary reproductive brain areas, including regions of the basal forebrain, hippocampus, thalamus, cerebral cortex, cerebellum and brainstem, where it is involved in regulating neural development, synaptic plasticity and cell survival (Azcoitia et al., 2011; Cui et al., 2013).

Under physiological conditions, neurons are the main site of E_2 synthesis in the brain, although elevated aromatase expression in astrocytes has also been found following brain injury, suggesting that neuronal impairment can induce E_2 production in these glial cells (Gatson et al., 2011). By contrast, microglia and oligodendrocytes fail to produce brain E_2 from cholesterol, although microglial cells do express 17β-HSD that can convert E_1 to E_2 and hypothetically, androstenedione to testosterone (Gottfried-Blackmore et al., 2008; Cui et al., 2013).

3. ESTROGEN RECEPTORS

Estrogen receptors (Figure 2) mediate the effects of estrogens and therefore, they participate in various cellular and physiological processes. Two subtypes of ERs are synthesized in distinct cell types: ER-α (Green et al., 1986) and ER-β (Kuiper et al., 1996; Tremblay et al., 1997). These are the products of separate genes located on chromosomes 6 and 14, which give rise to two proteins of 595 and 530 amino acids respectively, derived from the 8 exons of the ER genes. Recently, it became accepted that ER-α acts as a non-traditional G-protein coupled receptor (GPCR) at the plasma membrane (Adams et al., 2002; Micevych & Dominguez, 2010). Similarly, the GPCR GPR30, has been associated with specific estradiol binding at the cell membrane and with rapid estrogen-dependent signaling (Micevych & Dominguez, 2010; Cui et al., 2013).

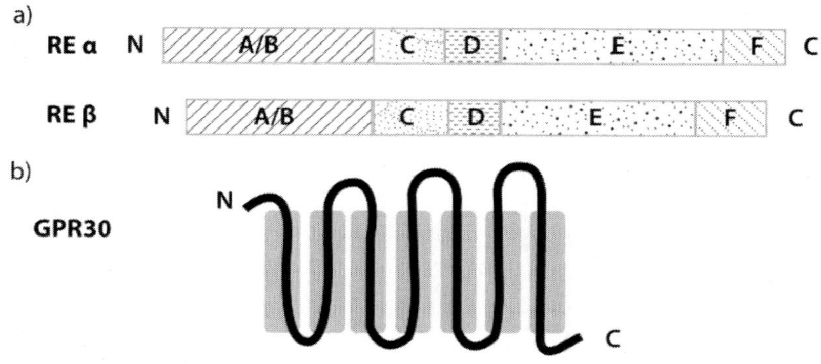

Figure 2. Estrogen receptors. a) The structure of 3 estrogen receptors is depicted. Two of them are the classical intracellular receptors known as ER-α and ER-β that have a modular structure. Both are similar but they differ in length; ER-α is longer than ER-β. b) GPR30 is a membrane estrogen receptor with seven transmembrane domains. Its N terminus lies outside the cell membrane and the C terminus is within the cell.

3.1. ER-α and ER-β Structure

ERs are members of the nuclear hormone receptor family that contain different functional domains with specific roles: 1) the N-terminal domain (NTD) located between amino acid 1 to 180, also called the A/B domain or activation function 1 (AF1). This region is responsible for protein-protein interactions and transactivation, as well as ligand independent AF1 function. In contrast to ER-α, the AF1 of ER-β contains a repressor domain that diminishes the overall transcriptional activity of the receptor by masking transactivation of the amino terminal domain, and it only functions in the context of a full length receptor (Hall & McDonell, 1999; Ellman et al., 2009); 2) the DNA binding domain, also called the C domain, is located between amino acids 181 and 263, and it contains two zinc-finger motifs that are responsible for both DNA-binding and receptor dimerization; 3) the D-domain located between amino acids 264 and 302 is also referred to as the Hinge-region, which allows receptor folding and is the region where the receptor can be phosphorylated; 4) the ligand binding domain (LBD) in the carboxyl terminal, also called the E and F domains, located between amino acid 303 and 552, and 553 and 595, respectively. The AF2 motif is located in the E domain and this domain not only binds the ligand but it is also an interaction site for co-activators and co-repressors. The F domain represents the last 45 amino acids of ER-α and approximately the last 30 amino acids of ER-β, where it potentially restrains ER dimerization and thereby protects against improper ligand activation (Skafar & Koide, 2006; Yang et al., 2008; Ellman et al., 2009).

ER-β is somewhat shorter than ER-α, containing 530 amino acids (Kuiper et al., 1996; Tremblay et al., 1997). The region of highest homology between ER-α and ER-β is in the DBD (95%), while the A/B, D and E domains are less well conserved. The two ER subtypes may also fulfill distinct physiological roles, as suggested by their somewhat different structures, especially in the crucial LBD where there is considerably less homology (53%). For instance, certain ligands are ER-β-selective agonists, such as the phytoestrogen genistein (Strissel & Strick, 2005; Ellman et al., 2009). Moreover, ER-β lacks a large portion of the carboxyl terminal F domain (Skafar & Koide, 2006; Yang et al., 2008), a region known to be important for the agonistic effect of anti-estrogens like tamoxifen (Norman et al., 2004). Since these sequence differences in the A/B and F domains can significantly alter protein function, it is possible that ER-β expression might contribute to clinical tamoxifen resistance by influencing the agonist effect of tamoxifen on breast tumor growth. This hypothesis is now under investigation.

3.1.1. Variant ER-α and ER-β Protein Isoforms

Several alternative mRNA splice variants of the wild-type ER-α66 and ER-β1 ERs are known to exist in cells, and three ER-α and five ER-β variants have been identified (e.g., ER-α36, ER-α46 and ER-β2–ER-β5) (Fluoriot et al., 2000; Hirata et al., 2003; Wang et al., 2005). ER-α46 lacks the first 173 amino acids (A/B or AF-1 domain) due to alternative splicing of the ER-α66 gene that produces skipping of exon 1 (Penot et al., 2005). A novel ER-α variant has been cloned and identified, ER-α36, which is located in the plasma membrane and cytoplasm, and that mediates rapid membrane-initiated non-genomic signaling pathway (Wang et al., 2005). Moreover, the subcellular distribution of ER-α36 differs from that of the wild-type receptor and it fulfills its own specific functions. Several groups have identified ER-α splice variants in a number of different tissues, such as human breast epithelium, endometrium and pituitary, as well as in a variety of tumors including breast cancer, endometrial carcinoma and meningiomas. Significantly, these mRNA variants are usually co-expressed along with the wild-type receptor (Bardin et al., 2004).

3.2. GPR30 (GPER1)

GPR30 is an orphan GPCR identified as an estrogen-sensitive receptor in cancer cells and that was renamed as G-protein estrogen receptor 1 (GPER1) (Funakoshi et al., 2006). GPR30 is characterized by the presence of seven transmembrane helices and it is predominantly expressed at the surface of the cell (Prossnitz et al., 2008). This receptor is comprised of 375 amino acids and it has a theoretical molecular mass of approximately 41 kDa. It is thought that its N-terminus is located outside of the cell and that the aspartic acid residues in the terminal region might be modified by glycosylation if GPR30 is situated in the plasma membrane. It has been speculated that its ligand associates with the N-terminal domain to activate the receptor. Based on its molecular structure, trimeric G proteins are presumed to bind to the 3rd loop of the intracellular domain (Mizukami, 2010).

4. ESTROGEN SIGNALING PATHWAYS (FIGURE 3)

4.1. ER-Dependent, Nuclear-Initiated Estrogen Signaling

Upon interacting with their ligand, ERs classically dimerize and translocate to the nucleus, acting as transcription factors by binding to specific EREs in promoter sequences or by interacting with other transcription factors (tethered actions). In addition, ligand-free ERs may be phosphorylated by activated kinases (e.g., through growth factor receptor activation)

(Kato et al., 1995) and they may then dimerize, bind to DNA and regulate gene transcription, contributing to the hormone-independence of certain tumors (Couts & Murphy, 1998; Shim et al., 2000).

ER-α and ER-β are mainly located within the nucleus (Edwards et al., 1980; Kampa et al., 2013), although their distribution is altered following ligand binding. For example, in a ligand-free state the distribution of the receptor is relatively homogeneous within the nuclear matrix, yet as the E_2-ER complex forms, the ER interacts with specific nuclear elements to drive gene transcription (Yamashita, 1998; Hager et al., 2000). Recently, it was found that these receptors constantly shuttle between the cytoplasm and the nucleus, while the binding of agonists and antagonists modifies this highly dynamic process (Dauvois et al., 1993).

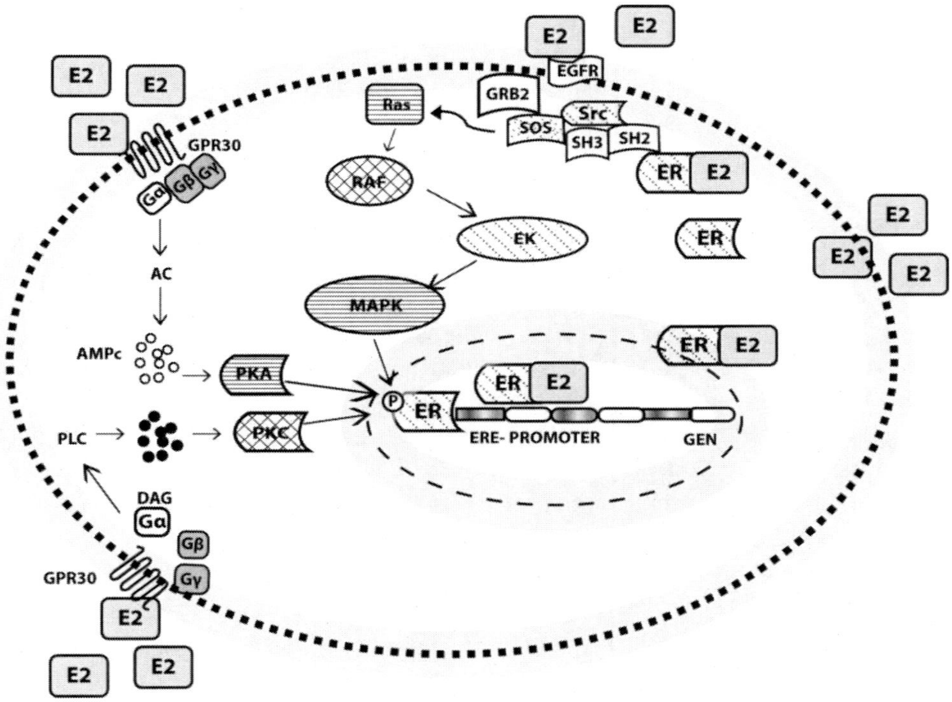

Figure 3. ER activation of transcription. There are 2 main pathways to activate transcription through ERs. Pathway 1: nuclear-initiated estrogen signaling mediated through classical ERs leads to the transcriptional changes in estrogen-responsive genes with or without EREs. Pathway 2: ligand independent genomic actions. Membrane initiated estrogen signaling activates protein-kinase cascades, leading to the phosphorylation (P) and activation of nuclear ERs at EREs.

The nuclear import of ERs is regulated by their binding to proteins that facilitate their transport through a specific sequence of basic amino acids (KRSKK in the case of ERs), a nuclear localization signal (Yamashita, 1998; Sebastian et al., 2004). ERs also interact with other proteins that contain nuclear export signals in order for them to be transported out to the cytoplasm as a protein complex (Castoria et al., 2009). In the nucleus, ligand- or phosphorylated-activated ERs bind to specific EREs to modify the transcription of estrogen-responsive genes, or alternatively, they interact with other transcription factors through protein-protein interactions in order to regulate genes lacking EREs (Rodriguez et al., 2004). This binding is enhanced or attenuated by the interaction of the ER with co-regulators (co-activators or co-repressors, respectively) (Edwards, 2000; Carlberg & Seuter, 2010). Co-activator binding and activity is relatively well characterized for the AF2 region of ER. Notably, these co-regulator proteins contain the characteristic LxxLL motif (Edwards et al., 1980; Savkur and Burris, 2004), and they bind to and activate (or phosphorylate) ERs by modifying their conformation. It is important to note that a platform (P295-T311) between the hinge (D) and the ligand binding domain (E/F) of the ER-α, which is well-conserved among all NR3 class receptors, participates actively in co-regulator binding and in modifying the activity of the receptor (Jacquot et al., 2007). By contrast, the AF1, ligand-independent co-regulator binding region is less well studied. It has been proposed that different domains of this AF1 region (amino acids 1-62, 80-113 and 118-149) represent the active platform for this function, while an interaction of AF1 and AF2 may also occur (Kato et al., 1995; Metzger et al., 1995). When the ERs are phosphorylated and they interact with DNA, the receptor molecule becomes polyubiquitinated, it dissociates from the DNA and it transiently accumulates in the nuclear matrix before being subsequently degraded by the action of the 26S proteasome (Laïos et al., 2005; Nonclercq et al., 2007).

4.2. ER-Dependent, Membrane-Initiated Estrogen Signaling (mERs)

In addition to the classical nuclear action of E_2, rapid membrane-initiated actions have been observed since the late 1960s (Toft & Gorski, 1966; Walter et al., 1985). Exposure to E_2 can rapidly induce the activation of many protein kinases and modulate ion flux across the plasma membrane (e.g., Ca^{2+}, K^+) (Valverde et al., 1999; Li et al., 2007). Since such transient events are not prevented by inhibitors of protein synthesis, specific mERs are involved. This is supported by the evidence that treatment with membrane impermeable estrogen, typically E_2 conjugated to bovine serum albumin (E_2-BSA) over a short time course (seconds to minutes), can mimic the rapid effects of E_2 on signal transduction pathways.

Extranuclear/membrane actions of estrogen have been defined and for example, a specific effect of E_2 on K^+-channels has been seen in the CNS (White et al., 1995; Wang et al., 2007). On the other hand, the activation of a number of kinases implicated in membrane signaling was one of the first E_2-related extranuclear actions observed. The kinases involved include cyclic nucleotide generating enzymes (cAMP, cGMP) and subsequently, activated protein lipid kinases like PI3K (Kim & Bender, 2009; Thomas, 2012) or Src (Ramseyet al.,2004; Alexaki et al., 2006), as well as their interaction with growth factor receptors (either direct as suggested for GPR30 or indirect through Src144). The most extensively studied interaction is that with the epidermal growth factor receptor (EGFR) (Filardo & Thomas, 2005; Filardo et al., 2007), particularly in view of its prominent role in cancer cell biology and its place as a therapeutic target. Indeed, an E_2-membrane binding component seems to interact with EGFR either physically (Filardo & Thomas, 2005; Filardo et al., 2007) or through Src kinases, transactivating it and inducing specific signaling cascades.

The activation of membrane-related kinases triggers or modifies a number of intracellular signaling cascades. Estrogens have been implicated in the modulation of all the major intracellular signaling cascades, those mediated by: MAP kinases (Shim et al., 2000; Wang et al., 2006); c-JUN/Jnk (Alexaki et al., 2006); JAK-STAT (Coutts & Murphy, 1998; Kampa et al., 2012); cAMP (that promotes CREB transcription initiation) (Coutts & Murphy, 1998; Kampa et al., 2012); and PI3K/Akt signaling (Kim & Bender, 2009; Kampa et al., 2012). This latter cascade may lead to both gene transcription and/or cytoskeletal modifications. Indeed, E_2 is an important regulator of the actin cytoskeleton in a variety of cell types (Simoncini et al., 2003; Kampa et al., 2011), producing effects ranging from axonal growth, endothelial remodeling, cell migration and synaptic plasticity.

4.3. Ligand-Independent Activation of ER

In contrast to the relatively well-characterized steroid-dependent activation of transcription, several nuclear receptors can be activated in the apparent absence of their cognate hormone by processes referred to as ligand-independent activation (e.g., ER, androgen receptor, progesterone receptor, etc.) (Blaustein, 2004). In general, the ability of intracellular signaling pathways (e.g., PKA, PKC, MAPK) to stimulate nuclear receptor-dependent transcription is thought to be due to the capacity of these signaling pathways to target the receptors and their associated proteins (e.g., co-activators, co-repressors, heat shock proteins), at least in part through specific phosphorylation-events (Blaustein, 2004).

4.3.1. Ligand-Independent Activation by Protein Kinase A

As well as the capacity of ER-α to be phosphorylated in response to hormone, it can also be activated by several intracellular signaling pathways. Interest in these alternative signaling mechanisms began with the observation that a protein kinase A (PKA) activator, 8-bromo-cAMP (8Br-cAMP), and a protein phosphatase inhibitor (okadaic acid) could apparently stimulate the transcriptional activity of the A form of the chicken progesterone receptor in the absence of hormone (Denner et al., 1990; Power et al., 1991). Transient transfection studies indicated that cAMP activation of ER-α does not require either Ser118 phosphorylation or that of the receptor's A/B domain (El-Tanani & Green, 1997). Indeed, an ER-α deletion mutant lacking its entire amino terminus can be phosphorylated to the same extent as the full-length receptor (Le Goff et al., 1994). Interestingly, the cAMP mediated signaling pathway enhances the association of cyclin D1 with the ER, suggesting that the receptor's enhanced activity is driven by its interaction with other co-activators (Lamb et al., 2000). Thus, cAMP-mediated receptor-dependent transcription may depend on protein-protein interactions, as well as the intrinsic modulation of co-activators.

4.3.2. Ligand-Independent Activation by MAP Kinases

Evidence that MAPK could stimulate ER transcriptional activity comes from observations that growth factors can stimulate ER reporter gene expression in cultured cells (e.g., EGF and IGF-1) (Ignar-Trowbridge et al., 1992; Bunone et al., 1996). Importantly, these responses were blocked by anti-estrogens. In contrast to the AF-2 domain of ER-α, the AF-1 domain is considered to have constitutive activity and it is strongly dependent on several of the mapped serine phosphorylation sites (Le Goff et al., 1994). Moreover, activation of the ER-α by growth factors leads to Ser118 phosphorylation (Kato et al., 1995; Bunone et al., 1996), a phosphorylation event that is probably mediated by MAPK since overexpression of a constitutively activated Ras or MAPK kinase resulted in enhanced AF-1 activity (Kato et al., 1995; Bunone et al., 1996). The Src/Jnk signaling pathway also stimulates ER-α AF-1 transcriptional activity, although this does not appear to require Ser118 phosphorylation (Feng et al., 2001). Likewise, the p38 and Jnk MAP kinases stimulate ER-α transcriptional activity independent of phosphorylation at the known receptor sites (Lee et al., 2000). Thus, multiple factors may mediate growth factor-dependent signaling via MAPKs.

4.3.3. Ligand-Independent Activation by Protein Kinase C

ER-α-dependent transcriptional responses can also be influenced by agents that stimulate the intracellular PKC signaling pathway (Ignar-Trowbridge et al., 1996; Guilbaud et al., 1998; Demay et al., 2001) and interestingly, gonadotropin releasing hormone (GnRH) activation of ER reporter genes can be blocked by PKC inhibitors (Demay et al., 2001). The phorbol ester that activates PKC augments the phosphorylation of the ER-α A/B domain and this is at least partially attributed to Ser118 phosphorylation (Le Goff et al., 1994; Joel et al., 1995). However, other PKC inhibitors reduce ER-α expression (Cho & Katzenellenbogen, 1993; Guilbaud et al., 1998) and its binding to EREs *in vitro* (Martin et al., 1995), such as 12-O-tetradecanoylphorbol-13-acetate (TPA). The implications of these TPA-mediated effects in relation to the transcriptional activity of ERs remain unknown. The ER-α can be activated by TPA alone or synergistically with E_2, while ER-α-dependent responses can also be inhibited by TPA in a promoter-dependent and cell type-dependent manner (Cho & Katzenellenbogen, 1993; Ignar-Trowbridge et al., 1996; Guilbaud et al., 1998). In contrast to the aforementioned signaling pathways, the ability of PKC to modulate ER-α-dependent transcription has received little attention and the significance of these effects on ER-α activation remains to be determined.

5. Neurobiological Mechanisms Involved in the Influence of Gonadal Steroids on Cognitive Functions

The cognitive processes in humans that are attributable to changes in the secretion of gonadal hormones like estradiol have been studied in experimental animal models that mimic physiological and pathological situations that arise in humans (Gasbarri & Tomaz, 2012).

How estradiol affects cognitive function clearly depends on the type of test used and/or the nervous structures involved in the integration of each of the different cognitive processes. For example, estradiol reduces efficiency in the performance of striatal-dependent behavioral tests in young women, whereas estradiol treatment improves the acquisition of hippocampal-dependent learning tasks. Furthermore, the improved performance in cognitive tests observed after infusion of estradiol into the hippocampus specifically reflects the functional activity of this structure, in which one of the actions of estradiol is to promote an increase in dendritic spine density of CA1 pyramidal neurons over a time course closely related to the efficient implementation of memory retention tests. However, it is possible that the effects of estradiol on hippocampal-mediated cognitive activities might involve interactions with other brain structures (Gould et al., 1990; Woolley et al., 1990; Berman et al., 1997; Sandstrom & Williams, 2001, 2004; Rapp et al., 2003; Davis et al., 2005; Xu & Zhang, 2006; Zurkovsky et al., 2006; Hao et al., 2007; Velázquez-Zamora et al., 2012a,b). Estrogens are not only able to modulate the processes in the nervous system leading to the formation of memory but also, they can determine the nature and direction of the strategies used to solve a particular test, considering not only the magnitude but also the characteristics of the information and how it was learned (Gasbarri et al., 2009; Pompili et al., 2010). Thus, rats with elevated concentrations of plasma estrogens preferably use allocentric strategies in which displacement and spatial orientation of the motor responses is derived from the configuration of spatial maps that take into account the visual signals in the surrounding environment. By contrast, rats with low plasma levels of estrogens tend to use egocentric strategies to resolve the task, based on learning from their own movements (Korol, 2004). Given the widespread distribution of ERs in brain structures involved in cognitive processes, estrogen could exert an important influence on the participation of the different memory systems (González-Burgos, 2015), both in terms of their time course as well as the preference for specific cognitive strategies during learning (McGaugh, 2000). However, they may not have the ability to influence all cognitive processes (Dohanich, 2002; Luine, 2007).

Several experimental studies have demonstrated that estrogen can modify the activity of some synaptic structures in the hippocampus. Indeed, in the rat the density of dendritic spines on pyramidal cells in Ammon's horn fluctuates during the estrous cycle in function of the variations in plasma estradiol, i.e., with a maximal density during proestrus when the concentrations of estradiol are highest. By contrast, ovariectomy provokes a decrease in the density of dendritic spines, which can be restored by treatment with estradiol. Moreover, estradiol administration to ovariectomized rodents is also associated with enhanced glutamatergic neurotransmission, and better performance in learning and memory tests. Thus, the induction of these changes in the hippocampus by estradiol appears to have important implications for the integration of memory-dependent activities by this structure (Gould et al., 1990; Woolley et al., 1990; Woolley & McEwen, 1992; Warren & Juraska, 1997; Woolley et al., 1997; Tang et al., 1999; Leranth et al., 2002; Leuner & Shors, 2004; González-Burgos et al., 2005; Prange-Kiel et al., 2009; Smith et al., 2009).

5.1. ER Involvement in Cognitive Functions Modulation

In the brain, estradiol's effects on organization and activation are the result of its interaction with ER-α and ER-β, which differ in their affinity for different ligands or compounds. As mentioned above, these receptors are nuclear receptors that act as ligand-activated transcription factors by interacting with components of the transcriptional complex to regulate gene expression, thereby affecting protein synthesis and the cell's phenotype (Lee & McEwen, 2001; Mellon et al., 2001; Osterlund & Hurd, 2001; Gruber et al., 2002; Rehman & Masson, 2005). This ability to regulate protein synthesis directly is associated with the lasting effects exerted by estrogen on developing systems, including the brain.

In addition to their genomic actions, estrogens may modify a neuron's activity by binding to membrane receptors associated with second messenger signaling pathways on neurites, the soma, dendritic spines and axon terminals (Lee & McEwen, 2001; Sherwin & Henry, 2008). In this way estrogen may influence the activity of pre- and postsynaptic structures related to cell communication and plasticity (Genazzani et al., 2007). There are many signaling pathways and genes regulated by estrogens through the activation of CREB, GABA-A receptors, NMDA receptors, glutamic acid decarboxylase (GAD), Choline acetyltransferase (ChAT), and synaptic and dendritic spine-associated proteins (McEwen et al., 2001; Frick et al., 2002; Rudick & Woolley, 2003). The interaction of estradiol with its receptors, which can affect cholinergic, serotonergic, catecholaminergic and GABAergic neurotransmission, can modify the activity of various brain structures that affect behavior, mood and cognitive functions (Hosil & Hosil, 1999; McEwen, 2002; Zhou et al., 2002; Smith & McMahon, 2005). In fact, the cholinergic system is activated by estrogens in some brain regions that are important for learning and memory, such as the basal forebrain and its cholinergic projections to the hippocampus and prefrontal cortex (Gibbs et al., 2004; Luine, 2008).

ERs have been identified in brain structures directly related with reproductive activity, such as the hypothalamus and pituitary. However, significant amounts of ERs are also found in different CNS regions that are not specifically involved in reproductive function, such as the hippocampus, neocortex, basal forebrain, brainstem, the midbrain raphe nuclei, caudate nucleus, putamen and locus coeruleus. Instead, in some of these areas ERs appear to be important for learning and memory (McEwen, 2002; Micevych & Mermelstein, 2008; Sherwin & Henry, 2008). The predominant distribution of ER-α transcripts in the hypothalamus and the amygdala complex is apparently related to the participation of estradiol in the regulation of autonomic functions, emotions and neuroendocrine phenomena associated with reproduction. By contrast, the predominance of ER-β in the thalamus, hippocampus, entorhinal cortex and neocortex, seems to reflect its involvement in cognitive and motor functions (Osterlund & Hurd, 2001).

It has been shown that ER-α and ER-β fulfill distinct roles in memory (Rhodes & Frye 2006; Hart et al., 2007). Selective agonists of ER-β increase the levels of proteins that are fundamental for synaptic processes in the hippocampus and they induce morphological changes in hippocampal neurons, such as increasing the proportion of mushroom-type dendritic spines that are related to the mnemonic storing of learned information (Liu et al., 2008; González-Burgos, 2009, 2012). ER-β agonists also improve performance in tests of hippocampal-dependent memory (Liu et al., 2008).

Rapid changes in cognitive functions may be mediated by membrane-associated ERs. These ERs would activate MAPK signaling pathways in specific neural structures (Bryant et al., 2006), as suggested by the rapid effects of estradiol (within 4 h) on performance in both inhibitory avoidance and object recognition paradigms. Moreover, memory consolidation may be modified by estrogen in function of the time at which it is administered, bearing in mind that this process takes place within 1-2 hours after learning (McGaugh, 2000). Indeed, this is the case for the enhanced memory consolidation observed in the inhibitory avoidance, spatial memory (Morris water maze), and object recognition and location tests (Rhodes & Frye, 2006; Walf & Frye, 2006; Frye et al., 2007, Luine, 2008).

5.2. Estrogen Modulates Synapses on Dendritic Spines Associated to the Integration of Mnemonic Information

Dendritic spines can be considered as bioelectrical compartments (Koch et al., 1992; Koch & Zador, 1993) that translate afferent synaptic inputs. Their capacity to interpret such inputs is due to their ability to undergo dynamic plastic changes, such as neo-formation, resorption, enlargement, growth, shrinkage and reshaping. Indeed, dendritic spines have been classified in function of their shape, mainly based on the geometric relationship between their head and neck, as thin, mushroom, stubby, wide, branched and double spines (González-Burgos, 2009, 2012; González-Burgos et al., 2015).

Synaptic transmission of mnemonic information has long been known to induce plastic changes in dendritic spines in several cognition-related brain regions, such as the hippocampus and prefrontal cortex (Kasai et al., 2010). Among others, the strengthening and weakening of pre-existing synapses (Martin et al., 2000; Neves et al., 2008) on thin spines has been related to the learning of new information, and mushroom spines are associated to the persistent formation of mnemonic traces in long-term memory (Kasai et al., 2003; Matsuzaki et al., 2004; Bourne & Harris, 2007; Hofer & Bonhoefer, 2010). Furthermore, the long-term potentiation (LTP) of synapses is associated with an increase in spine density and structural alterations to existing spines (Luine, 2014), including the enlargement of thin spines to mushroom spines (Toni et al., 2001; Lang et al., 2004). By contrast, long-term depression (LTD) provokes the shrinkage of pre-existing thin spines (Bosch & Hayashi, 2012), and a decrease in their number and size (Bastrikova et al., 2008). Thus, LTP would induce memory consolidation whilst LTD would be useful to verify and correct incorrect memories (Hojo et al., 2011).

Cognitive impairment in menopausal women has long been attributed to the decline in circulating estrogens, such as E_2. Exogenous restitution of E_2 through hormone replacement therapy leads to a reversion of such impairments, both humans and in mammalian experimental models (Smith et al., 2009). A significant increase in spine density on hippocampal CA1 pyramidal cells can be observed in proestrus (Woolley et al., 1990; González-Burgos et al., 2005) or in ovariectomized rats that receive exogenous E_2 (Gould et al., 1990), which is related to the memory enhancing effects of E_2 (Cordoba-Montoya & Carrer, 1997; Daniel & Dohanich, 2001; González-Burgos et al., 2012). In addition, plastic variations in the types of spines have been reported in both cycling female rats and after E_2 treatment of ovariectomized rats, such as an increase of thin, mushroom and stubby spines in hippocampal CA1 pyramidal neurons in the latter (Velázquez-Zamora et al., 2012a). Alternatively, along with a greater density of dendritic spines in proestrus compared to estrus, CA1 pyramidal cells of female rats in proestrus have more thin spines and less mushroom spines than in estrus (González-Burgos et al., 2005). Hence, the improved place learning performance of female estrus rats (Warren & Juraska, 1997) could be related to the fast, learning-related neurotransmission favored by the predominance of thin spines seen in proestrus.

Reference memory has long been thought to be organized chiefly in the hippocampus, whilst working memory is controlled by the prefrontal cortex. Different types of spines are increased selectively in response to estrogen treatment when behavioral tasks related to different memory systems are preformed (Cervantes-Alfaro et al., 2015). This phenomenon strongly suggests that while rapid actions of exogenous E_2 may increase spine density and enhance cognition (Phan et al., 2012; Luine, 2014) other phenomena could be implicated in the psychobiological effects of estrogens at the synaptic level.

The rapid effects of E_2 on dendritic spine-associated plastic changes are mainly mediated by cytosolic ERs, whilst those related to long-term memory are chiefly regulated by nuclear ERs. Indeed, E_2 can act through both cytosolic and nuclear ERs, ER-α or ER-β (Hojo et al., 2011), to modulate cognitive performance in a synergistic manner (Phan et al., 2012). ER-α predominates over ER-β in the hippocampus (Mitra et al., 2003). Moreover, ER-α accumulates in the cytosol of dendritic spines from CA1 pyramidal cells, in conjunction with the metabotropic glutamate receptor 1 (Boulware & Mermelstein, 2009). This co-localization could be related with both the concerted actions of intra-spine and nuclear ER receptors, as well as the effects on long-term memory consolidation mediated by E_2. Stimulation of hippocampal ER-α by E_2 promotes dendritic spine growth and the expression of NMDA receptors (Solum & Handa, 2002). However, ER-β is also thought to be involved in dendritic spine remodeling. In fact, both ER's have been proposed to act in concert to modulate LTP and LTD in order to organize the behavioral performance of hippocampal-related mnemonic processes (Smith et al., 2009).

6. Modulation of Mnemonic Functions by Estrogens Synthesized in the Brain

E_2 in the brain may be synthesized locally or it may originate in the periphery. The effect of E_2 proceeding from peripheral circulation depends on the cyclic biological rhythms, whereas E_2 synthesized in the brain has transient effects on neural excitation and its associated events (Hojo et al., 2011). Accordingly, and given that circulating E_2 levels are much lower than in brain tissue (Hojo et al., 2008, 2009), it was proposed that local synthesis may play a more important role than gonadal E_2 in the modulation of memory-associated and spine-mediated synaptic plasticity (Bian et al., 2014). When hippocampal slice cultures are exposed to letrozole, there is a loss of spines and spine synapses, similar to that observed in the hippocampus of female mice after systemic letrozole administration (Kretz et al., 2004; Rune & Frotscher, 2005). This is consistent with the impairment of LTP and the loss of mushroom spines and spine synapses induced by letrozole (Vierk et al., 2012). These findings are likely to be associated with the memory deficits seen in aromatase inhibitor-treated women (Shilling et al., 2005).

Aromatase is expressed strongly at synapses and particularly at presynaptic terminals in the cerebral cortex, suggesting a strong influence of E_2 on postsynaptic structures and that brain-synthesized estrogens act as neuromodulators of excitatory glutamatergic neurotransmission (Srivastava et al., 2010). As opposed to ER-α in the hippocampus, ER-β is more abundant in the cortex (Mitra et al., 2003), sustaining a key role for ER-β in the rapid effects of estrogen that induce plastic changes on dendritic spines. In addition, exposing cortical neurons to E_2 induces a rapid elevation in the number of dendritic spines (Srivastava et al., 2008), which could be modulated by ER-β but not ER-α. In fact, and as discussed, ER-α-induced dendritic spine plastic changes in the adult hippocampus in function of NMDA receptor activation after E_2 stimulation, whereas ER-β-dependent alterations to spines on cortical neurons initially depend on AMPA activation.

Previous behavioral studies reported improved egocentric working memory performance after aromatase inhibition by letrozole in male rats (Alejandre-Gómez et al., 2007), which seems to be discordant with the consensus that aromatase inhibition is detrimental to cognitive performance. However, these finding could be related to psychobiological factors such as gender, the cumulative Testosterone levels, as well as the test strategy used (i.e., egocentric but not allocentric) that might also involve other brain regions (Korol, 2004; Alejandre-Gómez et al., 2007). Indeed, recent experiments we performed (Velázquez-Zamora et al., in preparation) showed that ovariectomized and anastrozole-treated female rats performed worse than their ovariectomized controls in resolving a hippocampus-dependent allocentric working memory paradigm in the "Y" maze, and even worse than proestrus rats.

Concomitantly, anastrozole treatment of ovariectomized rats induced pruning of dendritic spines in CA1 pyramidal neurons, a decrease of thin spines and the emergence of filopodial structures. Such effects strongly suggest an impaired capability to efficiently acquire and process novel information at the synaptic level, and a compensatory plasticity that favors the *de novo* formation of dendritic spines (Fiala et al., 1998; Harris, 1999).

Conclusion

Both neuroactive steroids and neurosteroids are strongly involved in several physiological functions other than those of reproductive nature, including modulatory actions related with cognition in the brain. Particularly, E_2 has potent and specific activational effects both at nuclear and membrane estrogen receptors, leading to modulation of synaptic stimuli in several brain regions related with cognition such as prefrontal cortex and hippocampus.

The activational effects of ER-α and ER-β in dendritic spines have profound implications in the plastic changes that they may express. Plastic changes such as neoformation, resorption, and geometric interconversions of spines are crucial to process adequately the afferent information they convey, resulting in adaptive behavioral patterns under normal conditions.

References

Adams, M.M., Fink, S.E., Shah, R.A., Janssen, W.G., Hayashi, S., Milner, T.A., McEwen, B.S. & Morrison, J.H. (2002) Estrogen and aging affect the subcellular distribution of estrogen receptor-alpha in the hippocampus of female rats. *J. Neurosci.*, 22, 3608-3614.

Alejandre-Gómez, M., García-Segura, L.M., González-Burgos, I. (2007) Administration of an inhibitor of estrogen biosynthesis facilitates working memory acquisition in male rats. *Neurosci. Res.*, 58, 272-277.

Alexaki, V.I., Charalampopoulos, I., Kampa, M., Nifli, A.P., Hatzoglou, A., Gravanis, A. & Castanas, E. (2006) Activation of membrane estrogen receptors induce pro-survival kinases. *J. Steroid Biochem. Mol. Biol.*, 98, 97-110.

Azcoitia, I., Yague, J.G & Garcia-Segura, L.M. (2011) Estradiol synthesis within the human brain. *Neuroscience,* 191, 139-147.

Bardin, A., Boulle, N., Lazennec, G., Vignon, F. & Pujol, P. (2004) Loss of ERbeta expression as a common step in estrogen-dependent tumor progression. *Endocr. Relat. Cancer*, 11, 537-551.

Bastrikova, N., Gardner, G.A., Reece, J.M., Jeromin, A. & Dudek, S.M. (2008) Synapse elimination accompanies functional plasticity in hippocampal neurons. *PNAS*, 105, 3123-3127.

Berman, K.F., Schmidt, P.J., Rubinow, D.R., Danaceau, M.A., Van Horn, J.D., Esposito, G., Ostrem, J.L. & Weinberger, D.R. (1997) Modulation of cognition-specific cortical activity by gonadal steroids: a positron-emission tomography study in women. *Proc. Natl. Acad. Sci. USA, 94,* 8836-8841.

Bian, Ch., Zhu, H., Zhao, Y., Cai, W. & Zhang, J. (2014) Intriguing roles of hippocampus-synthesized 17β-Estradiol in the modulation of hippocampal synaptic plasticity. *J. Mol. Neurosci.*, 54, 271-281.

Blaustein, J.D. (2004) Minireview: Neuronal steroid hormone receptors: they're not just for hormones anymore. *Endocrinology,* 145, 1075-1081.

Bosch, M. & Hayashi, Y. (2012). Structural plasticity of dendritic spines. *Curr. Op. Neurobiol.*, 22, 383-388.

Boulware, M.I. & Mermelstein, P.G. (2009). Membrane estrogen receptors activate metabotropic glutamate receptors to influence nervous system physiology. *Steroids,* 74, 608-613.

Bourne, J. & Harris, K.M. (2007). Do thin spines learn to be mushroom spines that remember? *Curr. Op. Neurobiol.*, 17, 1-6.

Bryant, D.N., Sheldahl, L.C., Marriott, L.K., Shapiro, R.A. & Dorsa, D.M. (2006) Multiple pathways transmit neuroprotective effects of gonadal steroids. *Endocrinol.*, 29, 199-207.

Bunone, G., Briand, P.A., Miksicek, R.J. & Picard, D. (1996) Activation of the unliganded estrogen receptor by EGF involves the MAP kinase pathway and direct phosphorylation. *EMBO J.,* 15, 2174-2183.

Carlberg, C. & Seuter, S. (2010) Dynamics of nuclear receptor target gene regulation. *Chromosoma,* 119, 479-484.

Castoria, G., Migliaccio, A. & Auricchio, F. (2009) Signaling-dependent nuclear export of estradiol receptor controls cell cycle progression in breast cancer cells. *Mol. Cell. Endocrinol.*, 308, 26-31.

Cervantes-Alfaro, J.M., Velázquez-Zamora, D.A. & González-Burgos, I. (2015) Modulación estrogénica de las funciones cognitivas durante el ciclo menstrual y la menopausia, in: I. González-Burgos (Ed.). Psicobiología de la memoria. Un enfoque interdisciplinario. *Bios-Médica.* Guadalajara. pp. 263-290.

Cho, H. & Katzenellenbogen, B.S. (1993) Synergistic activation of estrogen receptor-mediated transcription by estradiol and protein kinase activators. *Mol. Endocrinol.*, 7, 441-452.

Cordoba-Montoya, D.A. & Carrer, H.F. (1997) Estrogen facilitates induction of long term potentiation in the hippocampus of awake rats. *Brain Res.,* 778, 430-438.

Coutts, A.S. & Murphy, L. C. (1998) Elevated mitogen-activated protein kinase activity in estrogen-nonresponsive human breast cancer cells. *Cancer Res.,* 58, 4071-4074.

Cui, J., Shen, Y. & Li, R. (2013) Estrogen synthesis and signaling pathways during aging: from periphery to brain. *Trends Mol. Med.*, 19, 197-209.

Daniel, J.M. & Dohanich, G.P. (2001). Acetylcholine mediates the estrogen-induced increase in nmda receptor binding in ca1 of the hippocampus and the associated improvement in working memory. *J. Neurosci.*, 21, 6949-6956.

Dauvois, S., White, R. & Parker, M.G. (1993) The antiestrogen ICI 182780 disrupts estrogen receptor nucleocytoplasmic shuttling. *J. Cell Sci.*, 106, 1377-1388.

Davis, D.M., Jacobson, T.K., Aliakbari, S. & Mizumori, S.J. (2005) Differential effects of estrogen on hippocampal- and striatal-dependent learning. *Neurobiol. Learn. Mem.*, 84, 132-137.

Demay, F., De Monti, M., Tiffoche, C., Vaillant, C. & Thieulant, M.L. (2001) Steroid-independent activation of ER by GnRH in gonadotrope pituitary cells. *Endocrinology*, 142, 3340-3347.

Denner, L.A., Weigel, N.L., Maxwell, B.L., Schrader, W.T. & O'Malley B.W. (1990) Regulation of progesterone receptor-mediated transcription by phosphorylation. *Science*, 250, 1740-1743.

Dohanich, G.P. (2002) Gonadal steroids, learning and memory, in: D.W. Pfaff, A.P. Arnold, A.M. Etgen, S.E. Fahrbach & R.I. Rubin (Eds.). Hormones, brain and behavior. Academic Press, San Diego. pp. 265-327.

Edwards, D.P. (2000) The role of coactivators and corepressors in the biology and mechanism of action of steroid hormone receptors. *J. Mammary Gland Biol. Neoplasia*, 5, 307-324.

Edwards, D.P., Martin, P.M., Horwitz, K.B., Chamness, G.C. & McGuire, W.L. (1980) Subcellular compartmentalization of estrogen receptors in human breast cancer cells. *Exp. Cell Res.,* 127, 197-213.

Ellmann, S., Sticht, H., Thiel, F., Beckmann, M.W., Strick, R. & Strissel, P.L. (2009) Estrogen and progesterone receptors: from molecular structures to clinical targets. *Cell Mol. Life Sci*., 66, 2405-2426.

El-Tanani, M.K. & Green, C.D. (1997) Two separate mechanisms for ligand-independent activation of the estrogen receptor. *Mol. Endocrinol*., 11, 928-937.

Feng, W., Webb, P., Nguyen, P., Liu, X., Li, J., Karin, M. & Kushner, P.J. (2001) Potentiation of estrogen receptor activation function 1 (AF-1) by Src/JNK through a serine 118-independent pathway. *Mol. Endocrinol*., 15, 32-45.

Fiala, J.C., Feinberg, M., Popov, V. & Harris, K.M. (1998). Sinaptogénesis via dendritic filopodia in developing hippocampal area CA1. J. Neurosci., 18, 8900-8911.

Filardo, E.J. & Thomas, P. (2005) GPR30: a seven-transmembrane-spanning estrogen receptor that triggers EGF release. *Trends Endocrinol. Metab.,* 16, 362-367.

Filardo, E.J., Quinn, J., Pang, Y., Graeber, C., Shaw, S., Dong, J. & Thomas, P. (2007) Activation of the novel estrogen receptor G protein-coupled receptor 30 (GPR30) at the plasma membrane. *Endocrinology*, 148, 3236-3245.

Flouriot, G., Brand, H., Denger, S., Metivier, R., Kos, M., Reid, G., Sonntag-Buck, V. & Gannon, F. (2000) Identification of a new isoform of the human estrogen receptor-alpha (hER-alpha) that is encoded by distinct transcripts and that is able to repress hER alpha activation function 1. *EMBO J.,* 19, 4688-4700.

Frick, K.M., Fernandez, S.M. & Bulinski, S.C. (2002) Estrogen replacement improves spatial reference memory and increases hippocampal synaptophysin in aged female mice. *Neuroscience,* 115, 547-558.

Frye, C.A., Duffy, C.A. & Walf, A.A. (2007) Estrogens and progestins enhance spatial learning of intact and ovariectomized rats in the object placement task. *Neurobiol. Learn. Mem*., 88, 208-216.

Funakoshi, T., Yanai, A., Shinoda, K., Kawano, M.M. & Mizukami, Y. (2006) G protein coupled receptor 30 is an estrogen receptor in the plasma membrane. *Biochem. Biophys. Res. Commun*., 346, 904-910.

Gasbarri, A. & Tomaz, C. (2012) Estrogen influences on cognition, in: S.M. Kahan (Ed.), *Sex steroids*. In Tech, Croatia. pp. 163-182.

Gasbarri, A., Pompili, A., Tavares M.C. & Tomaz, C. (2009) Estrogen and cognitive functions. *Exp. Rev. Endocrinol. Metab*., 4, 507-520.

Gatson, J.W., Simpkins, J.W., Yi, K.D., Idris, A.H. Minei, J.P. & Wigginton, J.G. (2011) Aromatase is increased in astrocytes in the presence of elevated pressure. *Endocrinology*, 152, 207-213.

Genazzani, A.R., Pluchino, N., Luisi, S. & Luisi, M. (2007) Estrogen, cognition and female geing. *Hum. Reprod. Update*, 13, 175-187.

Gibbs, R.B., Gabor, R., Cox, T. & Johnson, D.A. (2004) Effects of raloxifene and estradiol on hippocampal acetylcholine release and spatial learning in the rat. *Psychoneuroendocrinology,* 29, 741-748.

González-Burgos, I. (2009) Dendritic spines plasticity and learning / memory processes: Theory, evidence and perspectives, in: Louis R. Baylog, (Ed.). Dendritic spines. Biochemistry, modelling and properties. Neurosci. Res. Prog. Series, Nova Science Publishers, Inc. New York. pp. 163-186.

González-Burgos, I. (2012) From synaptic transmission to cognition: an intermediary role for dendritic spines. *Brain Cogn.*, 80, 177-183.

González-Burgos, I. (2015) Neuroanatomía funcional de los sistemas de memoria, in: I. González-Burgos (Ed.). Psicobiología de la memoria. Un enfoque interdisciplinario. *Bios-Médica*. Guadalajara. pp. 15-49.

González-Burgos, I., Alejandre-Gómez, M. & Cervantes, M. (2005) Spine-type densities of hippocampal CA1 neurons vary in proestrus and estrus rats. *Neurosci. Lett.*, 379, 52-54.

González-Burgos, I., González-Tapia, D. & Feria-Velasco, A. (2015). Plasticidad neuronal asociada al aprendizaje y la memoria, in: Ignacio González-Burgos (Ed.). Psicobiología de la memoria. Un enfoque interdisciplinario. *Bios-Médica*. Guadalajara. pp. 159-190.

González-Burgos, I., Rivera-Cervantes, M.C., Velázquez-Zamora, D.A., Feria-Velasco, A. & García-Segura, L.M. (2012). Selective estrogen receptor modulators regulate dendritic spine plasticity in the hippocampus of male rats. In special issue: Dendritic spine plasticity and cognition. I. González-Burgos, I. Nikonenko, V. Korz (Eds.). *Neural Plast.* Vol. 2012, Article ID 309494, 6 pages.

Gottfried-Blackmore, A., Sierra, A., Jellinck, P.H., McEwen, B.S. & Bulloch, K. (2008) Brain microglia express steroid-converting enzymes in the mouse. *J. Steroid. Biochem. Mol. Biol.*, 109, 96-107.

Gould, E., Woolley, C.S., Frankfurt, M. & McEwen, B. (1990). Gonadal steroids regulate dendritic spine density in hippocampal pyramidal cells in adulthood. *J. Neurosci.*, 10, 1286-1291.

Green, S., Walter, P., Greene, G., Krust, A., Goffin, C., Jensen, E., Scrace, G., Waterfield, M. & Chambon, P. (1986) Cloning of the human oestrogen receptor cDNA. *J. Steroid. Biochem.*, 24, 77-83.

Gruber, C.J., Tschugguel, W., Schneeberger, C. & Huber, J.C. (2002) Production and actions of estrogens. *N. Engl. J. Med.*, 346, 340-352.

Guilbaud, N., Pichon, M.F., Faye, J.C., Bayard, F. & Valette, A. (1998) Modulation of estrogen receptors by phorbol diesters in human breast MCF-7 cell line. *Mol. Cell Endocrinol.*, 56, 157-163.

Hager, G.L., Lim, C.S., Elbi, C. & Baumann, C.T. (2000) Trafficking of nuclear receptors in living cells. *J. Steroid Biochem. Mol. Biol.*, 74, 249-254.

Hall, J.M. & McDonnell, D.P. (1999) The estrogen receptor beta-isoform (ERbeta) of the human estrogen receptor modulates ERalpha transcriptional activity and is a key regulator of the cellular response to estrogens and antiestrogens. *Endocrinology,* 40, 5566-5578.

Hao, J., Rapp, P.R., Janssen, W.G., Lou, W., Lasley, B.L., Hof, P.R. & Morrison, J.H. (2007) Interactive effects of age and estrogen on cognition and pyramidal neurons in monkey prefrontal cortex. *Proc. Natl. Acad. Sci. USA,* 104, 11465-11470.

Harris, K.M. (1999) Structure, development, and plasticity of dendritic spines. Curr. Opin. Neurobiol., 9, 343-348.

Hart, S.A., Snyder, M.A., Smejkalova, T. & Woolley, C.S. (2007) Estrogen mobilizes a subset of estrogen receptor-alpha-immunoreactive vesicles in inhibitory presynaptic boutons in hippocampal CA1. *J. Neurosci.*, 27, 2102-2111.

Hillier, S.G., Whitelaw, P.F. & Smyth, C.D. (1994) Follicular oestrogen synthesis: the 'two-cell, two-gonadotrophin' model revisited. *Mol. Cell Endocrinol.*, 100, 51-54.

Hirata, S., Shoda, T., Kato, J. & Hoshi, K. (2003) Isoform/variant mRNAs for sex steroid hormone receptors in humans. *Trends Endocrinol. Metab.,* 14,124-129.

Hofer, S.B. & Bonhoeffer, T. (2010) Dendritic spines: the stuff that memories are made of? *Curr. Biol.,* 20, R157-R159.

Hojo, Y., Higo, S., Ishii, H., Ooishi, Y., Mukai, H., Murakami, G., Kominami, T., Kimoto, T., Honma, S., Poirier, D. & Kawato, S. (2009) Comparison between hippocampus-synthesized and circulation-derived sex steroids in the hippocampus. Endocrinology, 150, 5106-5112.

Hojo, Y., Higo, S., Kawato, S., Hatanaka, Y., Ooishi, Y., Murakami, G., Ishii, H., Komatsuzaki, Y., Ogiue-Ikeda, M., Mukai, H. & Kimoto, T. (2011) Hippocampal synthesis of sex steroids and corticosteroids: essential for modulation of synaptic plasticity. Front. Endocrinol., 2, 43.

Hojo, Y., Murakami, G., Mukai, H., Higo, S., Hatanaka, Y., Ogiue-Ikeda, M., Ishii, H., Kimoto, T. & Kawato, S. (2008) Estrogen synthesis in the brain--role in synaptic plasticity and memory. *Mol. Cell. Endocrinol.*, 290, 31-43.

Hosli, E. & Hosli, L. (1999) Cellular localization of estrogen receptors on neurones in various regions of cultured rat CNS: coexistence with cholinergic and galanin receptors. *Int. J. Dev. Neurosci.*, 17, 317-330.

Ignar-Trowbridge, D.M., Nelson, K.G., Bidwell, M.C., Curtis, S.W., Washburn, T. F., McLachlan, J.A. & Korach, K.S. (1992) Coupling of dual signaling pathways: epidermal growth factor action involves the estrogen receptor. *Proc. Natl. Acad. Sci. USA*, 89, 4658-4662.

Ignar-Trowbridge, D.M., Pimentel, M., Parker, M.G., McLachlan, J.A. & Korach, K.S. (1996) Peptide growth factor cross-talk with the estrogen receptor requires the A/B domain and occurs independently of protein kinase C or estradiol. *Endocrinology*, 137, 1735-1744.

Jacquot, Y., Laïos, I., Cleeren, A., Nonclercq, D., Bermont, L., Refouvelet, B., Boubekeur, K., Xicluna, A., Leclercq, G. & Laurent, G. (2007) Synthesis, structure, and estrogenic activity of 4-amino-3-(2-methylbenzyl)coumarins on human breast carcinoma cells. *Bioorg. Med. Chem.*, 15, 2269-2282.

Joel, P.B., Traish, A.M. & Lannigan, D.A. (1995) Estradiol and phorbol ester cause phosphorylation of serine 118 in the human estrogen receptor. *Mol. Endocrinol.,* 9, 1041-1052.

Kampa, M., Notas, G., Pelekanou, V., Troullinaki, M., Andrianaki, M., Azariadis, K., Kampouri, E., Lavrentaki, K. & Castanas, E. (2012) Early membrane initiated transcriptional effects of estrogens in breast cancer cells: First pharmacological evidence for a novel membrane estrogen receptor element (ERx). *Steroids*, 77, 959-967.

Kampa, M., Pelekanou, V., Gallo, D., Notas, G., Troullinaki, M., Pediaditakis, I., Charalampopoulos, I., Jacquot, Y., Leclercq, G. & Castanas, E. (2011) ERα17p, an ERα P295 -T311 fragment, modifies the migration of breast cancer cells, through actin cytoskeleton rearrangements. *J. Cell Biochem.,* 112, 3786-3796.

Kampa, M., Pelekanou, V., Notas, G., Stathopoulos, E.N. & Castanas, E. (2013) The estrogen receptor: two or more molecules, multiple variants, diverse localizations, signaling and functions. Are we undergoing a paradigm-shift as regards their significance in breast cancer? *Hormones* (Athens), 12, 69-85.

Kasai, H., Fukuda, M., Watanabe, S., Hayashi-Takagi, A. & Noguchi, J. (2010) Structural dynamics of dendritic spines in memory and cognition. *TINS,* 33, 121-129.

Kasai, H., Matsuzaki, M., Noguchi, J., Yasumatsu, N., Nakahara, H. (2003) Structure-stability-function relationships of dendritic spines. *TINS*, 26, 360-368.

Kato, S., Endoh, H., Masuhiro, Y., Kitamoto, T., Uchiyama, S., Sasaki, H., Masushige, S., Gotoh, Y., Nishida, E., Kawashima, H., Metzger, D. & Chambon, P. (1995) Activation of the estrogen receptor through phosphorylation by mitogen-activated protein kinase. *Science,* 270, 1491-1494.

Kim, K.H. & Bender, J.R. (2009) Membrane-initiated actions of estrogen on the endothelium. *Mol. Cell Endocrinol*., 308, 3-8.

Koch, C., Zador, A. (1993) The function of dendritic spines: devices subserving biochemical rather than electrical compartmentalization. J. Neurosci., 13, 413-422.

Koch, C., Zador, A., Brown, T.H. (1992) Dendritic spines: convergence of theory and experiment. Science, 256, 973-974.

Korol, D.L. (2004) Role of estrogen in balancing contributions from multiple memory systems. *Neurobiol. Learn. Mem*., 82, 309-323.

Kretz, O., Fester, L., Wehrenberg, U., Zhou, L., Brauckmann, S., Zhao, S., Prange-Kiel, J., Naumann, T., Jarry, H., Frotscher, M. & Rune, G.M. (2004) Hippocampal synapses depend on hippocampal estrogen synthesis. J. Neurosci., 24, 5913-5921.

Kuiper, G.G.J.M., Enmark, E., Peltohuikko, M. & Nilsson, S. (1996) Cloning of a novel estrogen receptor expressed in rat prostate and ovary. *Proc. Natl. Acad. Sci. USA,* 93, 5925-5930.

Laïos, I., Journé, F., Nonclercq, D., Vidal, D.S., Toillon, R.A., Laurent, G. & Leclercq, G. (2005) Role of the proteasome in the regulation of estrogen receptor alpha turnover and function in MCF-7 breast carcinoma cells. *J. Steroid Biochem. Mol. Biol., 94, 347-359.*

Lamb, J., Ladha, M.H., McMahon, C., Sutherland, R.L. & Ewen, M.E. (2000) Regulation of the functional interaction between cyclin D1 and the estrogen receptor. *Mol. Cell Biol.,* 20, 8667-8675.

Lang, C., Barco, A., Zablow, L., Kandel, E.R., Siegelbaum, S.A. & Zakharenko, S.S. (2004) Transient expansion of synaptically connected dendritic spines upon induction of hippocampal long-term potentiation. *PNAS*, 101, 16665-16670.

Le Goff, P., Montano, M.M., Schodin, D.J. & Katzenellenbogen, B.S. (1994) Phosphorylation of the human estrogen receptor. Identification of hormone-regulated sites and examination of their influence on transcriptional activity. *J. Biol. Chem*., 269, 4458-4466.

Lee, H., Jiang, F., Wang, Q., Nicosia, S.V., Yang, J., Su, B. & Bai, W. (2000) MEKK1 activation of human estrogen receptor alpha and stimulation of the agonistic activity of 4-hydroxytamoxifen in endometrial and ovarian cancer cells. *Mol. Endocrinol.*, 14, 1882-1896.

Lee, S.J. & McEwen, B.S. (2001) Neurotrophic and neuroprotective actions of estrogens and their therapeutic implications. *Annu. Rev. Pharmacol.* Toxicol., 41, 569-591.

Leranth, C., M., Shanabrough, D.E. & Redmond, Jr. (2002) Gonadal hormones are responsible for maintaining the integrity of spine synapses in the CA1 hippocampal subfield of female nonhuman primates, *J. Comp. Neurol.,* 447, 34-42.

Leuner, B., Shors, T.J. (2004) New spines, new memories. Mol. Neurobiol., 29, 117-130.

Li, C.J., Brake, W.G., Romeo, R.D., Dunlop, J.C., Gordon, M., Buzescu, R., Magarinos, A.M., Allen, P.B., Greengard, P., Luine, V. & McEwen, B.S. (2004) Estrogen alters hippocampal dendritic spine shape and enhances synaptic protein immunoreactivity and spatial memory in female mice. *PNAS,* 101, 2185-2190.

Li, L., Hisamoto, K., Kim, K.H., Haynes, M.P., Bauer, P.M., Sanjay, A., Collinge, M., Baron, R., Sessa, W.C. & Bender, J.R. (2007) Variant estrogen receptor-c-Src molecular interdependence and c-Src structural requirements for endothelial NO synthase activation. *Proc. Natl. Acad. Sci. USA,* 104, 16468-16473.

Liu, F., Day, M., Muñiz, L.C., Bitran, D., Arias, R., Revilla-Sanchez, R., Grauer, S., Zhang, G., Kelley, C., Pulito, V., Sung, A., Mervis, R.F., Navarra, R., Hirst, W.D., Reinhart, P.H., Marquis, K.L., Moss, S.J., Pangalos, M.N. & Brandon, N.J. (2008) Activation of estrogen receptor beta regulates hippocampal synaptic plasticity and improves memory. *Nat. Neurosci*., 11, 334-343.

Luine, V. (2014) Estradiol and cognitive function: Past, present and future. *Horm. Behav*., 66, 602-618.

Luine, V.N. (2007) The prefrontal cortex, gonadal hormones and memory. Horm. Behav., 51, 181-182.

Luine, V.N. (2008) Sex steroids and cognitive function. *J. Neuroend*., 20, 866-872.

Martin, M.B., Garcia-Morales, P., Stoica, A., Solomon, H.B., Pierce, M., Katz, D., Zhang, S., Danielsen, M. & Saceda, M. (1995) Effects of 12-O-tetradecanoylphorbol-13-acetate on estrogen receptor activity in MCF-7 cells. *J. Biol. Chem*., 270, 25244-25251.

Martin, S.J., Grimwood, P.D. & Morris, R.G. (2000) Synaptic plasticity and memory: an evaluation of the hypothesis. *Annu. Rev. Neurosci*., 23, 649-711.

Matsuzaki, M., Honkura, N., Ellis-Davies, G.C.R. & Kasai, H. (2004) Structural basis of long-term potentiation in single dendritic spines. *Nature,* 429, 761-766.

McEwen, B. (2002) Estrogen actions throughout the brain. *Recent. Prog. Horm. Res*., 57, 357-384.

McEwen, B., Akama, K., Alves, S., Brake, W.G., Bulloch, K., Lee, S., Li, C., Yuen, G. & Milner, T.A. (2001) Tracking the estrogen receptor in neurons: Implications for estrogen-induced synapse formation. *PNAS*, 13, 7093-7100.

McGaugh, J.L. (2000) Memory – A century of consolidation. *Science,* 287, 248-251.

Mellon, S.H., Griffin, L.D. & Compagnone, N.A. (2001) Biosynthesis and action of neurosteroids. *Brain Res. Rev.,* 37, 3-12.

Metzger, D., Ali, S., Bornert, J.M. & Chambon, P. (1995) Characterization of the amino-terminal transcriptional activation function of the human estrogen receptor in animal and yeast cells. *J. Biol. Chem*., 270, 9535-9542.

Micevych, P. & Dominguez, R. (2010) Membrane estradiol signaling in the brain. *Front. Neuroendocrinol.*, 30, 315-327.

Micevych, P.E. & Mermelstein, P.G. (2008) Membrane estrogen receptors acting through metabotropic glutamate receptors: an emerging mechanism of estrogen action in the brain. *Mol. Neurobiol.*, 38, 66-77.

Mitra, S.W., Hoskin, E., Yudkovitz, J., Pear, L., Wilkinson, H.A., Hayashi, S., Pfaff, D.W., Ogawa, S., Rohrer, S.P., Schaeffer, J.M., McEwen, B.S. & Alves, S.E. (2003) Immunolocalization of estrogen receptor beta in the mouse brain: comparison with estrogen receptor alpha. *Endocrinology,* 144, 2055-2067.

Mizukami, Y. (2010) In vivo functions of GPR30/GPER-1, a membrane receptor for estrogen: from discovery to functions in vivo. *Endocr. J.,* 57, 101-107.

Neves, G., Cooke, S.F. & Bliss, T.V. (2008) Synaptic plasticity, memory and the hippocampus: a neural network approach to causality. *Nat. Rev. Neurosci.,* 9, 65-75.

Nonclercq, D., Journé, F., Laïos, I., Chaboteaux, C., Toillon, R. A., Leclercq, G. & Laurent, G. (2007) Effect of nuclear export inhibition on estrogen receptor regulation in breast cancer cells. *J. Mol. Endocrinol.*, 39, 105-118.

Norman, A.W., Mizwicki, M.T. & Norman, D.P. (2004) Steroid-hormone rapid actions, membrane receptors and a conformational ensemble model. *Nat. Rev. Drug. Discov.*, 3, 27-41.

Osterlund, M.K. & Hurd, Y.L. (2001) Estrogen receptors in the human forebrain and the relation to neuropsychiatric disorders. *Prog. Neurobiol.,* 64, 251-267.

Penot, G., Le Peron, C., Merot, Y., Grimaud-Fanouillere, E., Ferriere, F., Boujrad, N., Kah, O., Saligaut, C., Ducouret, B., Metivier, R. & Flouriot, G. (2005) The human estrogen receptor-alpha isoform hERalpha46 antagonizes the proliferative influence of hERalpha66 in MCF7 breast cancer cells. *Endocrinology,* 146, 5474-5484.

Phan, A., Gabor, Ch.S., Favaro, K.J., Kaschack, S., Armstrong, J.N., MacLusky, N.J. & Choleris, E. (2012) Low doses of 17b-Estradiol rapidly improve learning and increase hippocampal dendritic spines. *Neuropsychopharmacology*, 37, 2299-2309.

Pompili, A., Tomaz, C., Arnone, B., Tavares, M.C. & Gasbarri, A. (2010) Working and reference memory across the estrous cycle of rat: a long term study in gonadally intact females. *Behav. Brain Res.*, 213, 10-18.

Power, R.F., Mani, S.K., Codina, J., Conneely, O.M. & O'Malley, B.W. (1991) Dopaminergic and ligand-independent activation of steroid hormone receptors. *Science,* 254, 1636-1639.

Prange-Kiel, J., Fester, L., Zhou, L., Jarry, H. & Rune, G.M. (2009) Estrus cyclicity of spinogenesis: underlying mechanisms. *J. Neural Transm.*, 116, 1417-1425.

Prossnitz, E.R., Oprea, T.I., Sklar, L.A. & Arterburn, J.B. (2008) The ins and outs of GPR30: a transmembrane estrogen receptor. *J. Steroid Biochem. Mol. Biol.*, 109, 350-353.

Ramsey, T.L., Risinger, K.E., Jernigan, S.C., Mattingly, K.A. & Klinge, C.M. (2004) Estrogen receptor beta isoforms exhibit differences in ligand-activated transcriptional activity in an estrogen response element sequence-dependent manner. *Endocrinology,* 145, 149-160.

Rapp, P.R., Morrison, J.H. & Roberts, J.A. (2003) Cyclic estrogen replacement improves cognitive function in aged ovariectomized rhesus monkeys. *J. Neurosci.*, 23, 5708-5714.

Rehman, H.U. & Masson, E.A. (2005) Neuroendocrinology of female aging. *Gend. Med.,* 1, 41-56.

Rhodes, M.E. & Frye, C.A. (2006) ERbeta-selective SERMs produce mnemonic enhancing effects in the inhibitory avoidance and water maze tasks. *Neurobiol. Learn. Mem.*, 85, 183-191.

Rodriguez, A.L., Tamrazi, A., Collins, M.L. & Katzenellenbogen, J.A. (2004) Design, synthesis, and in vitro biological evaluation of small molecule inhibitors of estrogen receptor alpha coactivator binding. *J. Med. Chem.,* 47, 600-611.

Rudick, C.N. & Woolley, C.S. (2003) Selective estrogen receptor modulators regulate phasic activation of hippocampal CA1 pyramidal cells by estrogen. *Endocrinology*, 144, 179-187.

Rune, G.M. & Frotscher, M. (2005) Neurosteroid synthesis in the hippocampus: role in synaptic plasticity. Neuroscience, 136, 833-842.

Sandstrom, N.J. & Williams, C.L. (2001) Memory retention is modulated by acute estradiol and progesterone replacement. *Behav. Neurosci.*, 115, 384-393.

Sandstrom, N.J. & Williams, C.L. (2004) Spatial memory retention is enhanced by acute and continuous estradiol replacement. *Horm. Behav.,* 45, 128-135.

Savkur, R.S. & Burris, T.P. (2004) The coactivator LXXLL nuclear receptor recognition motif. *J. Pept. Res.*, 63, 207-212.

Sebastian, T., Sreeja, S. & Thampan, R.V. (2004) Import and export of nuclear proteins: focus on the nucleocytoplasmic movements of two different species of mammalian estrogen receptor. *Mol. Cell Biochem.*, 260, 91-102.

Sherwin, B.B. & Henry, J.F. (2008) Brain aging modulates the neuroprotective effects of estrogen on selective aspects of cognition in women: A critical review. *Front. Neuroendocrinol.*, 29, 88-113.

Shilling, V., Jenkins, V., Morris, R., Deutsch, G. & Bloomfield, D. (2005) The effects of adjuvant chemotherapy on cognition in women with breast cancer--preliminary results of an observational longitudinal study. *Breast,* 14, 142-150.

Shim, W.S., Conaway, M., Masamura, S., Yue, W., Wang, J.P., Kmar, R. & Santen, R.J. (2000) Estradiol hypersensitivity and mitogen-activated protein kinase expression in long-term estrogen deprived human breast cancer cells in vivo. *Endocrinology,* 141, 396-405.

Simoncini, T., Rabkin, E. & Liao, J.K. (2003) Molecular basis of cell membrane estrogen receptor interaction with phosphatidylinositol 3-kinase in endothelial cells. *Arterioscler. Thromb. Vasc. Biol.*, 23, 198-203.

Skafar, D.F. & Koide, S. (2006) Understanding the human estrogen receptor-alpha using targeted mutagenesis. *Mol. Cell Endocrinol.*, 246, 83-90.

Smith, C.C. & McMahon, L.L. (2005). Estrogen-induced increase in the magnitude of long-term potentiation occurs only when the ratio of NMDA transmission to AMPA transmission is increased. *J. Neurosci.*, 25, 7780-7791.

Smith, C.C., Vedder, L.C. & McMahon, L.L. (2009) Estradiol and the relationship between dendritic spines, NR2B containing NMDA receptors, and the magnitude of long-term potentiation at hippocampal CA3-CA1 synapses. *Psychoneuroendocrinology,* 34S1, S130-S142.

Smith, R.G., Betancourt, L. & Sun, Y. (2005) Molecular endocrinology and physiology of the aging central nervous system. *Endo. Rev.*, 2, 203-250.

Solum, D.T. & Handa, R.J. (2002) Estrogen regulates the development of brain-derived neurotrophic factor mRNA and protein in the rat hippocampus. *J. Neurosci.*, 22, 2650-2659.

Srivastava, D.P., Woolfrey, K.M., Jones, K.A., Shum, C.Y., Lash, L.L., Swanson, G.T. & Penzes, P. (2008) Rapid enhancement of two-step wiring plasticity by estrogen and NMDA receptor activity. *PNAS,* 105, 14650-14655.

Srivastava, D.P., Woolfrey, K.M., Liu, F., Brandon, N.J. & Penzes, P. (2010) Estrogen receptor β (ERβ) activity modulates synaptic signaling and structure. *J. Neurosci.*, 30, 13454-13460.

Strissel, P.L. & Strick, R. (2005) Multiple effects of bioflavonoids on gene regulation, cell proliferation and apoptosis: natural compounds move into the lime light of cancer research. *Leuk. Res.,* 29, 859-861.

Tang, Y.P., Shimizu, E., Dube, G.R., Rampon, C., Kerchner, G.A, Zhuo, M., Liu, G. & Tsien, J.Z. (1999) Genetic enhancement of learning and memory in mice. *Nature,* 401, 63-69.

Thomas, P. (2012) Rapid steroid hormone actions initiated at the cell surface and the receptors that mediate them with an emphasis on recent progress in fish models. *Gen. Comp. Endocrinol.*, 175, 367-383.

Toft, D. & Gorski, J. (1966) A receptor molecule for estrogens: isolation from the rat uterus and preliminary characterization. *Proc. Natl. Acad. Sci. USA,* 55, 1574-1581.

Toni, N., Buchs, P.A., Nikonenko, I., Povilaitite, P., Parisi, L. & Muller, D. (2001) Remodeling of synaptic membranes after induction of leng-term potentiation. *J. Neurosci.*, 21, 6245-6251.

Tremblay, G.B., Tremblay, A., Copeland, N.G., Gilbert, D.J., Jenkins, N.A., Labrie, F. & Giguere, V. (1997) Cloning, chromosomal localization, and functional analysis of the murine estrogen receptor. *Mol. Endocrinol.*, 11, 353-365.

Valverde, M.A., Rojas, P., Amigo, J., Cosmelli, D., Orio, P., Bahamonde, M.I., Mann, G.E., Vergara, C. & Latorre, R. (1999) Acute activation of Maxi-K channels (hSlo) by estradiol binding to the beta subunit. *Science,* 285, 1929-1931.

Velázquez-Zamora, D.A., García-Segura, L.M. & González-Burgos, I. (2012a) Effects of selective estrogen receptor modulators on allocentric working memory performance and on dendritic spines in medial prefrontal cortex pyramidal neurons of ovariectomized rats. *Horm. Behav.*, 61, 512-517.

Velázquez-Zamora, D.A., González-Tapia, D., González-Ramírez, M.M., Flores-Soto, M.E., Vázquez-Valls, E., Cervantes, M. & González-Burgos, I. (2012b) Plastic changes in dendritic spines of hippocampal CA1 pyramidal neurons from ovariectomized rats after estradiol treatment. *Brain Res.,* 1470, 1-10.

Vierk, R., Glassmeier, G., Zhou, L., Brandt, N., Fester, L., Dudzinski, D., Wilkars, W., Bender, R.A., Lewerenz, M., Gloger, S., Graser, L., Schwarz, J. & Rune, G.M. (2012) Aromatase inhibition abolishes LTP generation in female but not in male mice. *J. Neurosci.*, 32, 8116-8126.

Walf, A.A. & Frye, C.A. (2006) A review and update of mechanisms of estrogen in the hippocampus and amygdala for anxiety and depression behavior. *Neuropsychopharm.*, 31, 1097-1111.

Walter, P., Green, S., Greene, G., Krust, A., Bornert, J. M., Jeltsch, J.M., Staub, A., Jensen, E., Scrace, G., Waterfield, M. & Chambon, P. (1985) Cloning of the human estrogen receptor cDNA. *Proc. Natl. Acad. Sci. USA*, 82, 7889-7893.

Wang, Y.J., Lin, M.W., Wu, S.N. & Sung, R.J. (2007) The activation by estrogen receptor agonists of the BK(Ca)-channel in human cardiac fibroblasts. *Biochem. Pharmacol.*, 73, 1347-1357.

Wang, Z., Zhang, X., Shen, P., Loggie, B.W., Chang, Y. & Deuel, T.F. (2005) Identification, cloning, and expression of human estrogen receptor-alpha36, a novel variant of human estrogen receptor alpha 66. *Biochem. Biophys. Res. Commun.*, 336, 1023-1027.

Wang, Z., Zhang, X., Shen, P., Loggie, B.W., Chang, Y. & Deuel, T.F. (2006) A variant of estrogen receptor-α, hER-α36: transduction of estrogen- and antiestrogen-dependent membrane-initiated mitogenic signaling. *Proc. Natl. Acad. Sci. USA*, 103, 9063-9068.

Warren, S.G. & Juraska, J.M. (1997) Spatial and nonspatial learning across the rat estrous cycle. *Behav. Neurosci.*, 111, 259-266.

White, R.E., Darkow, D.J. & Lang, J.L. (1995) Estrogen relaxes coronary arteries by opening BKCa channels through a cGMP-dependent mechanism. *Circ. Res.*, 77, 936-942.

Woolley, C.S. & McEwen, B.S. (1992) Estradiol mediates fluctuation in hippocampal synapse density during the estrous cycle in the adult rat. *J. Neurosci.*, 12, 2549-2554.

Woolley, C.S., Gould, E., Frankfurt, M. & McEwen, B. (1990) Naturally occurring fluctuation in dendritic spine density on adult hippocampal pyramidal neurons. *J. Neurosci.*, 10, 4035-4039.

Woolley, C.S., Weiland, N.G., McEwen, B.S. & Schwartzkroin, P.A. (1997) Estradiol increases the sensitivity of hippocampal CA1 pyramidal cells to NMDA receptor-mediated synaptic input: correlation with dendritic spine density. *J. Neurosci.*, 17, 1848-1859.

Xu, X. & Zhang, Z. (2006) Effects of estradiol benzoate on learning-memory behavior and synaptic structure in ovariectomized mice. *Life Sci.*, 79, 1553-1560.

Yamashita, S. (1998) Localization and functions of steroid hormone receptors. *Histol. Histopathol.*, 13, 255-270.

Yang, J., Singleton, D.W., Shaughnessy, E.A. & Khan, S.A. (2008) The F-domain of estrogen receptor-alpha inhibits ligand induced receptor dimerization. *Mol. Cell Endocrinol.*, 295, 94-100.

Young, W.C., Goy, R.W. & Phoenix, C.H. (1964) Hormones and sexual behavior. *Science,* 143, 212-218.

Zhou, W., Koldzic-Zivanovic, N., Clarke, C.H., De Beun, R., Wassermann, K., Bury, P.S., Cunningham, K.A. & Thomas, M.L. (2002) Selective estrogen receptor modulator effects in the rat brain. *Neuroendocrinology,* 75, 24-33.

Zurkovsky, L., Brown, S.L. & Korol, D.L. (2006) Estrogen modulates place learning through estrogen receptors in the hippocampus. *Neurobiol. Learn. Mem.*, 86, 336-343.

In: Synaptic Fundamentals of Memory Performance
Editor: Ignacio González-Burgos
ISBN: 978-1-63483-279-3

Chapter 3

THE MOLECULAR BIOLOGY OF DENDRITIC SPINE PLASTICITY IN MEMORY PROCESSING

***David González-Tapia*[1,2]*, Dulce A. Velázquez-Zamora*[1,2] *and Ignacio González-Burgos*[1,*]

[1]Laboratorio de Psicobiología, División de Neurociencias, Centro de Investigación Biomédica de Occidente, IMSS, Guadalajara, Jalisco, México

[2]Universidad Politécnica de la Zona Metropolitana de Guadalajara, Tlajomulco de Zúñiga, Jalisco, México

ABSTRACT

The functional organization of neural circuits that underlies learning and memory is defined by very specific synaptic contacts. Under normal conditions, the synaptic contacts between neurons can be modified by experience in order to establish other brain responses. In most cases such modifications tend to promote re-adaptation, although they can also lead to aberrant behaviour. Whatever the case, a wide range of changes can occur in nerve tissue at different levels of organization, tending to maintain an adequate balance between the individual's activity and their environmental demands. The adaptation of nerve cells to novel or adverse conditions, whether effective or not, is known as neuroplasticity. Experimental studies of plasticity in the nervous system have shown that the ability to acquire new information from the environment (learning) and to evoke stored information (memory) is closely related to structural changes in neuronal cytoarchitecture, specifically in the synaptic contacts mediated by dendritic spines. Dynamic modifications to the molecular components of both pre- and post-synaptic synaptic elements involved in plasticity underlie and define these cytoarchitectonic changes.

---

* Send correspondence to: Ignacio González-Burgos, PhD; Laboratorio de Psicobiología, División de Neurociencias, Centro de Investigación Biomédica de Occidente, IMSS. Guadalajara, Jalisco, México. Email: igonbur@hotmail.com.

1. INTRODUCTION

The plasticity of the Nervous System can be witnessed through essentially adaptive events associated with the neuropsychological processes, including learning and memory. The transmission of information at the level of the synapse is important for both the psychoneural organization of these cognitive processes and for the expression of plastic phenomena related to them. It is conventionally accepted that excitatory synaptic transmission is linked to the input of "new" information, the bioelectrical characteristics of which are transmitted at synaptic junctions established by dendritic spines. The capacity of individuals to respond to environmental demands that require effective mnemic capacity is defined by the afferent information in question, the type of synaptic potentials that are activated and the brain regions involved in the formation of the relevant memory traces.

Excitatory synaptic contacts predominantly involve dendritic spines, whose morphofunctional characteristics determine how the afferent information is translated. In the case of mnemic information at least, spines are capable of experiencing plastic phenomena that are presumed to be an adaptation to the changing conditions of the environment. These adaptations occur both when these conditions are normal, such as experience-based learning, or atypical, such as the adaptive changes that ensue after brain damage.

2. DENDRITIC SPINES

Dendritic spines are 0.1 - 2 μm long cytoplasmic protuberances observed occasionally on the soma of neurons (Mugnaini et al., 1967) and on the axon hillock (Westrum, 1970), although they are mainly found on dendrites (which is why they are generically known as "dendritic" spines). These spines protrude more or less perpendicularly with respect to the longitudinal axis of their parent dendrite and significantly, they are responsible for establishing most excitatory synaptic contacts whenever excitatory and inhibitory synapses exist. At the beginning of the 1970's, pioneering electrophysiology studies showed that experimentally potentiated excitatory synapses exhibit synaptic effects that persisted for prolonged periods of time, a phenomenon that was termed long-term potentiation (LTP). This phenomenon was later linked to the induction and consolidation of memory (Bliss & Lømo, 1970, 1973).

Dendritic spines have two distinctive morphological features: a head and a neck (Rao et al., 1998). Based on the geometric proportions of these two components, spines have been classified into at least six basic types: thin, stubby, mushroom, wide, branched and double (Harris et al., 1989; Tarelo-Acuña et al., 2000; González-Burgos, 2009, 2012). Thin spines are characterized by having a neck which is longer than the head and the diameter of the neck itself is smaller than that of the head. Alternatively, mushroom spines have a narrow and relatively short neck (shorter than that of thin spines). In fact the neck of these spines is shorter than the length of the head which is incidentally, much larger in terms of diameter than the neck and the head of thin spines. In stubby spines there is no distinction between the head and the neck, and the total length of the spine is similar to or even smaller than its diameter. Wide spines are similar to stubby spines whereby the only morphological difference between them is that the length of the wide spines is greater than that of stubby spines and it exceeds their diameter. Branched spines are distinguished by having two heads, the short necks of which also converge to form a short, narrow neck that is a continuation of the parent dendrite. Finally, double spines have a distal head that is joined longitudinally to another head of similar proportions by a small, narrow neck. The head closest to the dendrite is connected to the latter by an equally narrow and short neck (González-Burgos, 2009, 2012). The proportional density of the different types of spines varies on neurons, although thin and mushroom spines predominate, followed by stubby spines and in a much lower proportion, the wide, and finally the branched and double spines (Lee et al., 2005; González-Burgos, 2012).

Following their morphological characterization, at the beginning of the 1990's it was demonstrated that the diameter of the spine neck is directly related to their resistance to the passage of Ca^{2+}-mediated electrical current. Hence, dendritic spines would appear to play a role in modulating the synaptic currents that are related to the excitatory afferent information to be relayed to neurons (Koch et al., 1992; Koch & Zador, 1993). Based on these findings and a wide range of complementary evidence, we now know that the role of each type of spine in the transmission of the synaptic impulses is also different. Indeed, there is a close connection between the shape of spines and the differential processing of the excitatory synaptic information that is relayed to them, their plastic capacity and the transmission of synaptic information related to learning and memory (Kasai et al., 2010a, Kasai et al., 2010b; González-Burgos, 2009, 2012).

3. Excitatory Synaptic Transmission

Excitatory transmission in the Central Nervous System (CNS) is primarily mediated by glutamate. This neurotransmitter activates postsynaptic ionotropic and metabotropic receptors, receptors associated with ion channels or coupled to intracellular second-messenger systems and G proteins, respectively (Meldrum, 2000). The majority of the rapid glutamate-mediated chemical excitation in dendritic spines occurs through ionotropic N-methyl-D-aspartate (NMDA), alpha-amino-3-hydroxy-5-methyl-isoxazolepropionic acid (AMPA) and kainate (KA) receptors (Salinska et al., 2005). NMDA receptors are cation channels that allow the passage of Na^+, K^+ and Ca^{2+} ions, and that show particularly high permeability to Ca^{2+} ions (Ascher & Nowak, 1988). In their resting state, NMDA receptors are blocked by physiological concentrations of Mg^{2+}, making them voltage-dependent (Nowak et al., 1984; Mayer & Westbrook, 1987). They also have a long open time (Nowak et al., 1984), and a relatively slow kinetic profile of activation and deactivation (Lester et al., 1990). As for AMPA receptors, their participation in rapid transmission and phenomena related to synaptic plasticity occurs in coordination with NMDA receptors (Fox, 1996). There are two sub-families of kainate receptors: one includes GluR5, GluR6 and GluR7 subunits; and the other includes KA1 and KA2. Kainate receptors are widely distributed throughout the entire CNS, although the distinct subtypes are have quite heterogeneous distributions (Bahn et al., 1994), which explains the relatively limited knowledge we have of these receptors from a pharmacological point of view.

There are eight different subtypes of metabotropic receptors and they have been classified into three groups. The first includes the mGluR1 and mGluR5 subtypes, which are coupled to the phosphatidylinositol pathway, whereas the members of the second group, mGluR2 and mGluR3, and those of the third group (mGluR4, mGluR6, mGluR7 and mGluR8), are negatively coupled to adenylyl cyclase. In a typical excitatory synapse, ionotropic receptors are more abundant than metabotropic receptors and they are strongly involved in rapid impulse transmission. By contrast, metabotropic receptors regulate the activity of the former and they mediate the slow effects of glutamate (Cooper et al., 2003), which is facilitated by their localization at the periphery of synapses on dendritic spines (Luján et al., 1996). In general, both ionotropic and metabotropic receptors have been linked to both transitory and longer lasting synaptic plasticity and in particular, to the induction and maintenance of LTP (Bennett, 2000; Bortolotto et al., 2005). mGluR1 receptors are mainly localized at the periphery of synapses, which favours the modulation of the activity of ionotropic AMPA and NMDA receptors (Bessis et al., 2001), and consequently, the excitability of the postsynaptic neuron (Niswender & Conn, 2010). As for mGluR2 and mGluR3, they are both located pre- and postsynaptically, while those of the third group of metabotropic receptors (mGluR4, mGluR6, mGluR7 and mGluR8) are localized presynaptically and they act as inhibitory autoreceptors (Niswender & Conn, 2010).

Given that a high percentage of excitatory synaptic contacts occur on dendritic spines, they have all the metabolic machinery required to process afferent information, including glutamate receptors. Accordingly, they are regarded as quasi-independent compartments of the parent dendrite that regulate the flow of afferent excitatory information (Koch et al., 1992).

The process of glutamate-mediated information transmission begins with the transmission of an excitatory potential to the axon terminal. The glutamate concentration in a synaptic vesicle is approximately 100 mmol/l and the release of its content generates an excitatory postsynaptic potential that primarily corresponds to the activation of ionotropic AMPA receptors (Meldrum, 2000). AMPA receptors located on the external surface of the dendritic spine are permeable to reciprocal flux, which occurs against Na^+ and K^+ gradients. The small increase in potential caused by this ion current flow gives rise to microenvironments that promote the removal of the Mg^{2+} ion from the inside of the voltage-sensitive NMDA receptor channel, which opens as a result. Like the AMPA receptor, the NMDA receptor is also permeable to Na^+ and K^+, and it is also permeable to ions (Bear et al., 1998). Under certain conditions, metabotropic receptors can be activated secondarily (Luján et al., 1996) and they induce the release of calcium, either from the so-called "spine apparatus" (formed by the lamellae of smooth endoplasmic reticulum) found in large spines (Spacek & Harris, 1997) or from the Ca^{2+} chelating systems in smaller spines (Ellisman et al., 1990). This process is reversible, such that the systems involved in the release of Ca^{2+} are the same as those responsible for its capture, thereby avoiding damage as a result of an abnormal intracellular increase in the concentration of Ca^{2+} (Ellisman et al., 1990). Thus, there is a system for regulating the Ca^{2+} concentration inside the spine that naturally protects the cell from the possible excitotoxic damage caused by neurotransmitter activity and an abnormal increase in Ca^{2+}, not just in the spine but also in the parent dendrite (Kostyuk, 1998). This regulatory system is further enhanced by the presence of Ca^{2+} pumps in spines, which participate in the extrusion of these ions (Majewska et al., 2000) and thereby avoid increased Ca^{2+} accumulation in the parent dendrite during their diffusion towards the latter (Volfovsky et al., 1999). Once the effects of neurotransmission have desisted, glutamate is recaptured from the intersynaptic space by transporter proteins in the presynaptic terminal or in glial cells (Danblot, 2001).

4. Plasticity of Dendritic Spines

The different forms of dendritic spines respond distinctly to the excitatory synaptic impulse, which under certain stimulation conditions can in turn induce modifications in the geometric structure of the spines themselves (Harris & Kater, 1994). After the action of a synaptic stimulus, spines may alter their geometric structure in a matter of minutes (Muller et al., 2000). Furthermore, when such modifications occur, the distribution of glutamate receptors is also modified. Thus, if the head of the spine increases in size, the area occupied by ionotropic receptors expands with respect to that occupied by metabotropic receptors, although the area that the latter occupy also increases as does their number (Luján et al., 1996).

Both ionotropic and metabotropic receptors are involved in short- (transitory) and long- (persistent) term synaptic plasticity (Bennett, 2000; Bortolotto et al., 2005). If the synaptic stimulation is intense, the metabotropic receptors are activated secondarily due, amongst other things, to the fact that they are predominantly located on the periphery of the synapse (Luján et al., 1996). As part of the transmission of nerve impulse at the synaptic level, the flow of Ca^{2+} ions towards the parental dendrite encounters greater physical and electrical resistance in spines with a narrower neck (Volfovski et al., 1999; Majewska et al., 2000). The electrical resistance of the neck of a dendritic spine depends on its length, the transversal space it occupies, its cytoplasmic resistivity and the activity of the organelles it contains (Wickens, 1988). In fact, 95% of the total Ca^{2+} that enters a typical spine is captured by intracellular buffering systems, whereas the remaining 5% resides freely inside the spine exerting a signalling effect. About 70% of this latter fraction is expelled from the spine through the action of Ca^{2+} pumps located in the lateral membrane of the spine, while the remaining 30% is taken up by the smooth endoplasmic reticulum. Thus, in terms of signalling, only 0.01% flows towards the parent dendrite through the neck of the spine (Nimchinsky et al., 2002).

The concentration of Ca^{2+} inside the spine is a determining factor in its plastic geometrical transformation (Koch & Zador, 1993; Kovalchuk et al., 2000). In fact, a moderate increase in Ca^{2+}, within normal limits, causes spine elongation, while an excessive increase in the concentration of this ion produces a contraction of the spine or even its disappearance (Segal et al., 2000). Coinciding with these findings, it has been reported that small pulses of glutamate lengthen spines and that pulses of greater magnitude induce their retraction or loss (Korkotian & Segal, 1999). Similarly, excessive experimental excitatory stimulation of synapses on dendritic spines produces a reduction in their density (Jiang et al., 1998), whereas weak stimulation augments their number (Kirov and Harris, 1999).

Spines in adults are less plastic and they remain plastic for shorter periods of time than in younger individuals (Grutzendler et al., 2002). In fact, in the course of brain development, the proportion of spines that can express plastic transformations is gradually reduced. These transitory spines are predominantly thin (Holtmaat et al., 2005) and since they are the most efficient in transmitting synaptic impulses (Koch et al., 1992), they enable adjustments in the processing of information to be made. In experimental studies performed on rodents, it has been reported that the proportion of persistent spines (which are less plastic than their transitory counterparts) ranges from 35% in young rodents to as high as 73% in mature adults (Holtmaat et al., 2005).

5. The Plasticity of Dendritic Spines Associated with Learning and Memory

The plasticity of dendritic spines in response to different conditions is based on modifications that occur at the molecular, sub-cellular and cellular level of organization. The cognitive information that a neuron receives varies in accordance with its origin and its eventual confluence with other afferent systems, as well as its bioelectric pattern, amongst other additional factors. This information largely determines the nature of the plastic changes that dendritic spines might undergo. In general terms, these changes tend to tailor the eventual psychoneural response to the adaptive demands that this information implies. Therefore, it is relevant to analyse the morphofunctional changes in dendritic spines as they probably underlie the organization of mnemic information at the synaptic level.

There is no distinction between the head and neck of stubby and wide spines, which means that the passage of electrical current from the head of the spine to the parent dendrite encounters virtually no resistance. Consequently, it has been proposed that stubby and wide spines could act as cellular shock absorber designed to cushion neuron excitability (González-Burgos, 2009, 2012), especially in virtue of the fact that their density increases when excitatory synaptic stimulation becomes more intense (Perez-Vega et al., 2000; González-Burgos et al., 2011). On the other hand, spines with a well-differentiated neck and head more efficiently transmit the synaptic impulse (Koch et al., 1992) and their participation -at least that of the more predominant spines (thin and mushroom spines)- in plasticity related to the transmission of mnemic information is well documented (Bourne and Harris, 2007; González-Burgos, 2009, 2012; Kasai et al., 2010a; Segal, 2010).

Presynaptic activity is an indispensable prerequisite for the expression of the structural plasticity of dendritic spines, particularly in terms of the geometric inter-conversions they can undergo as a result of afferent stimulation related to adaptive phenomena like learning and memory (Muller et al., 2000; Kasai et al., 2003; González-Burgos et al., 2005; Lee et al., 2005;). It has been reported that LTP induction occurs in small (presumably thin spines: Matsuzaki et al., 2004) and silent (Geinisman, 2000) spines (Fifkova & Van Harreveld, 1977), through the activation of ionotropic AMPA (Isaac et al., 1995) and NMDA (Bennett, 2000) glutamate receptors, as well as through the secondary activation of metabotropic receptors located at the periphery of the synapse (Petrozzino & Connor, 1994). Such neurochemical events enable both the initial induction and sustainment of potentiation (Muller et al., 2002), and they encourage the subsequent consolidation of mnemic information (Lamprecht & LeDoux, 2004).

The capacity to induce LTP is strongly determined by both presynaptic and postsynaptic factors. The concurrence of synaptically active axons on a group of spines in close proximity strongly enhances their potentiation (McNaughton et al., 1978) as a result of the transfer of electrical charge between these neighbouring spines (Harris & Kater, 1994; Sorra & Harris,

2000). Furthermore, different groups of spines can be potentiated distinctly because they are in different dendritic regions, their population density is different, the proximity amongst them differs or even because the relative proportions of their geometric forms vary. In addition, if individual spines in the same vicinity have a narrow neck this facilitates LTP induction even further (Matsuzaki et al., 2004), thereby enhancing the association between synaptic stimuli, the specificity of a given type of presynaptic activity, and the durability of the postsynaptic effect and its integration in the neuron in question (Harris & Kater, 1994). It is worth mentioning that even despite the above, LTP is not induced or consolidated if the spine is stimulated presynaptically below the threshold, if Ca^{2+} is chelated inside the spine or if the ionotropic NMDA receptors are neurochemically antagonized (Bennett, 2000).

After LTP induction, the number of axon terminals that are in synaptic contact with more than one spine increases (Toni et al., 1999). Indeed, both the number of synapses and the complexity of the dendritic cytoarchitecture are enhanced after the recent acquisition of information (Moser et al., 1994; Kleim et al., 1997). What is more, after several days after LTP induction spine turnover in the vicinity of potentiated spines is seen, new spines replacing those that were not stimulated. This encourages the stabilization of the postsynaptic effects of potentiation in the group of spines that were initially stimulated (De Roo et al., 2008) although we must consider that this stabilization may perhaps be related to processes of homeostatic plasticity. Thus, the increase in spines observed as a result of the learning process would in fact only be represented by those spines that have been potentiated (Fedulov et al., 2007).

LTP induction provokes plastic changes in the geometric structure of potentiated spines. A few hours after potentiation, the head of the spine enlarges (Toni et al., 2001; Lang et al., 2004) in a manner that remains stable over a period of several days (Harris et al., 2003; De Roo et al., 2008), which presumably could correspond to the transformation of a thin spine into a mushroom spine. During this process, various neurochemical events contribute to the maintenance of LTP once it has been induced (Williams et al., 1989), such that the enlargement of the spine head could have more to do with sustaining and consolidating LTP than with its induction (Bennett, 2000; Lang et al., 2004; Yang et al., 2008). The expansion of the spine head resulting from the consolidation of LTP usually precedes a series of additional plastic changes that succeed one another, such as the formation of a perforated synapse (Geinisman et al., 1993; Toni et al., 2001) from macular synapses (Hering & Sheng, 2001). Synapse perforation in large (mushroom) spines can lead to the transitory formation of a branched spine, finally giving rise to two thin spines (Moser et al., 1994; Muller et al., 2000). This implies that there is a causal link between LTP induction and a high incidence of perforated spines that can transform themselves into double spines. In turn, such events may be related to learning and subsequently remembering a task, for example, one involving spatial memory (Geinisman, 2000; Muller et al., 2000).

There is evidence that the density of spines on neurons in the CA1 region of the hippocampus increases as a result of the formation of associative memory traces (Leuner et al., 2003). Moreover, several reports have suggested that the activity of thin spines is related to the acquisition of information, in other words, to the learning process. By contrast, mushroom spines are apparently linked to the retention, storage and retrieval of previously learned information, in other words to memory (Kasai et al., 2003; Matsuzaki et al., 2004; Bourne & Harris, 2007). In relation to this, studies into spatial reference memory performance have been conducted on female mice during the stages of the estrous cycle in which the circulating estrogen concentration is highest (proestrus) or lowest (estrus). The premise was that the modulation of the density of hippocampal dendritic spines by estrogens is associated with cognitive task performance (González-Burgos et al., 2012; Velázquez-Zamora et al., 2012a,b). However, despite the higher spine density during proestrus than during the oestrus (Woolley et al., 1990), and the enhanced capacity to integrate synaptic signals associated with this increase in density (Harris & Kater, 1994), behavioural efficiency is greater during the estrus (Warren & Juraska, 1997). This behavioural manifestation could reflect the higher proportion of thin spines (González-Burgos et al., 2005), which might produce a compensatory plastic phenomenon that would mean hippocampal neurons have a greater capacity for the acquisition of contextual information.

In another series of experimental studies, an increase in the dendritic spine density of pyramidal neurons in cortical layer III was detected after improved behavioural performance in short-term memory tests as a result of prefrontal serotonin (inhibitory neurotransmitter) depletion. This was accompanied by a proportional increase in thin spines in regions distant from the neuronal soma, as well as an increase in stubby spines in the proximal region of the apical dendrite (Perez-Vega et al., 2000). There was also a concomitant plastic increase in the density of 5-HT2A serotonin receptors (Soria-Fregoso et al., 2008) that could provoke hypersensitivity as a result of denervation. Following serotonergic denervation, the increase in spine density and in the proportion of thin spines - which has been linked to the rapid synaptic transmission (Bennett, 2000; Bortolotto et al., 2005) of recently acquired information (Kasai et al., 2003; Matsuzaki et al., 2004; Bourne & Harris, 2007)- suggests that the excitability of the neurons involved must also be enhanced. This supposition was subsequently confirmed in electrophysiological studies in which multiunitary activity of these neurons increased during the execution of working-memory related behavioural tests (Lopez-Vázquez et al., 2006). These findings would be consistent with the increase in serotonin receptors and stubby spines in the dendritic zone close to the soma, such that both phenomena would constitute plastic events that regulate the increase in neuronal excitability caused by the decrease in serotonin-mediated inhibitory transmission. This assertion is also supported by previous reports showing that inhibitory synaptic contacts are chiefly established in the dendritic vicinity of the soma and on the soma itself (Edwards, 1995).

6. Molecular Events Underlying the Plasticity of Dendritic Spines

6.1. General Structure of the Synapse

As already indicated, dendritic spines are anatomical structures on neurons that establish the vast majority of excitatory synaptic contacts in the brain. In general terms, excitatory synapses are comprised of the presynaptic and postsynaptic components of neurons, as well as by the inter-synaptic space or synaptic cleft. Presynaptic buttons, approximately 40 nm in diameter, are found at the end of axons (Sudhof, 2004) and they contain the so-called synaptic vesicles that carry neurotransmitters, in this case glutamate. The synaptic cleft is the site where proteins that play a key role in the establishment and proper functioning of the synapse act. This region measures about 22 nm, and it "separates" the pre- and postsynapse, representing the extraplasmatic zone into which neurotransmitters are released from the presynapse so that they can then bind to the receptors anchored postsynaptically in the spine membrane (Lucic et al., 2005). Adhesion proteins can also be found in this intersynaptic space, the activity of which ensures the junction between the pre- and postsynapse is maintained (Bukalo & Dityatev, 2012). Finally, the postsynaptic region (which for the purposes of this Chapter will be represented by the dendritic spines) contains complex "molecular machinery" that provides support and shapes the spine. This 'machinery' reacts to the interactions between specific proteins and the actin cytoskeleton that, when anchored to the inner apical surface of the spines' plasma membrane, forms what is known as the postsynaptic density (Ethell & Pasquale, 2005). The proteins involved in this machinery are associated with actin filaments and they have been linked to the translation of the chemical signals transmitted by glutamate, as well as to the structural changes in spine geometry that underlie normal and pathological synaptic plasticity (Sheng & Hoogenraad, 2007; Cingolani & Goda, 2008). Thus, actin not only serves as the building block of the dendritic spine's cytoskeleton but it also serves as the molecular substrate on which the structural transformation undergone by dendritic spines is based (Hering & Sheng, 2001).

6.2. Synaptic Adhesion Proteins

Once it is clear what dendritic spines are, what role they play in neuronal plasticity and what the basic components of a synapse are, it is time to look at the proteins involved in the processes that underlie the plasticity associated with these structures as a whole.

There are proteins in the synaptic cleft that are mainly involved in providing support and in strengthening the synaptic contact that has been established. These proteins are known as neuronal cell adhesion molecules (NCAMs), which include α-catenin, β-catenin, δ-catenin, N-caderin, neurexin and neuroligin (Sheng & Hoogenraad, 2007). N-cadherin is a transmembrane protein located in the presynapse that forms a bridge between this and the postsynapse, conferring stability and strength to the synaptic junction. This requires the coupling of the extramembrane portion of N-cadherin in the synaptic cleft with the extramembrane portion of β-catenin located in the postsynaptic membrane. Recently, it has been elucidated the role of these synaptic adhesion proteins (N-cadherin and β-catenin) in the development of synaptic cones in bipolar cells and in the transmission of visual information to the CNS (Nuhn & Fuerst, 2014).

Besides coupling with N-cadherin, the β-catenin protein also binds to the peripheral α-catenin protein within the postsynapse, which is linked directly to the actin filaments of the postsynaptic density. N-cadherin couples indirectly with the spine cytoskeleton by binding to δ-catenin, which also binds directly to actin filaments (Calabrese et al., 2006). In attempting to elucidate the role of cell adhesion proteins in specific synaptic events, N-cadherin was seen to associate directly with AMPA receptors in the postsynaptic region in manner that was dependent on extracellular calcium (Nuriya & Huganir, 2006). However, it has also been reported that overexpression of α-catenin accelerates the maturation of dendritic spines and reduces their motility, which suggests that its activity promotes the stability of dendritic spine as well as spinogenesis (Abe et al., 2004). As for neurexin and neuroligin, they form a protein complex which is particularly important to establish synapses. Indeed, it has been demonstrated that both proteins have an anchorage site that corresponds, on the one hand, to the presynaptic region to which neurexin binds itself and on the other, to the postsynaptic region in which neuroligin is found (Graf et al., 2004). Thus, the evidence available shows that cell adhesion molecules are implicated in the formation and establishment of the synapse. Consequently, the distribution of these and other proteins that will be referred to later in this chapter will have important implications for plasticity in normal and atypical circumstances.

6.3. Postsynaptic Proteins

The presynaptic region is the region in which the vesiculation of specific neurotransmitters takes place, and from which these and other vesiculated molecules from the neuronal soma are released into the intersynaptic space. This involves various processes, in which a considerable number of molecules located in the presynapsis participate, the most abundant of these being actin (Kavalali & Jorgensen, 2014; Rust & Maritzen, 2015).

Despite the activity of presynaptic proteins, the proteins found in the postsynaptic region are believed to be responsible for the structural changes that dendritic spines undergo and which decide how neuronal excitability is regulated. The postsynaptic density is defined as the region immediately underlying the head of the dendritic spine. This region contains a wide range of proteins, actin filaments and other molecules that have a specific affinity for the AMPA and NMDA receptors in excitatory synapses (Rao et al., 1998). As already mentioned, morphological distinct dendritic spines exist that may undergo plastic structural changes, switching between one type and another. Their shape and any geometric modification is determined by physiological events associated with plasticity, and at the molecular level, by structural modifications to actin and through the dynamics of the proteins involved in the polymerization of this protein into filaments (F-actin) (Woodrum et al., 1975; Koskinen & Hotulainen, 2014).

The proteins associated with the cytoskeleton of dendritic spines have been linked to changes in the geometric structure of the latter. This association is principally due to their participation in the addition of actin monomers (G-actin) and in the binding of previously formed filaments, which results in the creation of molecular conditions that ensure dynamic stability (Sekino et al., 2007; Sala et al., 2008). The dynamics of the proteins associated with the actin cytoskeleton are complex. First of all, they compete with one another in their efforts to bind to the actin complex that constitutes the postsynaptic density. Hence, the competition between these proteins in binding to F-actin represents a challenge to our understanding of the molecular machinery that triggers plastic phenomena at the level of the dendritic spine.

Amongst others, these actin binding proteins include cofilin, drebrin, α-actinin, profilin, gelsolin and myosin (Calabrese et al., 2006). Cofilin is a small, approximately 20 KDa protein that is found beneath the postsynaptic density where it plays a key role in the rate at which actin filament phosphorylation occurs (Bamburg et al., 1999; DesMarais et al., 2005). The activity of cofilin depends on its own phosphorylation state and when phosphorylated, its ability to bind to actin filaments is inhibited and it is considered to be in an inactive state. However, when cofilin is unphosphorylated, it becomes active, a state that arises as a result of the action of specific phosphatases. This active state of cofilin is enhanced when the synapse is exposed to LTP (Pontrello & Ethell, 2009), which promotes the stabilization of mature dendritic spines (Andrianantoandro & Pollard, 2006; Frotscher et al., 2014). This situation is consistent with the fact that this type of synaptic stimulation can induce structural changes in dendritic spines, changes that may dependent on the structural modification of actin filaments and their interaction with other cytoskeleton associated proteins in the spine (Okamoto et al., 2004). Hence, cofilin appears to play an important role in dendritic spine dynamics and consequently, in the synaptic plasticity associated with cognitive processes (Pontrello & Ethell, 2009) such as reference memory in successful aging (González-Ramírez et al., 2014). In fact, some studies have described changes in the expression and phosphorylation of cofilin and other proteins in the postsynaptic density in pathologies such as Alzheimer's disease (AD), in which a very clear deterioration in memory can be seen (Zhu et al., 2014; Barone et al., in press).

Drebrin also appears to be involved in stabilization of the cytoskeleton, by virtue of its selective competitive binding to actin filaments, along with proteins, including α-actinin, tropomyosin, gelsolin, fascin and cofilin (Ishikawa et al., 1994; Ishikawa et al., 2007). The drebrin protein has been linked to various plastic phenomena, ranging from the development of dendritic spines to synaptogenesis, and it has even been demonstrated that the distribution of NMDA and AMPA receptors in the cell membrane of dendritic spines varies in accordance with drebin expression (Takahashi et al., 2003; Takahashi et al., 2006; Takahashiet al.,2009). Moreover, drebrin promotes dendritic spine elongation in neuronal cultures through its inhibitory effect on the activity of myosin, which is responsible for contracting actin filaments (Hayashi & Shirao, 1999). Drebrin also has important implications in various diseases, and weak drebrin expression has been reported in the hippocampus of patients with AD (Harigaya et al., 1996), as in the temporal cortex of individuals with Down's Syndrome (Shim & Lubec, 2002). A more recent study has shown that changes in diet and the consumption of specific antioxidants, such as resveratrol, increases the expression of drebrin and other molecules, enhancing neuroprotection in experimental models of AD (Varamini et al., 2014).

Profilin is a protein that is regulated by the activity of Rho GTPases and that binds to free actin monomers in the cytoplasm of spines, ensuring they are available to bind to the terminal regions of filaments and elongate them (Wolven et al., 2000). The actin networks established inside dendritic spines can also be formed in such a way that it is not only actin monomers that bind to filaments. The cytoskeletal mesh can also be formed by the addition of complete filaments, and the ARP2/3 protein complex collaborates in this task by adding actin filaments to other previously established ones. In turn, the activity of this protein complex is controlled by other types of protein found inside the spine, such as WASP and cortactin (Millard et al., 2004). Cortactin is a protein that plays a key role in the internal dynamics of dendritic spines, since it represents a nexus between the synaptic stimulus at metabotropic receptors and the actin cytoskeleton.

The Shank and Homer protein complex ensures that groups of topographically circumscribed postsynaptic glutamate receptors are stabilized (Tu et al., 1999). During synaptogenesis, at least, this complex binds to cortactin and the latter to the actin cytoskeleton, modulating the polymerization of filaments (Pontrello & Ethell, 2009). In addition, cortactin is also linked to some proteins involved in cell adhesion, such as δ-catenin, an association that appears to have a positive influence on the elongation of actin filaments when cortactin is in its active state, in other words, when it is dephosphorylated (Martínez et al., 2003). It has also been confirmed that cortactin has implications in plasticity, as it influences the morphogenesis of dendritic spines. Indeed, the inhibition of cortactin synthesis by siRNA (silencing RNA) results in a drastic reduction in spine density, whereas its overexpression leads to spine elongation (Hering & Sheng, 2003). Furthermore, cortactin binds to the PSD95 protein, which is found in the postsynaptic density, encouraging the anchorage of the proteins closest to the postsynaptic density to the regions closest to the actin cytoskeleton (Yoshii & Constantine-Paton, 2007). In addition, the acetylation levels of cortactin appear to determine its capacity to bind to other molecules, as well as influencing the motility of dendritic spines (Catarino et al., 2013). This makes this protein a target molecule to study the plastic events that, at the molecular level, determine the establishment of stable, long-term synaptic contacts, possibly promoting the consolidation of implicit information in the memory.

As well as cytoskeleton associated proteins, the Rho GTPases constitute a family of proteins involved in regulating the morphology of dendritic spines. These proteins include Rho A, Rac 1 and Cdc42 (Luo, 2000; Tashiro & Yuste, 2004; Saneyoshi et al., 2010), and they regulate the activity of other proteins, such as profilin and cofilin. As mentioned previously, the interaction of different protein families results in the correct establishment of synaptic contacts and it has even been confirmed that certain interactions encourage neuroprotection under unfavourable circumstances. This has been seen in studies that show how the expression of proteins like Rho GTPases and cell adhesion proteins, is important in the functional recovery of the nervous system following cerebrovascular accidents and in experimental models of ischaemia (Gibson et al., 2014; Posada-Duque et al., 2014).

The role played by Rho GTPases is subject to the activity, albeit inhibitory or excitatory, of GAPs (GTPase-activating proteins), a function that is the responsibility of GEFs (guanine exchange factors). The latter group of proteins includes kalirin, a protein that has been the focus of extensive research given its implications in the synaptic plasticity of dendritic spines. Kalirin also fulfils a key role in processes that involve the consolidation of information in the memory, as well as in certain psychiatric conditions, such as schizophrenia and AD (Ma et al., 2008a). Moreover, kalirin overexpression provokes the sprouting of dendritic spines on inhibitory hippocampal interneurons that normally lack these structures, and the normal levels of kalirin found in this same region could well be involved in the maintenance of the synapses formed in the dendritic trunk of neurons (Maet al., 2008b). In addition, overexpression of kalirin in cortical neurons causes an increase in the density of dendritic spines (Penzes et al., 2001), which demonstrates its importance in certain plastic phenomena and, in particular, in *de novo* spinogenesis.

The activation of signalling pathways that result in the coupling of actin monomers or F-actin stabilization may be triggered by the coupling of specific proteins located in the postsynaptic density with ionotropic glutamate receptors found in the cell membrane. In general, the activity of Rho GTPases (proteins like PSD-95 and the Shank proteins that form the postsynaptic density), kinases and intracellular Ca^{2+} (which drives the opening of synaptic channels) are some of the factors that promote the structural adjustment of the actin cytoskeleton following glutamate receptor activation (Schubert & Dotti, 2007). The activation of these elements -which form part of specific signalling pathways- ultimately encourages other proteins to activate cofilin, such as Rac-1, PAK, LIMK-1 and second messengers (Penzeset al., 2003). Alternatively, they ensure that the action of the spinophilin protein, derived from CaMKII driven phosphorylation (see Nurrish, 2014) can be completed, in order to regulate F-actin polymerization (Hsieh-Wilsonet al., 2003). Thus, variations in the relationship between the aforementioned proteins are associated with plastic changes, such as spine morphogenesis and synapse formation (Penzes et al., 2003).

In addition, the molecular events that lead to plastic phenomena in dendritic spines can be initiated as a result of the phosphorylation of other proteins that interact with cell adhesion molecules or tyrosine-kinase receptors, such as TrkB located in the postsynaptic membrane (Schubert & Dotti, 2007). TrkB receptors are phosphorylated upon interacting with brain-derived neurotrophic factor (BDNF), which is a crucial molecule for synaptic transmission and some plasticity (Bramham & Messaoudi, 2005; Nagappan & Lu, 2005). As a result of this phosphorylation cortactin and other proteins are activated (e.g., the Arp2/3 complex and WASP), which regulates actin polymerization and filament elongation, in collaboration with other cytoskeleton associated proteins like gelsolin (Mullins et al., 1998; Lua & Low, 2005).

In the postsynaptic membrane we find ephrin receptors, which as well as being involved in neuronal differentiation and synaptic plasticity processes (Klein, 2004), also promote the activation of proteins within dendritic spines, one of which is kalirin. Through the mediation of Rac and PAK, kalirin activates myosin, a protein that has been linked to spinogenesis and that is also closely linked to F-actin contractibility (Penzes et al., 2003; Zhang et al., 2005).

Conclusion

Dendritic spines are cytoplasmic protrusions that modulate synaptic excitatory activity depending on their density and geometric shape. It is well established that the processing of memory information is a complex series of psychoneural phenomena useful for the individual adaptive capabilities. When environmental demands require of memory traces' retrieval, certain events like neurotransmitter release and changes in receptors activity—among others—are strongly involved. The synaptic stimulation trigger several molecular cascades in dendritic spines, changing in turn the cytoskeleton-associated proteins activity, which determines the shape of the spine and drives the molecular machinery for spinogenesis in dendrites. Such plastic remodelling of dendritic spine's shape depends therefore on polymerization / depolymerization of actin filaments. Altogether, these neurobiological events modify the synaptic information processing. This chapter describes the participation of several spine-associated proteins in the maintenance of synapses and their strength, through their concerted actions in the dynamics of actin filaments, under normal or atypical circumstances.

References

Abe, K., Chisaka, O., Van Roy, F. & Takeichi, M. (2004) Stability of dendritic spines and synaptic contacts is controlled by alpha N-catenin. *Nat. Neurosci.,* 7, 357-363.

Andrianantoandro, E. & Pollard, T.D. (2006) Mechanism of actin filament turnover by severing and nucleation at different concentrations of ADF/cofilin. *Mol. Cell.,* 24, 13-23.

Ascher, P. & Nowak, L. (1988) The role of divalent cations in the N-methyl-D-aspartate responses of mouse central neurons in culture. *J. Physiol.,* 399, 247-266.

Bahn, S., Volk, B. & Wisden, W. (1994) Kainate receptor gene expression in the developing rat brain. *J. Neurosci.,* 14, 5525-5547.

Bamburg, J.R., McGrough, A. & Ono, S. (1999) Putting a new twist on actin: ADF/cofilins modulate actin dynamics. *Trends Cell Biol.*, 9, 364-370.

Barone, E., Mosses, S. &Fraering, P.C. (in press) Inactivation of brain Cofilin-1 by age, Alzheimer´s disease and γ-secretase. *Biochim. Biophys. Acta,* 1842, 2500-2509.

Bear, M.F., Connors, B.W. & Paradiso, M.A. (1998) Neurociencia. Explorando el cerebro. *MASSON-Williams & Wilkins,* Barcelona.

Bennett, M.R. (2000) The concept of long-term potentiation of transmission at synapses. *Prog. in Neurobiol.*, 60, 109–137.

Bessis, A.S., Acher, F. & Pin, J.P. (2001) Metabotropic glutamate receptor: exciting possibilities in excitatory transmission. *Cell Trans.,* 17, 3-9.

Bliss, T.V. & Lømo, T. (1970) Plasticity in a monosynaptic cortical pathway. *J. Physiol.,* 207, p. 61.

Bliss, T.V. & Lømo, T. (1973) Long-lasting potentiation of synaptic transmission in the dentate area of the anesthetized rabbit following stimulation of the perforant path. *J. Physiol.,* 232, 331-356.

Bortolotto, Z.A., Collett, V.J., Conquet. F., Jia, Z., van der Putten, H. & Collingridge, G.L. (2005) The regulation of hippocampal LTP by the molecular switch, a form of metaplasticity, requires mGlu5 receptors. *Neuropharmacology*, 49, 13-25.

Bourne, J. & Harris, K.M. (2007) Do thin spines learn to be mushroom spines that remember? *Curr. Op. Neurobiol.,* 17, 381-386.

Bramham, C.R. & Messaoudi, E. (2005) BDNF function in adult synaptic plasticity: the synaptic consolidation hypothesis. *Prog. Neurobiol.*, 76, 99-125.

Bukalo, O. & Dityatev, A. (2012) Synaptic cell adhesion molecules. *Adv. Exp. Med. Biol.,* 970, 97-128.

Calabrese, B., Wilson, M.S. & Halpain, S. (2006) Development and regulation of dendritic spine synapses. *Physiology*, 21, 38-47.

Catarino, T., Ribeiro, L., Santos, S.D. & Carvalho, A.L. (2013) Regulation of synapse composition by protein acetylation: the role of acetylated cortactin. *J. Cell Sci.,* 126, 149-162.

Cingolani, L.A. & Goda, Y. (2008) Actin in action: the interplay between the actin cytoskeleton and synaptic efficacy. *Nat. Rev. Neurosci.,* 9, 344-356.

Cooper, J.R., Bloom, F.E. & Roth, R.H. (2003) The biochemical basis of neuropharmacology. 8th ed. *Oxford University Press,* New York.

Danbolt, N.C. (2001) Glutamate uptake. *Prog. Neurobiol.,* 65, 1-105.

De Roo, M., Klauser, P. & Muller, D. (2008) LTP promotes a selective long-term stabilization and clustering of dendritic spines. *Plos Biol.*, 6, 1850-1860.

DesMarais, V., Ghosh, M., Eddy, R. & Condeelis, J. (2005) Cofilin takes the lead. *J. Cell Sci.,* 118, 19-26.

Edwards, F.A. (1995) Anatomy and electrophysiology of fast synapses lead to a structural model for long-term potentiation. *Physiol. Rev.*, 75, 759-787.

Ellisman, M.H., Deering, T.J., Ouyang, Y., Beck, C.F., Tanksley, S.J., Walton, P.D., Airey, J.A. & Sutko, J.L. (1990) Identification and localization of ryanodine binding proteins in the avian central nervous system. *Neuron,* 5, 135-146.

Ethell, I.M. & Pasquale, E.B. (2005) Molecular mechanisms of dendritic spine development and remodeling. *Prog. Neurobiol.,* 75, 161-205.

Fedulov, V., Rex, Ch.S., Simmons, D.A., Palmer, L., Gall, Ch.M. & Lynch, G. (2007) Evidence that long-term potentiation occurs within individual hippocampal synapses during learning. *J. Neurosci*., 27, 8031-8039.

Fifkova, E. & Van Harreveld, A. (1977) Long-lasting morphological changes in dendritic spines of dentate granular cells following stimulation of the entorhinal area. *J. Neurocytol.,* 6, 211-230.

Fox, K. (1996) The role of excitatory amino acid receptors in developmental plasticity of sensory neocortex, in: Conti, F., Hicks, Ph. (Eds.), Excitatory amino acids in the cerebral cortex. *MIT*, USA, pp. 229-244.

Frotscher, M., Studer, D., Graber, W., Chai, X., Nestel, S. & Zhao, S. (2014) Fine structure of synapses on dendritic spines. *Front. Neuroanat.,* 8, 94.

Geinisman, Y. (2000) Structural synaptic modifications associated with hippocampal LTP and behavioural learning. *Cereb. Cortex,* 10, 952-962.

Geinisman, Y., de Toledo-Morrell, L., Morrell, F., Heller, R.E., Rossi, M. & Parshall, R.F. (1993) Structural synaptic correlate of long-term potentiation: formation of axospinous synapses with multiple, completely partitioned transmission zones. *Hippocampus,* 3, 435-446.

Gibson, C.L., Srivastava, K., Sprigg, N., Bath, P.M. & Bayraktutan, U. (2014) Inhibition of Rho-kinase protects cerebral barrier from ischaemia-evoked injury through modulations of endothelial cell oxidative stress and tight junctions. *J. Neurochem.,* 129, 816-826.

González-Burgos, I. (2009) Dendritic spines plasticity and learning / memory processes: Theory, evidence and perspectives, in: Baylog, L.R. (Ed.), Dendritic spines. Biochemistry, modelling and properties. Neuroscience Research Progress Series, *Nova Science Publishers,* New York, pp. 163-186.

González-Burgos, I. (2012) From synaptic transmission to cognition: an intermediary role for dendritic spines. *Brain Cogn.,* 80, 177-183.

González-Burgos, I., Alejandre-Gómez, M. & Cervantes, M. (2005) Spine-type densities of hippocampal CA1 neurons vary in proestrus and estrus rats. *Neurosci. Let*., 379, 52-54.

González-Burgos, I., González-Tapia, D., Velázquez Zamora, D.A., Feria-Velasco, A. & Beas-Zárate, C. (2011) Guided motor training induces dendritic spine plasticity in adult rat cerebellar Purkinje cells. *Neurosci. Lett.,* 491, 216-220.

González-Burgos, I., Rivera-Cervantes, M.C., Velázquez-Zamora, D.A., Feria-Velasco, A. & García-Segura, L.M. (2012) Selective estrogen receptor modulators regulate dendritic spine plasticity in the hippocampus of male rats, in: González-Burgos, I., Nikonenko, I., Korz, V. (Eds.), Special Issue: Dendritic Spine Plasticity and Cognition, *Neural Plast.* Vol. 2012, artículo 309494, 6 pages.

González-Ramírez, M.M., Velázquez-Zamora, D.A., Olvera-Cortés, M.E. & González-Burgos, I. (2014) Changes in the plastic properties of hippocampal dendritic spines underlie the attenuation of place learning in healthy aged rats. *Neurobiol. Learn. Mem.,* 109, 94-103.

Graf, E.R., Zhang, X., Jin, S.X., Linhoff, M.W. & Craig, A.M. (2004) Neurexins induce differentiation of GABA and glutamate postsynaptic specializations via neuroligins. *Cell,* 119, 1013-1026.

Grutzendler, J., Kasthuri, N. & Gan, W.B. (2002) Long-term dendritic spine stability in the adult cortex. *Nature,* 420, 812-816.

Harigaya, Y., Shoji, M., Shirao, T. & Hirai, S. (1996) Disappearance of actin-binding protein, drebrin, from hippocampal synapses in Alzheimer's disease. *J. Neurosci. Res.,* 43, 87-92.

Harris, K.M., Fiala, J.C. & Ostroff, L. (2003) Structural changes at dendritic spine synapses during long-term potentiation. *Phil. Trans. R. Soc. Lond.,* 358, 745-748.

Harris, K.M., Jensen, F.E. & Tsao, B.H. (1989) Ultrastructure, development, and plasticity of dendritic spine synapses in area CA1 of the rat hippocampus: extending our vision with serial electron microscopy and three-dimensional analyses, in: Chan-Palay, V., Kohler, Ch. (Eds.), The hippocampus – new vistas, *Alan R. Liss,* USA, pp. 33-52.

Harris, K.M. & Kater, S.B. (1994) Dendritic spines: Cellular specializations imparting both stability and flexibility to synaptic function. *Ann. Rev. Neurosci.,* 17, 341-371.

Hayashi, K. & Shirao, T. (1999) Change in the shape of dendritic spines caused by overexpression of drebrin in cultured cortical neurons. *J. Neurosci.,* 19, 3918-3925.

Hering, H. & Sheng, M. (2001) Dendritic spines: structure, dynamics and regulation. *Nat. Rev. Neurosci.*, 2, 880-888.

Hering, H. & Sheng, M. (2003) Activity-dependent redistribution and essential role of cortactin in dendritic spine morphogenesis. *J. Neurosci.*, 23, 11759-11769.

Holtmaat, A.J.G.D., Trachtenberg, J.T., Wilbrecht, L., Shepherd, G.M., Zhang, X., Knott, G.W. & Svoboda, K. (2005) Transient and persistent dendritic spines in the neocortex in vivo. *Neuron,* 45, 279-291.

Hsieh-Wilson, L.C., Benfenati, F., Snyder, G.L., Allen, P.B., Nairn, A.C. & Greengard, P. (2003) Phosphorylation of spinophilin modulates its interaction with actin filaments. *J. Biol. Chem.*, 278, 1186-1194.

Isaac, J.T.R., Nicoli, R.A. & Malenka, R.C. (1995) Evidence for silent synapses: implications for the expression of LTP. *Neuron,* 15, 427-434.

Ishikawa, R., Hayashi, K., Shirao, T., Xue, Y., Takagi, T., Sasaki, Y. & Kohama, K. (1994) Drebrin, a development-associated brain protein from rat embryo, causes the dissociation of tropomyosin from actin filaments. *J. Biol. Chem.,* 1994. 269, 29928-29933.

Ishikawa, R., Katoh, K., Takahashi, A., Xie, C., Oseki, K., Watanabe, M., Igarashi, M., Nakamura, A. & Kohama, K. (2007) Drebrin attenuates the interaction between actin and myosin-V. *Biochem. Biophys. Res. Commun.,* 359, 398-401.

Kasai, H., Fukuda, M., Watanabe, S., Hayashi-Takagi, A. & Noguchi, J. (2010a) Structural dynamics of dendritic spines in memory and cognition. *TINS,* 33, 121-129.

Kasai, H., Hayama, T., Ishikawa, M., Watanabe, S., Yagishita, S. & Noguchi, J. (2010b). Learning rules and persistence of dendritic spines. *Eur. J. Neurosci.*, 32, 241-249.

Kasai, H., Matsuzaki, M., Noguchi, J., Yasumatsu, N. & Nakahara, H. (2003) Structure-stability-function relationships of dendritic spines. *TINS*, 26, 360-368.

Kavalali, E.T. & Jorgensen, E.M. (2014) Visualizing presynaptic function. *Nat. Neurosci.,* 17, 10-16.

Kirov, S.A. & Harris, K.M. (1999) Dendrites are more spiny on mature hippocampal neurons when synapses are inactivated. *Nat. Neurosci.*, 2, 878-883.

Kleim, J.A., Vij, K., Ballard, D.H. & Greenough, W.T. (1997) Learning-dependent synaptic modifications in the cerebellar cortex of the adult rat persists for at least four weeks. *J. Neurosci.,* 17, 717-721.

Klein, R. (2004) Eph/ephrin signaling in morphogenesis, neural development and plasticity. *Curr. Opin. Cell Biol.,* 16, 580-589.

Koch, Ch. & Zador, A. (1993) The function of dendritic spines: devices subserving biochemical rather than electrical compartmentalization. *J. Neurosci.,* 13, 413-422.

Koch, Ch., Zador, A. & Brown, T.H. (1992) Dendritic spines: convergence of theory and experiment. *Science,* 256, 973-974.

Korkotian, E. & Segal, M. (1999) Bidirectional regulation of dendritic spine dimensions by glutamate receptors. *Neuroreport.,* 10, 2875-2877.

Koskinen, M. & Hotulainen, P. (2014) Measuring F-actin properties in dendritic spines. *Front. Neuroanat.*, 8, 74.

Kostyuk, P. (1998) Plasticity in nerve cell function. *Oxford University Press,* New York.

Kovalchuk, Y., Eilers, J., Lisman, J. & Konnerth, A. (2000) NMDA receptor-mediated subthreshold Ca($^{2+}$) signals in spines of hippocampal neurons. *J. Neurosci.,* 20, 1791-1799.

Lamprecht, R. & LeDoux, J. (2004). Structural plasticity and memory. *Nat. Rev. Neurosci.,* 5, 45-54.

Lang, C., Barco, A., Zablow, L., Kandel, E.R., Siegelbaum, S.A. & Zakharenko, S.S. (2004) Transient expansion of synaptically connected dendritic spines upon induction of hippocampal long-term potentiation. *Proc. Natl. Acad. Sci.,* 101, 16665-16670.

Lee, K.J., Kim, H. & Rhyu, I.J. (2005) The roles of dendritic spine shapes in Purkinje cells. *The Cerebellum,* 4, 97-104.

Lester, R.A., Clements, J.D., Westbrook, G.L. & Jahr, C.E. (1990) Channel kinetics determine the time course of NMDA receptor-mediated synaptic currents. *Nature,* 346, 565-567.

Leuner, B, Falduto, J. & Shors, T.J. (2003) Associative memory formation increases the observation of dendritic spines in the hippocampus. *J. Neurosci.,* 23, 659-665.

López-Vázquez, M.A., Olvera-Cortés, M.E. & González-Burgos, I. (2006) Multiunitary activity of prefrontal piramidal neurons increases Turing spatial working memory performance, alter serotonina depletion. *Int. J. Devl. Neurosci.*, 24, 502-503.

Lua, B.L. & Low, B.C. (2005) Cortactin phosphorylation as a switch for actin cytoskeletal network and cell dynamics control. *FEBS Lett.,* 579, 577-585.

Lucic, V., Yang, T., Schweikert, G., Forster, F. & Baumeister, W. (2005) Morphological characterization of molecular complexes present in the synaptic cleft. *Structure, 13*, 423-434.

Luján, R., Nusser, Z., Roberts, D.B., Shigemoto, R. & Somogyi, P. (1996) Perisynaptic location of metabotropic glutamate receptors mGluR1 and mGluR5 on dendrites and dendritic spines in the rat hippocampus. *Eur. J. Neurosci.,* 8, 1488-1500.

Luo, L. (2000) Rho GTPases in neuronal morphogenesis. *Nat. Rev. Neurosci.,* 1, 173-180.

Ma, X., Kiraly, D.D., Gaier, E.D., Wang, Y., Kim, E., Levine, E.S., Eipper, B.A. & Mains, R.E. (2008a) Kalirin-7 is required for synaptic structure and function. *J. Neurosci.,* 28, 12368-12382.

Ma, X., Wang, Y., Ferraro, F., Mains, R.E. & Eipper, B.A. (2008b) Kalirin-7 is an essential component of both shaft and spine excitatory synapses in hippocampal interneurons. *J. Neurosci.*, 28, 711-724.

Majewska, A., Brown, E., Ross, J. & Yuste, R. (2000) Mechanisms of calcium decay kinetics in hippocampal spines: role of spine calcium pumps and calcium diffusion through the spine neck in biochemical compartmentalization. *J. Neurosci.,* 20, 1722-1734.

Martínez, M.C., Ochiishi, T., Majewski, M. & Kosik, K.S. (2003) Dual regulation of neuronal morphogenesis by a delta-catenin-cortactin complex and Rho. *J. Cell Biol.,* 162, 99-111.

Matsuzaki, M., Honkura, N., Ellis-Davies, G.C.R. & Kasai, H. (2004) Structural basis of long-term potentiation in single dendritic spines. *Nature,* 429, 761-766.

Mayer, M.L. & Westbrook, G.L. (1987) Permeation and block of N-methyl-D-aspartic acid receptor channels by divalent cations in mouse cultured central neurons. *J. Physiol.*, 394, 501-527.

McNaughton, B.L., Douglas, R.M. & Goddard, G.V. (1978) Synaptic enhancement in fascia dentate: cooperativity among coactive afferents. *Brain Res.,* 157, 277-293.

Meldrum, B. (2000) Glutamate as a neurotransmitter in the brain: Review of physiology and pathology. *J. Nutr.*, 130, 1007-1015.

Millard, T.H., Sharp, S.J. & Machesky, L.M. (2004) Signalling to actin assembly via the WASP (Wiskott-Aldrich syndrome protein)-family proteins and the Arp2/3 complex. *Biochem. J.,* 380, 1-17.

Moser, M.B., Trommald, M. & Andersen, P. (1994) An increase in dendritic spine density on hippocampal CA1 pyramidal cells following spatial learning in adult rats suggests the formation of new synapses. *Proc. Natl. Acad. Sci. USA.,* 91, 12673-12675.

Mugnaini, E., Walberg, F. & Hauglie-Hanssen, E. (1967) Observations on the fine structure of the lateral vestibular nucleus (Deiters' nucleus) in the cat. *Exp. Brain Res.,* 4, 146-186.

Muller, D., Nikonenko, I., Jourdain, P. & Alberi, S. (2002) LTP, memory and structural plasticity. *Curr. Mol. Med.,* 2, 605-611.

Muller, D., Toni, N. & Buchs, P.A. (2000) Spine changes associated with long-term potentiation. *Hippocampus*, 10, 596-604.

Mullins, R.D., Heuser, J.A. & Pollard, T.D. (1998) The interaction of Arp2/3 complex with actin: nucleation, high affinity pointed end capping, and formation of branching networks of filaments. *Proc. Natl. Acad. Sci.,* 95, 6181-6186.

Nagappan, G. & Lu, B. (2005) Activity-dependent modulation of the BDNF receptor TrkB: mechanisms and implications. *TINS,* 28, 464-471.

Nimchinsky, E.A., Sabatini, B.L. & Svoboda, K. (2002) Structure and function of dendritic spines. *Annu. Rev. Physiol.,* 64, 313-353.

Niswender C.M. & Conn P.J. (2010) Metabotropic glutamate receptors: physiology, pharmacology, and disease. *Annu. Rev. Pharmacol. Toxicol.,* 50, 295-322.

Nowak, L., Bregestovski, P., Ascher, P., Herbet, A. & Prochiantz, A. (1984) Magnesium gates glutamate-activated channels in mouse central neurons. *Nature,* 307, 462-465.

Nuhn, J.S. & Fuerst, P.G. (2014) Developmental localization of adhesion and scaffolding proteins at the cone synapse. *Gene Expr. Patt.,* 16, 36-50.

Nuriya, M. & Huganir, R.L. (2006) Regulation of AMPA receptor trafficking by N-cadherin. *J. Neurochem.,* 97, 652-661.

Nurrish, S. (2014) Dense core vesicle release: controlling the where as well as the when. *Genetics,* 196, 601-604.

Okamoto, K., Nagai, T., Miyawaki, A. & Hayashi, Y. (2004) Rapid and persistent modulation of actin dynamics regulates postsynaptic reorganization underlying bidirectional plasticity. *Nat. Neurosci.*, 7, 1104-1112.

Penzes, P., Beeser, A., Chernoff, J., Schiller, M.R., Eipper, B.A., Mains, R.E. & Huganir, R.L. (2003) Rapid induction of dendritic spine morphogenesis by trans-synaptic ephrinB-EphB receptor activation of the Rho-GEF kalirin. *Neuron,* 37, 263-274.

Penzes, P., Johnson, R.C., Sattler, R., Zhang, X., Huganir, R.L., Kambampati, V., Mains, R.E. & Eipper, B.A. (2001) The neuronal Rho-GEF Kalirin-7 interacts with PDZ domain-containing proteins and regulates dendritic morphogenesis. *Neuron,* 29, 229-242.

Pérez-Vega, M.I., Feria-Velasco, A. & González-Burgos, I. (2000) Prefrontocortical serotonin depletion results in plastic changes of prefrontocortical pyramidal neurons, underlying a greater efficiency of short-term memory. *Brain Res. Bull.,* 53, 291-300.

Petrozzino, J.J. & Connor, J.A. (1994) Dendritic Ca^{2+} accumulations and metabotropic glutamate rceptor activation associated with an N-methyl-D-aspartate receptor-independent long-term potentiation in hippocampal CA1 neurons. *Hippocampus,* 4, 546-558.

Pontrello, C.G. & Ethell, I.M. (2009) Accelerators, brakes, and gears of actin dynamics in dendritic spines. *Open Neurosci. J.,* 3, 67-86.

Posada-Duque, R.A., Barreto, G.E. & Cardona-Gomez, G.P. (2014) Protection after stroke: cellular effectors of neurovascular unit integrity. *Front. Cell Neurosci.,* 8, 231.

Ramón y Cajal, S. (1952) Neuronismo o Reticularismo? Instituto Cajal, CSIC, Madrid.

Rao, A., Kim, E., Sheng, M. & Craig, A.M. (1998) Heterogeneity in the molecular composition of excitatory postsynaptic sites during development of hippocampal neurons in culture. *J. Neurosci.,* 18, 1217-1229.

Rust, M.B. & Maritzen, T. (in press). Relevance of presynaptic actin dynamics for synapse function and mouse behavior. *Exp. Cell Res.*

Sala, C., Cambianica, I. & Rossi, F. (2008) Molecular mechanisms of dendritic spine development and maintenance. *Acta Neurobiol. Exp.,* 68, 289-304.

Salinska, E., Wojciech, D., Lazerewicz, J.W., 2005. The role of excitotoxicity in neurodegeneration. *Folia Neuropathol.,* 43, 322-339.

Saneyoshi, T., Fortin, D.A. & Soderling, T.R. (2010) Regulation of spine and synapse formation by activity-dependent intracellular signaling pathways. *Curr. Opin. Neurobiol.,* 20, 108-115.

Schubert, V. & Dotti, C.G. (2007) Transmitting on actin: synaptic control of dendritic architecture. *J. Cell Sci*., 120, 205-212.

Segal, M. (2010) Dendritic spines, synaptic plasticity and neuronal survival: activity shapes dendritic spines to enhance neuronal viability. *Eur. J. Neurosci.,* 31, 2178-2184.

Segal, M., Korkotian, E. & Murphy, D.D. (2000) Dendritic spine formation and pruning: common cellular mechanisms? *TINS*, 23, 53-57.

Sekino, Y., Kojima, N. & Shirao, T. (2007) Role of actin cytoskeleton in dendritic spine morphogenesis. *Neurochem. Int.,* 51, 92-104.

Sheng, M. & Hoogenraad, C.C. (2007) The postsynaptic architecture of excitatory synapses: a more quantitative view. *Annu. Rev. Biochem*., 76, 823-847.

Shim, K.S. & Lubec, G. (2002) Drebrin, a dendritic spine protein, is manifold decreased in brains of patients with Alzheimer's disease and Down syndrome. *Neurosci. Lett*., 324, 209-212.

Soria-Fregozo, C., Pérez-Vega, M.I., González-Burgos, I., Feria-Velasco, A. & Beas-Zárate, C. (2008) Prefrontal serotonergic denervation induces increase in the density of $5\text{-}HT_{2A}$ receptors in adult rat prefrontal cortex. *Neurochem. Res.,* 33, 2350-2357.

Sorra, K.E. & Harris, K.M. (2000) Overview on the structure, composition, function, development, and plasticity of hippocampal dendritic spines. *Hippocampus,* 10, 501-511.

Spacek, J. & Harris K.M. (1997) Three-dimensional organization of smooth endoplasmic reticulum in hippocampal CA1 dendrites and dendritic spines of the immature and mature rat. *J. Neurosci.*, 17, 190-203.

Sudhof, T.C. (2004) The synaptic vesicle cycle. *Annu. Rev. Neurosci.* 27, 509-547.

Takahashi, H., Sekino, Y., Tanaka, S., Mizui, T., Kishi, S. & Shirao, T. (2003) Drebrin-dependent actin clustering in dendritic filopodia governs synaptic targeting of postsynaptic density-95 and dendritic spine morphogenesis. *J. Neurosci.*, 23, 6586-6595.

Takahashi, H., Yamazaki, H., Hanamura, K., Sekino, Y. & Shirao, T. (2009) Activity of the AMPA receptor regulates drebrin stabilization in dendritic spine morphogenesis. *J. Cell Sci.*, 122, 1211-1219.

Tarelo-Acuña, L., Olvera-Cortés, E. & González-Burgos, I. (2000) Prenatal and postnatal exposure to etanol induces changes in the shape of the dendritic spines from hippocampal CA1 pyramidal neurons of the rat. *Neurosci. Lett.*, 286, 13-16.

Tashiro, A. & Yuste, R. (2004) Regulation of dendritic spine motility and stability by Rac1 and Rho kinase: evidence for two forms of spine motility. *Mol. Cell. Neurosci.*, 26, 429-440.

Toni, N., Buchs, P.A., Nikonenko, I., Bron, C.R. & Muller, D. (1999) LTP promotes formation of multiple spine synapses between a single axon terminal and a dendrite. *Nature,* 402, 421-425.

Toni, N., Buchs, P.A., Nikonenko, I., Povilaitite, P., Parisi, L. & Muller, D. (2001) Remodeling of synaptic membranes after induction of leng-term potentiation. *J. Neurosci.,* 21, 6245-6251.

Tu, J.C., Xiao, B., Naisbitt, S., Yuan, J.P., Petralia, R.S., Brakeman, P., Doan, A., Aakalu, V.K., Canahan, A.A., Sheng, M. & Worley, P.F. (1999) Coupling of mGluR/Homer and PSD-95 complex by the Shank family of postsynaptic density proteins. *Neuron*, 23, 583-592.

Varamini, B., Sikalidis, A.K. & Bradford, K.L. (2014) Resveratrol increases cerebral glycogen synthase kinase phosphorylation as well as protein levels of drebrinand transthyretin in mice: an exploratory study. *Int. J. Food Sci. Nutr.*, 65, 89-96.

Velázquez-Zamora, D.A., González-Tapia, D., González-Ramírez, M.M., Flores-Soto, M.E., Vázquez-Valls, E., Cervantes, M. & González-Burgos, I. (2012a) Plastic changes in dendritic spines of hippocampal CA1 pyramidal neurons from ovariectomized rats after estradiol treatment. *Brain Res.,* 1470, 1-10.

Velázquez-Zamora, D.A., García-Segura, L.M. & González-Burgos, I. (2012b) Effects of selective estrogen receptor modulators on allocentric working memory performance and on dendritic spines in medial prefrontal cortex pyramidal neurons of ovariectomized rats. *Horm. Behav.,* 61, 512-517.

Volfovsky, N., Parnas, H., Segal, M. & Korkotian, E. (1999) Geometry of dendritic spines affects calcium dynamics in hippocampal neurons: theory and experiments. *J. Neurophysiol.,* 81, 450-462.

Warren, S.G. & Juraska, J.M. (1997) Spatial and nonspatial learning across the rat estrous cycle. *Behav. Neurosci.,* 111, 259-266.

Westrum, L. E. (1970) Observations on initial segments of axons in the prepyriform cortex of the rat. *J. Comp. Neurol.,* 139, 337-356.

Wickens J. (1988) Electrically coupled but chemically isolated synapses: dendritic spines and calcium in a rule for synaptic modification. *Prog. Neurobiol.,* 31, 507-528.

Williams, J.H., Errington, M.L., Lynch, M.A. & Bliss, T.V. (1989) Arachidonic acid induces a long-term activity-dependent enhancement of synaptic transmission in the hippocampus. *Nature,* 341, 739-742.

Wolven, A.K., Belmont, L.D., Mahoney, N.M., Almo, S.C. & Drubin, D.G. (2000) In vivo importance of actin nucleotide exchange catalyzed by profilin. *J. Cell Biol.,* 150, 895-904.

Woodrum, D.T., Rich, S.A. & Pollard, T.D. (1975) Evidence for biased bidirectional polymerization of actin filaments using heavy meromyosin prepared by an improved method. *J. Cell Biol.*, 67, 231-237.

Woolley, C.S., Gould, E., Frankfurt, M. & McEwen, B.S. (1990) Naturally occurring fluctuation in dendritic spine density on adult hippocampal pyramidal neurons. *J. Neurosci.,* 10, 4035-4039.

Yang, Y., Wang, X., Frerking, M. & Zhou, Q. (2008) Spine expansion and stabilization associated with long-term potentiation. *J. Neurosci.*, 28, 5740-5751.

Yoshii, A. & Constantine–Paton, M. (2007) BDNF induces transport of PSD-95 to dendrites through PI3K-AKT signaling after NMDA receptor activation. *Nat. Neurosci.,* 10, 702–711.

Zhang, H., Webb, D.J., Asmussen, H., Niu, S. & Horwitz, A.F. (2005) AGIT1/PIX/Rac/PAK signaling module regulates spine morphogenesis and synapse formation through MLC. *J. Neurosci.,* 25, 3379-3388.

Zhu, H., Luo, L., Hu, S., Dong, K., Li, G. & Zhang, T. (2014) Treating Alzheimer's disease with Yizhijiannao granules by regulating expression of multiple proteins in temporal lobe. *Neural Regen. Res.,* 9, 1283-1287.

In: Synaptic Fundamentals of Memory Performance
Editor: Ignacio González-Burgos
ISBN: 978-1-63483-279-3

Chapter 4

LONG-TERM POTENTIATION AND LONG-TERM DEPRESSION IN SPATIAL MEMORY: AN UPDATE

María Esther Olvera-Cortés[1,*], Miguel Ángel López-Vázquez[1,2], Blanca Érika Gutiérrez-Guzmán[1] and J. Jesús Hernández-Pérez[1]

[1]Centro de Investigación Biomédica de Michoacán,
Instituto Mexicano del Seguro Social, Morelia, Michoacán, México
[2]Instituto de Física y Matemáticas,
Universidad Michoacana de San Nicolás de Hidalgo, Morelia, Michoacán, México

ABSTRACT

Synaptic plasticity has been proposed as the main consequence of experience-induced learning and as a possible mechanism of information storage for memory. The principal learning-related expressions of synaptic plasticity are long-term potentiation (LTP) and long-term depression (LTD). LTP in the pyramidal neurons of the hippocampal Ammon's horn has been extensively proposed as a key mechanism in the establishment of learning and memory and as an essential pre-requisite for spatial learning. Hippocampal LTP has been associated with spatial learning through different behavioural paradigms; however, the establishment of links between place representations, learning, and LTP has required experimental evidence showing that LTP is facilitated by exposure to novel environments, the influence of LTP on spatial representations, as well as evidence of LTP induced by behavioural experiences producing spatial learning. However, LTD is an intrinsic hippocampal electrical phenomenon that takes place when the afferent stimulation is paired with a novel spatial circumstance, leading to the assumption that LTD is required for reversal learning and consolidation of spatial memory. In fact, it has been suggested that LTD may underlie the novelty-induced learning facilitation, accounting with LTP for the learning of novel environments. However, LTP and LTD involved in spatial learning show differences

* Send correspondence to: María Esther Olvera Cortés. Laboratorio de Neurofisiología Experimental, División de Neurociencias, Centro de Investigación Biomédica de Michoacán, IMSS. Morelia, Mich. México. Email: maesolco@yahho.com.

among hippocampal regions, suggesting that both types of potentiation participate in different components of spatial learning. This chapter deals with the main bodies of evidence linking LTP and LTD to spatial learning and memory, to hippocampal regions activity (CA1, CA3 and dentate gyrus), and to cognitive processes (learning, consolidation, reversion, spatial novelty detection), with both acting in hippocampal neural circuits and in concert with other cerebral regions.

1. Introduction

Synaptic plasticity refers to the modification of the strength of synapse as a result of its previous activity, thereby implying a form of neuronal memory. However, can the phenomenon of synaptic plasticity account for the memory of individuals? Many efforts from the 1970s until now support this notion, although absolute confirmation remains elusive. Donald Hebb was the proponent of a theory indicating that synaptic plasticity could indeed sustain memory processes. Hebbian plasticity states that changes in synaptic strength occur when the synapse between two neurons is repeatedly activated. The induction of Hebbian plasticity requires the correlated firing of both pre- and post-synaptic neurons and a rapid change in synaptic strength that is specific to the active inputs (Bliss & Collingridge, 1993; Bliss & Lomo, 1973). Both long-term potentiation (LTP) and long-term depression (LTD) are mechanisms that satisfy all the Hebbian postulates.

Terje Lomo discovered LTP at hippocampal synapses. Influenced by the work of Per Andersen on frequency potentiation, Lomo studied the synaptic mechanisms of the dentate gyrus (Lomo, 1971a, 1971b, 2003) during his doctoral work; however, the relevance of LTP as a memory mechanism of synaptic plasticity was established later from research in collaboration with Tim Bliss (Bliss & Lomo, 1973). Bliss and Lomo described the changes in synaptic efficiency after stimulation of the perforant pathway (pp) with 20 Hz trains of 15 seconds in duration, showing the increased amplitude and the reduced latency of the evoked population of spikes, characteristic of LTP (Bliss & Lomo, 1973). Subsequent studies contributed evidence showing how LTP evoked under different conditions could persist not only for minutes but also for days and months (Bliss & Gardner-Medwin, 1973; Douglas & Goddard, 1975). Following these results, the first works appeared in which a link between synaptic plasticity and memory was explicitly addressed. Four characteristics sustaining the synaptic plasticity-memory relation had been stated: (1) The ease of inducing LTP in the hippocampus, a region with a principal role in memory processes, (2) the similarity between the rhythmic bursts of stimulation used to induce LTP and the naturally occurring patterns of hippocampal activity (theta rhythm), (3) the adverse effect of inhibitors of hippocampal LTP on learning and retention of tasks, and (4) the similarity of the biochemical changes that occur both after LTP and after learning (Lynch, 2004).

As was mentioned previously, the main mechanisms of synaptic plasticity to be widely studied are LTP and LTD. LTD was first observed in non-stimulated synapses as a heterosynaptic phenomenon as a consequence of HFS stimulation of one branch of the pp (Abraham & Goddard, 1983; Doyere et al., 1997). Both LTP and LTD can be evoked widely throughout the cerebral areas, and both involve pre-synaptic and postsynaptic mechanisms. LTP has been induced throughout the limbic system, prefrontal cortex, cerebellum, and other regions (Racine et al., 1983; Teskey & Valentine, 1998), whereas LTD has been induced in the cerebellum, hippocampus, striatum, and cortex. These forms of synaptic plasticity occur at inhibitory and excitatory synapses and may lead to an increase or decrease in the amount of neurotransmitter released as a consequence of their previous history of neuronal activity, which ultimately results in potentiated or depressed synaptic strength (Castillo, 2012). In addition, postsynaptic mechanisms sustain LTD and LTP phenomena, frequently including changes in the number of receptors and in their activation properties at the post-synapse level. In the context of spatial memory, we will refer to synaptic plasticity related to spatial behaviour, specifically in the hippocampus.

Although synaptic plasticity has been considered the underlying neural mechanism of learning and memory, it is necessary to consider that learning-related changes in synaptic strength would be specific and localized to some synapses, thereby making it nearly impossible to locate and observe the naturally occurring synaptic changes in distributed circuits of the hippocampus. Thus, LTP and LTD are experimental strategies that permit us to observe changes in synaptic responses, which likely are related to changes in the natural plasticity of the cerebral substrate. Therefore, one important body of evidence linking plastic changes and spatial learning comes from studies in which the learning experience can induce changes in synaptic potentials that are similar to those observed after LTP or LTD induction protocols or can potentiate the changes induced with weak stimulation protocols. Examples of this are the studies of inhibitory avoidance learning, which induces changes like LTP in CA1 (Whitlock et al., 2006).

In an effort to discover the relationships between learning and LTP, studies were initiated to evaluate the development of learning ability and LTP in rodents. The rat hippocampus reaches its mature state by the third postnatal week, which is equivalent to approximately 3 years in a human being (Diamond, 1990). Post-tetanic potentiation (PP) is present at 1 week postnatal, whereas LTP emerges at the second postnatal week, both in the dentate gyrus and in CA1 (Harris & Teyler, 1984; Wilson, 1984). However, despite the similar trajectory of maturation, LTP possesses different characteristics in different hippocampal regions. Further, the proposed role in spatial processing for each hippocampal region could be somewhat different, thus implying that localized alterations in LTP related to place learning sub-processes would induce different deficits. Unfortunately, few works have evaluated the consequences of precise alterations of LTP and LTD in one hippocampal region on specific spatial learning sub-processes.

2. LTP in the Hippocampus

2.1. LTP in the Dentate Gyrus

LTP could be associative, in fact high frequency stimulation (HFS) of the pp induces LTP in the dentate gyrus but requires the co-activation of many synapses (McNaughton et al., 1978). Also, the concurrent HFS of lateral and medial perforant pathways induces LTP, whereas individually activating each one fails to induce LTP. Thus, the cooperative requirement of learning is fulfilled by LTP of the dentate gyrus, whereas the associative nature in dentate gyrus LTP which depends on NMDA receptors and requires post-synaptic depolarization to remove the magnesium block from the NMDA channels, thereby constituting a mechanism of coincidence detection between pre- and post-synaptic activity (Nowak et al., 1984; Wigstrom & Gustafsson, 1986), for a review see: (Bennett, 2000). The induction of LTP by stimulation of the pp induces a prolonged increase in glutamate release in the dentate gyrus (Bliss et al., 1990; Dolphin et al., 1982; Lynch et al., 1990), which is mediated by an elusive retrograde messenger generated in the arachidonic acid cascade sustaining the latter stage of LTP induction (Blundon & Zakharenko, 2008; Williams et al., 1989); the incorporation of AMPA receptors to the synapses determines the stability of the potentiated synapses.

2.2. LTP in CA3

The CA3 hippocampal region processes information through two synaptic systems, the mossy fiber-CA3 synapses and the commissural input (CA3-CA3) synapses. The mossy fibber (mf) afferents from the dentate gyrus make contact on the stratum lucidum of CA3 and express a kainate dependent fast excitatory transmission (Acsady et al., 1998; Contractor et al., 2001). Early research suggested that mf synapses on CA3 neurons could undergo LTP; however, several differences were apparent between the LTP of the commissural input (CA3-CA3), pp-dentate gyrus LTP and CS-CA1 LTP. For example, CA3 LTP was observed to be independent of the activity of NMDA receptors, involving a mechanism that was pre-synaptically initiated and required voltage dependent Ca^{+2} channels (Harris & Cotman, 1986; Johnston et al., 1992; Nicoll & Schmitz, 2005; Zalutsky & Nicoll, 1990). Additionally, Huanget al., (1994) showed that both the induction and the maintenance of LTP of the CA3 mossy fibres depended on cyclic AMP through cAMP-dependent PKA; whereas, commissural/ associative fibres were shown to project to the pyramidal neurons of the CA3 stratum radiatum through fast-AMPA mediated excitatory transmission and to display NMDA-dependent forms of synaptic plasticity (Harris & Cotman, 1986; Kakegawa et al., 2004). Moreover, CA3 receives direct inputs from neurons of layer II of the entorhinal cortex (Amaral & Witter, 1989).

2.3. LTP in CA1

LTP can be produced at Schaffer collaterals-CA1 synapses after HFS trains and theta burst stimulation (TBS) protocols. CA1 LTP is widely considered a non-unitary phenomenon that includes two phases: one unstable phase showing a decline within a half to one hour (t-LTP; transitory-LTP), and a late phase of stable and enduring LTP (Gustafsson et al., 1989; Gustafsson & Wigstrom, 1990; Hess & Gustafsson, 1990). Late and early LTP have been considered as the neural representations of long and short-term memory, respectively (Bach et al., 1999; Jones et al., 2001).

Although CA3-CA1 LTP was initially considered NMDA-dependent, more recent data suggest that LTP at CA3-CA1 in fact consists of both NMDA-dependent and NMDA-independent forms of LTP (Bayazitov et al., 2007; Bliss & Collingridge, 1993). The existence of forms of LTP that are dependent and independent of NMDA receptors is now well accepted, and it implies important functional differences in relation to behavioural performance. NMDA dependent LTP is necessary for learning and memory in certain types of tasks, whereas the inhibition of these receptors only partially impairs spatial learning (Bannerman et al., 1995). The NMDA independent LTP appears to depend on voltage dependent calcium channels (L-VGCCs) since their pharmacological blockade or genetic manipulations impairing this type of LTP severely impair spatial memory (Borroni et al., 2000; Grover & Teyler, 1990a, 1990b; Moosmang et al., 2005). Subsequently, it was proposed that multiple forms of LTP induced at a single synapse constitute a composite LTP. In CA1-CA3 synapses, composite LTP could be induced both by HFS and long TBS protocols (Morgan & Teyler, 2001). NMDA dependent LTP requires the activation of serine/threonine kinases, whereas the expression of NMDA independent LTP also requires the activation of tyrosine kinases, brain derived neurotrophic factor, mitogen-activated protein kinase, and protein kinase A (Cavus & Teyler, 1996; Moosmang, et al., 2005; Zakharenko et al., 2003). The Zakharenko's group have demonstrated the pre-synaptic nature of NMDA-independent LTP (Bayazitov, et al., 2007; Zakharenko et al., 2001). Behaviourally, NMDA dependent LTP has been associated with memory retention over short periods of time, whereas NMDA independent LTP is necessary for the retention of information for long periods of time (Borroni, et al., 2000). Calcium entry through NMDA activates protein kinases leading to the redistribution of AMPA receptors in dendritic spines and eventually increases the sensitivity of the spines to glutamate, increasing the response of the synapses and activating silent synapses. Additionally, NMDA dependent LTP occurs through post-synaptic mechanisms, but NMDA-independent LTP can be sustained by changes at the pre-synaptic terminals. Zakharenko et al., argue that the LTP generated in most of the research evaluating learning could in fact be a composite LTP. Moreover, and more interestingly, they suggest that the changes in spines associated with LTP could be related to the process of short-term memory but not long-term memory processes because changes at the presynaptic level are fundamental to long-term memory traces (Bayazitov, et al., 2007; Blundon & Zakharenko, 2008; Zakharenko, et al., 2001).

3. Hippocampal LTD

LTD is a decrease in the synaptic efficacy that has a long duration (hours to days), and it can be induced at CA1, CA3 and dentate gyrus synapses (Dudek & Bear, 1992; Kobayashi et al., 1996) as well as in other cerebral regions. Similar to LTP, LTD could be mediated by activation of NMDA receptors or by metabotropic glutamatergic receptors (mGluRs) (Bashir et al., 1993; Dudek & Bear, 1992). LTD could be induced by electrical stimulation and through the administration of agonists to NMDA and type I mGluRs receptors (Lee et al., 1998; Palmer et al., 1997). This last LTD is mediated by the internalization of AMPA receptors triggered by mGluRs activation (for a review, see: Gladding et al., 2009). The induction of NMDA-dependent LTP could occur without cooperative interactions, on single SC-pyramidal cell contacts (Debanne et al., 1996), whereas the mGluRs-dependent LTD requires the multiple activity of SC on a pyramidal cell, at least under *in vitro* conditions (Fan et al., 2010). After the induction of LDT, both forms of LTD are induced simultaneously in most of the cases (Poschel & Stanton, 2007).

CA1 homosynaptic LTD could be induced by repeated stimulation of the SC pathway with a low frequency (1-2 Hz) and long duration (10-15 min); it is called homosynaptic because only the stimulated via develops the LTD (Dudek & Bear, 1992). Heterosynaptic LTD implies interactions between groups of synapses that converge on the same neuron. In CA1, heterosynaptic LTD could be induced in a non-stimulated via by stimulating a parallel convergent via (Lynch et al., 1977) (for a review, see: Poschel & Stanton, 2007).

In the dentate gyrus, LTD could also be homosynaptic after stimulation of the medial perforant path (MPP) (Poschel & Manahan-Vaughan, 2007), whereas heterosynaptic LTD was observed at medial and lateral pp after HFS of the other synaptic input (Abraham & Goddard, 1983; Doyere, et al., 1997). Associative LTD can be induced in the lateral pp by different stimulation protocols (for a review, see Poschel & Stanton, 2007). LTD was initially proposed as a mechanism for erasure or forgetting of memory traces (Bear et al., 1987; Bear & Malenka, 1994); however, accumulating evidence involves LTD in the coding of novel information. Low-frequency stimulation of the collateral fibres system (CA3-CA3) induces NMDA-dependent LTD through the internalization of AMPA receptors, whereas LTD that is induced at mf-CA3 synapses is NMDA independent (Kobayashi, et al., 1996; Montgomery & Madison, 2002).

4. Hippocampus and Spatial Memory

The participation of the hippocampal formation in spatial memory has been the subject of extensive research by many research groups through the years. Next, we describe the participation of the different hippocampal regions in the organization of spatial information in order to understand a theory that was developed based on the cumulative evidence in support of the function of hippocampal regions in spatial memory and the experimental results concerning LTP and learning processes sustained at each relay of the hippocampal circuit.

Declarative memory is defined as the recall of facts and events and encompasses autobiographical information (i.e., the what, where and when of the events). One important property of declarative memory is the ability to recall a whole memory from a single element; this has been called pattern completion and is defined as the process of reconstructing a complete pattern from a partial version (Myers & Scharfman, 2011). The ability to discriminate between the memories for two very similar events is defined as pattern separation (Cohen & Squire, 1980). Another relevant function of episodic memory traces is place representation. Furthermore, allocentric place memory is a central component of an episodic memory since it constitutes the contexts of the events stored in memory (Gaffan, 1991). Research has shown that this contextual information depends on the spatial encoding of place cells in the rodent hippocampus (O'Keefe & Conway, 1978; Wilson & McNaughton, 1993).

4.1. Dentate Gyrus and Spatial Memory

It has been proposed that the dentate gyrus participates in pattern separation, enabling the hippocampus to store as different memories of very similar events (For revision of the theme see the Rollset al., works), which is a principal characteristic of episodic memory (Rolls, 2013; Rolls & Kesner, 2006). Rolls proposed that dentate neurons could implement a competitive network able to form place cells in which each dentate cell learns to respond to a particular combination of entorhinal cortex grid cells relaying information about the constituents of places. Thus, combinations of grid cells specifically relaying to dentate cells could specify a granular place cell (Rolls et al., 2006).

4.2. CA3 and Spatial Memory

CA3 has been proposed to act as an auto-association network, which would permit all elements of one episode first to be linked and then to be recalled as a whole memory. In the context of this theory, CA3 operates as a single network that can allow arbitrary associations between cortical inputs of very different origin and subcortical regions providing information relative to the components of the episode (Rolls, 2013; Rolls & Kesner, 2006). Auto-associative networks, as are proposed to exist in CA3, store input patterns in the form of modifiable connections between neurons, which can be activated together when an element or elements of the pattern are experienced, leading to the activation of the complete pattern (Kohonen, 1984). A group of researchers have found evidence for the participation of CA3 (sub-regions a, b) in the retrieval of information from memory when short delay periods are introduced (Rolls & Kesner, 2006). Also based on their proposed role as an auto-association network, it was suggested that CA3 could be crucial in short-term memory tasks requiring the encoding of novel information and pattern completion (Kesner, 2013). When a short delay is imposed in tasks in which the animals had to choose a response, CA3 function is required; however, CA1 became essential when delay periods were longer (i.e., minutes or hours) (Lee & Kesner, 2003). Kesner and co-workers showed the participation of NMDA mediated CA3 a,b plasticity in spatial learning; in delayed not matching to place tasks, when the rats were tested in a new environment (novel maze or novel testing room) or in the same environment but with delay (ten seconds), the blockade of NMDA receptors impaired their performance, whereas no deficiencies were produced by injections into CA1 or the dentate gyrus in this task (Lee & Kesner, 2003). These authors maintain a role for CA3 a,b in the rapid encoding of place-object associations, which are impaired by lesions of this region as evaluated by place cued recall and object cued recall tasks (Kesner et al., 2008). Based on this body of evidence, it was proposed that plastic changes mediated by NMDA receptors are central for CA3 a,b network encoding of novel information relative to associations between places and odours, visual landmarks and spatial locations. Accordingly, results from aged rats with deficiencies in memory revealed elevated firing rates in CA3 associated with the failure to rapidly encode novel information, which was assumed to predominantly reflect pattern completion through the associative commissural projection excitatory drive (Wilson et al., 2005).

4.3. CA1 and Spatial Memory

CA1 constitutes the main output pathway for the hippocampal processed information and sends its projections to the subiculum, entorhinal cortex, and parahipppocampal structures; the prefrontal cortex is also a target of hippocampal afferents (Delatour & Witter, 2002; Witter, 1993).

The connection between CA3 sc and CA1 neurons could represent a way to combine sub-components of episodic memory coded separately in CA3, which could produce an efficient retrieval cue for recall through the back-projection pathways to the neocortex where memories are stored. Thus, CA1 would be involved in the retrieval of information from the neocortex through these pathways; the connection between CA3 and CA1 would permit a generalization process when the pattern completion at CA3 produced ambiguous results, and CA1 generalization toward the closest representation would occur.

Therefore, the whole episode can be represented by CA1 neurons, which could activate the parahippocampal cortical areas and these in turn activate the areas of the association cortex that originally provided the inputs to the hippocampus. Thus, the recall would be produced in multimodal cortical areas and areas of unimodal association. The back projections, recalling previous episodic events, could provide information useful to the construction of new representations in the multi- and unimodal association cortices in order to build new well-structured long-term representations, useful in organizing actions (Rolls, 2013).

4.4. Intermediate Hippocampus and Spatial Learning

As was mentioned previously, the hippocampus has been proposed as a crucial structure for the rapid encoding of one trial events and other fast forms of learning, such as place learning, a fact that is evident from the rapid development of the place fields after exposure to a novel environment (Wilson & McNaughton, 1993). Different sub-regions have been related to different learning and memory processes (see below), but a gradient also exists in the precision along the hippocampal transverse and longitudinal axes from the septal pole to the temporal pole, with anatomical differences in three partially overlapping regions: the septal, temporal and intermediate areas (Bast et al., 2009). In regard to visuospatial coding, the septal to intermediate hippocampus has strong connectivity to the dorsolateral entorhinal cortex, this region in turn receives strong visuospatial neocortical inputs and contains neurons that represent visuospatial information named grid cells (Fyhn et al., 2004). In circumstances in which changing information must be applied to emit a behavioural response based on spatial information, the prefrontal cortical areas take relevance, and hippocampal-prefrontal communication is required to achieve working spatial memory computation (Churchwell & Kesner, 2011; Wang & Cai, 2006). It has been proposed that hippocampal links with the prelimbic and infralimbic cortices could sustain the translation of the spatial information to actions spatially directed. Based on the input connectivity patterns, the septal and intermediate hippocampus are proposed to sustain accurate place encoding through their connectivity with the dorsolateral entorhinal cortex, whereas the intermediate to temporal hippocampus participate in behavioural control through their connectivity with the prefrontal cortex and subcortical regions, which are critical for translating rapid place learning into behaviour (Bast, et al., 2009).

In a study with hippocampal lesions, Bast et al., (2009) showed the participation of the intermediate hippocampus in a task based on the rapid performance of place learning in the water maze. Specifically, the rats had to locate a novel platform position in trial one, and in the second trial a reduction in swimming distance or an increased time in the quadrant where the platform was placed during the first trial indicated that a rapid place learning memory was achieved. The two remaining trials served as win-stay strategy enforcement. Only rats with an intact intermediate hippocampus performed as well as control rats in this task. They also observed that incremental learning (i.e., spatial reference memory trained with eight daily trials for five days, with the platform position fixed) was eventually achieved by all groups except the complete hippocampal lesioned group. When evaluated on rapid one trial learning after the incremental learning, only the sham and the spared intermediate hippocampus groups successfully searched in the location of the platform, the rest of the groups were deficient (Bast, et al., 2009). Importantly, the septal pole of the hippocampus of animals with lesions to the rest of the hippocampus showed unimpaired CA1 plasticity (LTP). Also, the effect of novel experiences on synaptic plasticity of the intermediate hippocampus was evaluated in freely moving rats. HFS alone induced LTP of 4 hours of duration, whereas HFS coupled with the exploration of a novel environment induced LTP that lasted for at least 24 hours. LFS produced short-term depression (STD), which was enhanced by exposure to large novel cues (orientation landmarks), but LTD was not enabled (Kenney & Manahan-Vaughan, 2013a, 2013b). Thus, there exist clear differences between the intermediate hippocampus and the dorsal hippocampus (see below) in their participation in spatial learning and plasticity modulation of novelty exposure.

5. Exploration and Synaptic Plasticity

Exploration serves as the principal behavioural strategy for an animal to acquire knowledge of its environment and implies the collection and storage of spatial information into episodic representations. Changes in hippocampal synaptic responses have been observed during the exploration of new environments (Erickson et al., 1993; Moser, 1995). Novelty detection occurs when changes in previously experienced information are detected. CA1 neurons receive direct input from the entorhinal cortex as well as information previously processed in the tri-synaptic circuit. One hypothesis put forward states that pyramidal neurons could detect mismatches between previously experienced information (DG-CA3), relayed through the Schaffer collaterals and cortical sensory inputs (Lisman & Otmakhova, 2001). It has been proposed that LTP and LTD encode different aspects of novelty acquisition. As previously mentioned, exploration facilitates SC-CA1 late-LTD both when an animal is exposed to a new environment and when old objects occur in a novel configuration; however, late- LTP is facilitated by the exploration of an empty novel environment (Kemp & Manahan-Vaughan, 2004; Manahan-Vaughan & Braunewell, 1999).

Sharp et al., (1985) observed increased synaptic efficiency in the dentate gyrus after rats were exposed to a new complex environment. In other results, the exposure of rats to a different environment lead to the increased population of EPSPs, decreased amplitude and peak latency of the population of spikes; these changes were a result of alterations in synaptic efficacy in granule cells, which outlast by hours the behavioural display of exploration (Green et al., 1990a, 1990b). Andersen and Moser observed significant changes to EPSPs at dentate gyrus synapses that were associated with exploration related learning after subtracting the effects of temperature changes on the evoked potentials associated with behavioural activity (Andersen et al., 1996). Furthermore, Moser et al., reported an inhibition of the dentate input during spatial exploration associated with the reduction of inhibition at granular somas. The authors proposed that these changes served as mechanisms of amplification of the entorhinal inputs arriving at the dentate gyrus during exploration related learning (Moser, 1996).

There is a general consensus that LTP can be divided into two phases: an early LTP phase lasting about 4-6 hours that is independent of protein synthesis, and a late LTP phase of longer duration that depends on protein synthesis (Frey et al., 2001; 1988; Krug et al., 1984). Different approaches and experimental results lead to the idea that early-LTP can be reinforced and transformed into late-LTP and that this could be a process underlying the consolidation of memory.

Weak tetanic stimulation of the perforant path induces an early LTP in dentate gyrus spike populations that decays to basal levels within the next eight hours. However, the exploration of a novel environment 30 minutes before tetanic stimulation lead to LTP lasting more than eight hours with a decay to basal levels within twenty four hours, whereas the exploration of a novel environment fifteen minutes earlier lead to LTP that persisted for at least twenty four hours. Similarly, the fEPSPs were potentiated by the exploration of a novel environment relative to non-exploring controls. Both of these effects were specific to the maintenance of LTP, since the evoked responses were unchanged when measured at one minute post-tetanic stimulation. The exploration of a familiar box had no effect on the early LTP. The authors controlled factors such as brain temperature, corticosterone levels and locomotor activity and did not find a relationship between these variables and the duration of LTP. Both the application of a beta-adrenergic antagonist (propranolol) and anisomycin prevented the reinforcement of early LTP, which decayed within 8 h, whereas the administration of a beta-adrenergic agonist 30 minutes before the LTP induction induced the late-LTP with a duration of at least 24 h (Straube et al., 2003). Similar results have been reported for CA1 LTP, although the time required to facilitate the induction of LTP was ten minutes between the exploration of the novel environment and the start of the tetanic stimulation protocol (Li et al., 2003). Sacchetti et al., (2001) observed increased responses of CA1 cells to the increasing stimulation of the Schaffer collateral pathway in animals exposed to contextual fear conditioning that persisted for seven hours after the conditioning paradigm, whereas rats that received only shocks and naive rats did not show this increase. Furthermore, the group of rats experiencing only exploration in the conditioning context showed enhanced responses but only when recorded immediately after the exploration session. In addition, LTP in CA1 was found to be reversed by the exposure to a novel non-threatening environment whose exploration induced increased theta activity. Consequently, increased theta activity was proposed to induce the depotentiation of the previously potentiated synapses (Xu et al., 1998). In contrast, the exploration of a novel environment induces LTP facilitation at the perforant path-dentate gyrus synapses, SC-CA1 synapses, Mossy Fibers-CA3 synapses, and commissural-Ca3 synapses (Hagena & Manahan-Vaughan, 2011; Kemp & Manahan-Vaughan, 2004, 2008).

LTD is also facilitated by the exploration; however, the effect of exploration on LTD in each hippocampal field is related to different characteristics of the environment. Specifically, LTD at the perforant path-dentate gyrus is facilitated by exploration in an environment with large novel orientational landmarks (Kemp & Manahan-Vaughan, 2004, 2008), whereas LTD facilitation occurs in CS-CA1 synapses when small cues are contained in the environment and there is no possibility of using orientational cues (Manahan-Vaughan & Braunewell, 1999). At CA3, LTD of commissural- associational fibres is facilitated by small spatial cues possibly associated with learned information during exploration of the novel environment, but absent when rats are re-exposed to the environment (Hagena & Manahan-Vaughan, 2011; Kemp & Manahan-Vaughan, 2007). LTD has also been associated with spatial memory (see below), as manipulations that abolish learning also abolish learning LTD facilitation (Kemp & Manahan-Vaughan, 2005; Lemon & Manahan-Vaughan, 2006). These works are noteworthy for showing how behavioural experiences demanding information processing cause plastic changes that are reflected in the modification of artificially induced plastic changes; this modification acts as an amplifier of the naturally occurring synaptic plasticity.

6. LTP and Spatial Learning

Hippocampal cells have been recognized as place cells based on their selective increased rate discharges in a defined place of an environment (Place field) (O'Keefe & Conway, 1978). The place representations of place cells undergo modifications after LTP with the extinction of previous place fields and the creation of new place fields (Dragoi et al., 2003). Thus, synaptic plasticity appears to be involved in the establishment of spatial maps.

Initial observations suggested an integral role for NMDA receptors (NMDAR) in place learning, which was evident from the profound spatial learning deficits following the infusion of NMDAR antagonists; however, many of these studies employed doses that were high enough to alter sensory-motor processing, which profoundly affected the performance of rats in, for example, the water maze (Cain et al., 1996). Morris et al., (1986) chronically infused rats intra-cerebro-ventricullary (i.c.v.) with D(-)-2-amino-5-phosphonovaleric acid (AP5) and observed an impairment in place learning ability, whereas an infusion of AP5-L (L-isomer) did not produce this effect on place learning. However, when the rats were pre-trained in the Morris maze spatial task in a different room and maze in order to investigate spatial searching strategies, the AP5 infusion had a small effect on the escape latencies, which were still longer (group effect) but showed that the rats were able to significantly reduce their escape latencies and directed more search time in the quadrant of the platform position. The rats were able to learn the spatial reference information under chronic AP5 action (administered each day before training), despite the absence of pp LTP. When rats were pre-trained in a non-spatial procedure (a curtain was used to surround the maze and to prevent the use of hippocampal spatial learning) and then in the spatial task under the influence of AP5, the animals did not learn the platform position in the first four training days (none spent more time in the quadrant containing the platform during a probe trial applied after four training days), but they did reduce their escape latencies in the last four training days. Therefore, non-spatial training had a modest but still protective effect on place learning ability (Bannerman, et al., 1995). This finding indicates that place learning could occur in rats without the use of NMDAR, although the performance was less efficient than in control rats, possibly through hippocampal dependent and hippocampal independent processes. In this research, LTP of synapses in the dentate gyrus was impaired by the antagonist infusion; however, as it was not selective to the dentate gyrus, the function of the CA3 and CA1 regions may also have been affected. Similar to this work, many others aimed to test if non-spatial pretraining could provide the rats access to the use of searching strategies developed during the pretraining while training in the place learning tasks, whose lack could be responsible for the deficient performance observed in naive animals after blockade of NMDAR (and NMDAR-dependent

LTP). In many of these studies, pretraining was determinant of the ability of the animals to solve the place learning tests after NMDAR blockade (Cain, et al., 1996; Saucier & Cain, 1995; Saucier et al., 1996). However, in the Hoh et al., (1999) study, rats were trained in a non-spatial procedure under the influence of a systemically applied NMDAR antagonist [6]cis-4-phosphono-methyl-2-piperidine carboxylic acid [CGS19755 (CGS)] at doses that do not interfere with motor activity and observed that the rats administered the antagonist learned the strategies used in the Morris maze during the non-spatial training as well as the control rats. Moreover, no deficit was observed in the spatial training or in spatial reversal learning of the animals under the effect of the NMDAR antagonist. However, in this study the researchers used a one day training task with ten consecutive trials; thus, some differences in collapsed training tasks may occur in the results obtained in the short term in comparison to the long-term training in which consolidation processes take place daily after the training. Only naive rats trained under the drug condition were deficient in place learning. The authors also evaluated the expression of LTP under the action of the antagonist and observed a blockade of LTP at the dentate gyrus and CA1 synapses. Thus, the learning of the behavioural strategies needed to solve the Morris tasks were independent of NMDAR mediated LTP. The authors also observed that reversal learning was easily achieved by non-spatial pretrained rats under the action of the NMDAR antagonist, contrasting with the severe impairment reported in other works in naive rats during reversal learning after hippocampal damage (Whishaw et al., 1995; Whishaw & Jarrard, 1996). The possibility was discussed of the participation of NMDAR-independent LTP as well as the potential of a determinant role for the complexity of the tasks, implying the participation of NMDAR-dependent LTP only in tasks of greater complexity.

Further evidence for the role of NMDAR in spatial learning comes from the observation that both the chronic i.c.v. infusion and the acute intrahippocampal infusion of AP5 caused a delay dependent impairment in spatial memory in a delayed matching to place task (DMPT) developed to test the one trial acquisition of spatial information in the water maze (Steele & Morris, 1999). No effects of the antagonist were observed in the memory of the spatial information or in the memory for the position of the platform on the last day before the administration of AP5. The chronic antagonist infusion also impaired dentate gyrus LTP induction in vivo. Given that the observed deficiencies were delay dependent (i.e., they appeared only with fifteen minutes and two hours delays between trial one, when a new position of the platform was acquired by the rat, and the second trial, when the rat had to remembered the information acquired in the first trial), the NMDAR antagonists and LTP impairment did not affect the short-term memory (fifteen seconds) of spatial information or the recovery of reference spatial memory. Since the contents of a recently visited place that is temporarily held in mind to guide behaviour constitutes a spatial working memory problem (Goldman-Rakic, 1995), the delay-dependent impairment observed could imply that working memory processing is deficient in rats under NMDAR antagonists.

Along these lines, Zhang and co-workers (Zhang et al., 2013) evaluated the role of the NR2 subunit containing NMDAR in spatial working memory tasks, based on previous research showing an enhancement of spatial memory in adult mice overexpressing NR2B subunits and impaired fear memory by the pharmacological inhibition of NR2A and NR2B subunit containing NMDARs (Tang et al., 1999; Zhao et al., 2005). The authors used the Morris maze and applied a similar task to the one previously described, in which the hidden platform was placed in a novel location each training day (four daily trials). In this manner, the localization of the platform must be achieved in trial 1, the working memory of the new position in the second trial (retain the information during a period of time to emit a response, 30 seconds and 10 minutes were the delays applied between trial 1 and 2), and the 3-4 trials to sustain the win-stay strategy. NR2B-NMDAR inhibition via CA1 infusion of (α*R*,β*S*)-α-(4-Hydroxyphenyl)-β-methyl-4-(phenylmethyl)-1-piperidinepropanol maleate (Ro 25-6981), or ifenprodil before trial 1 was ineffective when a delay of 30 seconds was imposed, but produced a deficit when a ten minute delay was imposed between trials 1 and 2. Since the rats learned the spatial reference memory during the pre-training, the deficiency observed after ten minutes of delay could be related to the inability to maintain the new position information on line for later use. During the short delay, antagonists infused into CA1 had no effect on the recovery of information maintained in working memory. In the same work, spatial working memory was evaluated in a T-maze delayed alternation task. After reaching a criterion performance level of 80% correct responses in three consecutive days, the rats were infused in CA1 with Ro 25-6981, ifenprodil or [(R)-[(S)-1-(4-bromophenyl)-ethylamino]-(2, 3-dioxo-1,2,3,4-tetrahydroquinoxalin-5-yl)-methyl]-phosphonic acid (NVP-AAM077) an NR2A-NMDAR containing blocker, and tested using delays of 5 or 30 seconds. The treatment with NVP-AAM077 produced an increase in errors for both the 5- and 30-second delays, whereas Ro 25-6981 and ifenprodil only increased the total errors under the 30 second delay condition. When the rat repeated a previously correct response it was considered as a win shift failure; when the rat committed an error and repeated the response, a second error was considered a lose-shift failure. Dividing the errors in this way, the NVP-AAM077 administration induced both types of errors yet without delay period, whereas Ro and ifenprodil caused increased errors only when a ten-minute delay was interposed. Taken together, these results support several issues: first, the spatial learning could be realized without NMDAR (and NMDAR dependent LTP) participation; second, there are NMDAR dependent and NMDAR independent components of spatial learning; and third, the use of spatial information in working memory for long delays is dependent of NMDAR function and possibly also NMDAR dependent LTP.

The subcutaneous administration of the NMDAR antagonist dizocilpine (MK-801) before exposure to a T-maze or training in a task that can be solved using place or response strategies, did not produce changes in the use of the place strategy except when it was administered both during maze exposure and during training. These results appear to support the NMDAR-independence of the use of previously acquired spatial information (Mackes & Willner, 2006). In addition, the use of MK-801 in rats pre-trained in the Morris maze had no effect when the rats were observed in a familiar ambient, but deficiencies were found using the same task in a new environment (Uekita et al., 2006).

Morris & Frey (1997) recapitulated previous research using NMDAR antagonists in spatial memory encoding and retrieval, employing chronic i.c.v. infusions of AP5, acute intrahippocampal infusions and ibotenate mediated hippocampal dentate lesions. LTP in vivo in the dentate gyrus was blocked in the chronically infused D-AP5 rats. The authors indicated that short-term memory for spatial information is independent of NMDAR, whereas the rapid consolidation of spatial information into long-term memory requires activation of hippocampal NMDAR receptors. In this sense, the authors refer to rapid consolidation with respect to the memory for the spatial position of the platform after long delays in the DMPT as a model of episodic information occurring as a discrete event that is rapidly consolidated in memory. The authors also showed that NMDA receptors are not involved in memory retrieval. These findings are related to the idea that hippocampal synaptic plasticity is involved in events-memory by its episodic nature, that is LTP could be related to spatial learning not because the nature of the information is "spatial," but by the character of the episode that involved the spatial information (Morris & Frey, 1997). Many other studies have shown results similar to these. For example, Bas et al., (2005) studied a form of one-trial memory for the spatial representation of the position of a reward in an arena and infused NMDAR and AMPA/Kainate receptor antagonists in the dorsal hippocampus. The antagonist AP5 was infused before the learning trial when the place position of the reward was acquired by the rat (like a sample trial), or before retrieval when the rat searched again after a variable delay the same rewarded place (like a test trial). The AMPA/Kainate receptor antagonist 6-cyano-7-nitroquinoxaline-2,3-dione (CNQX) was infused only before retrieval. The NMDAR antagonist impaired the encoding but not the retrieval of the spatial information, whereas CNQX impaired the retrieval of the information.

Additionally, mice with impaired CaMKII-GluN2B binding were trained in three different tests of learning: the Barnes maze training through five days, massed Morris maze learning through one day with 12 consecutive trials, and contextual fear conditioning. The mice showed very mild differences in escape latency, principally on trials 7-8 and 11-12 (collapsed by comparisons), and an effect of interaction (genotype X trial) but not for the genotype, reflecting a mild effect on the last two trials of training more than a general deficit in the acquisition of the task. However, clear differences in the memory tests were observed in these mice at 1 and 7 days after the training. No differences occurred in the Barnes maze test in any measured parameter (Stein et al., 2014). Although sc-CA1 NMDAR-dependent LTP is blunted in these mice, this effect appears related to short-term acquisition but not to long-term learning and memory (Barnes Maze); however, it is possible that NMDAR dependent LTP through all hippocampal fields was blunted in the mutant mice, in accordance with the proposed dissociation of NMDAR-dependent and NMDAR-independent LTP, for short and long-term memory, respectively.

An extensive body of evidence has implicated a principal role for Ca^{+2}/calmodulin-dependent protein kinase II (CaMKII) and NMDAR in the establishment of LTP (Barria & Malinow, 2005; Halt et al., 2012). CaMKII mutant mice exhibit no hippocampal NMDAR dependent LTP and show impaired learning in the Morris maze (Giese et al., 1998). Also, CaMKII-Asp-286 mutant mice, which when stimulated with a TBS protocol showed LTD instead of LTP, were very deficient in a Barnes maze test when spatial learning was required but not for the cued version of the task. Furthermore, these mutant mice showed normal LTP and LTD induced by 100Hz (HFS) and 1Hz (LFS), implying a critical role more physiologically evoked plasticity (induced by theta burst stimulation) (Bach et al., 1995). Other mutations impairing CaMKII function also reduced LTP and produced spatial memory deficits in the Morris maze task, whereas the acquisition in the same maze and working memory in the radial arm maze were unaffected by the mutation (Halt, et al., 2012). It was suggested that the more difficult place learning task requires NMDA dependent LTP, whereas the easier tasks do not require this plastic change (Hoh, et al., 1999).

From the previous research, it is evident that a weak relationship exists between NMDAR- mediated LTP and the learning of spatial memory. Some works suggest the participation of NMDAR in spatial working memory or a role is proposed for NMDARs in the one trial-learning processing of spatial information as part of an automatic learning system engaged in declarative memory processes (Morris and Frey); nevertheless, NMDAR do not appear to have a clear or relevant role in long-term reference spatial learning and memory.

Regarding spatial learning and LTP modulation without NMDARs, the Manahan-Vaughan group have demonstrated a relevant role for metabotropic glutamate receptors (mGluR) in hippocampal plasticity and spatial memory (Manahan-Vaughan, 1997; Manahan-Vaughan et al., 1998; Naie & Manahan-Vaughan, 2005). These researchers tested spatial learning after the i.c.v. administration of the group I mGluR antagonist (S)4-carboxyphenylglycine (4-CPG) (Balschun et al., 1999). LTP was evoked at cs-CA1 synapses in vivo in the 4-CGP group, but decayed 100 min after the induction, whereas the control group maintained the LTP for at least 240 minutes. The antagonist induced a weak deficit in spatial working memory when tested in the radial maze. Subsequent work by the authors asked if differences in the expression of the different subtypes of metabotropic receptors could contribute to differences in learning and plasticity. The authors have extensively evaluated the mGluR5 receptors in relation to their influence on synaptic plasticity and learning. In this work, they also uncovered working and reference memory deficits in the radial arm maze by the i.c.v. administration of the mGluR5 antagonist 2-methyl-6-(phenylethynyl)pyridine (MPEP), and impaired late LTP in the dentate gyrus in conjunction with an increased CA1 LTP; the spatial memory deficits in this case were severe, however the effects were mediated by alterations in mGluR I and NMDAR (Bikbaev et al., 2008). Moreover, it was reported that the systemic administration of the positive allosteric modulators of mGluR5, such as 3-ciano-N-(1,3-difenil-1H-pirazol-5-il)benzamid (CDPPB) and [S-(4-Fluoro-phenyl)-{3-[3-(4-fluoro-phenyl)-[1,2,4]-oxadiazol-5-yl]-piperidin-1-yl}-methanone] (ADX47273), produced increased LTP and LTD at sc-CA1 synapses and enhanced learning in the Morris maze in mice (Ayala et al., 2009). Furthermore, mice mutant for mGluR5 showed reduced LTP in CA1 and the dentate gyrus, without alterations in mf-CA3 LTP (which is principally NMDAR independent), such that these receptors were hypothesized to exert a modulatory role on NMDAR dependent LTP. The mutant mice displayed impaired spatial learning in the Morris maze and also in a context fear-conditioning test (Lu et al., 1997).

Thus, both NMDA and metabotropic receptors influence LTP and are involved in spatial learning and memory. However, it remains difficult to know the specific participation of each class of receptor to LTP, since, as mentioned previously, many studies have likely evoked a composite form of LTP through HFS. Furthermore, because the pharmacological alteration of one kind of receptor affects the expression and activity of other classes of glutamate receptors, it is very difficult to dissect the specific contribution of each receptor to the plastic phenomenon.

6.1. Dentate Gyrus LTP and Spatial Learning

Barnes (1979), comparing mature and old rats, was among the first to search for correlations between spatial memory and synaptic plasticity. Rats implanted with electrodes to stimulate the pp and to record the dentate gyrus were tested in a circular maze task, and it was observed that old rats showed reduced memory for a rewarded place relative to mature rats. Afterwards, the author gave one session of HFS to the pp of both groups and observed similar increased synaptic efficacy with also a similar decay time. However, after three repetitions of HFS, the synaptic efficacy at the dentate gyrus of the young rats remained increased during the 14 days of the test whereas the old rats showed an immediate decay. These results were also correlated with the behavioural performance, such that increased synaptic efficacy was observed in rats displaying better performance in a place preference test. Thus, the rapid decay of LTP could be related to the reduced spatial memory in the rats. However, Brun et al., (2001) tested the animals in the Morris maze but used a more efficient stimulation protocol (through the stimulation of the angular bundle) in order to exclude the possibility that a minimal number of activated fibres with the tetanisation could explain the lack of effect on long-term memory. The authors trained rats over several days to find a submerged platform located in a constant position in the Morris maze. After training, they stimulated the angular bundle to induce LTP in CA1 until no further LTP could be induced, and submitted the rats to the retention test. When HFS was applied two hours before the retention tests, the rats spent a similar amount of time in the four zones of the maze, such that the LTP induction had an amnesic effect on these rats; in contrast, low frequency stimulation had not effect. However, LTP was not saturated, as some residual LTP could be induced after the HFS through the angular bundle by stimulating one electrode. Thus, an amnesic effect was obtained after LTP induction in distributed synapses, which could alter the pattern of synaptic weights related to the memory trace of the platform position. An additional group was tested in a similar experiment with the modification that the NMDAR antagonist 3-(2-carboxypiperazin-4-yl)propyl-1-phosphonic acid (CPP) was intraperitoneal administered before the HFS, and they observed that the amnesic effect was blocked. The authors suggest that HFS leading to LTP disrupts memory retention by altering the spatial pattern of synaptic weights through the NMDAR receptors.

Other early attempts to show a causal relationship between LTP and learning included studies employing the saturation of LTP to test if learning could be achieved in conditions of impaired behavioural related synaptic plasticity. Moseret al., (1998) trained rats in a place learning task after inducing cumulative rounds of pp-dentate gyrus LTP, which caused saturation in some rats and preserved some residual capacity of LTP in other rats; only rats with a saturated capacity for LTP were deficient in place learning. McNaughtonet al., (1986) induced maximal bilateral LTP in the dentate gyrus by pp stimulation and then trained the rats in a task requiring the establishment of spatial maps using the Barnes and radial arm mazes. No learning occurred in rats that had the maximal LTP response induced prior to the test. Moreover, recently acquired spatial information was lost, whereas no deficiencies were observed when the animals used previously acquired spatial information in a working memory task. Thus, the authors proposed a link between spatial map formation and synaptic plasticity of the dentate gyrus. Although initially questioned, the results of saturation LTP studies in which adequate controls were run showed impaired spatial learning in conditions of artificial synaptic enhancement of the neuronal learning substrate.

In another experimental strategy, a weak HFS stimulation protocol was applied to rats pre-trained in the water Morris maze (four trials one day) and classified as poor learners, good learners and one untrained control group, before a fifth trial was applied on the following day. After the weak HFS protocol, no differences were observed in the induction of early LTP, but in the late phase (8-24h) higher population spike amplitudes (PSA) were observed for both poor learners and good learners compared with the untrained controls. Furthermore, the excitatory post-synaptic potentials (EPSPs) differed between all groups in induction (good learners had minor potentiation compared to poor learners), early LTP (higher potentiation for poor learners compared with good learners) and in late LTP (poor learners had higher potentiation than both good learners and controls). The escape latencies achieved in the fifth trial were correlated with the synaptic potentiation observed 24 hours later (Schulz & Korz, 2010). The authors proposed that once the memory is established in the good learner group further synaptic potentiation with a weak HFS is impaired due to the storage and retrieval of information. Thus, the synapse could be protected against the new encoding through a "homeostatic shutdown" of the EPSP-LTP (Roth-Alpermann et al., 2006; Schulz & Korz, 2010).

Uzacovet al., (2005) observed changes in synaptic responses of the dentate gyrus after training rats in a hole-board task requiring both reference and working memory, and compared it with a pseudo-trained group. The rats that were trained for ten trials (five trials on day one, four trials on the second day, and the tenth trial on the third day of training) made fewer reference memory errors compared with the pseudo-trained rats, whereas no differences were observed in working memory errors. The last trial of training in the hole-board was achieved fifteen minutes after the induction of early LTP and tested 24 hours after the persistence of LTP. Only the groups of rats that showed a significant reduction in reference memory errors compared to pseudo-trained animals had enhanced populations of spikes compared to the chamber control animals. Moreover, the authors observed that the pseudo-trained animals that were impaired at forming a reference memory of the baited holes did not exhibit an enhancement of the population of spikes but showed reduced amplitude of the population of spikes (depotentiation) compared with chamber control rats. The authors controlled for the factors of food reinforcement, novelty reaction, and stress response for different trials of training, and were able to exclude all these factors as related to the observed LTP differences. After testing one group of rats that was administered a protein synthesis inhibitor (anisomycin) before the second session of training (day two, trials four to eight) considered critical for the establishment of reference memory (implying pattern recognition), and 24 hours before the tetanisation, it was found that no reinforcement of LTP occurred in the group treated with anisomycin compared with a saline group. Furthermore, deficiencies in the consolidation of reference memory were also evident in the higher number of errors in trials eight to ten compared with saline group, whereas neither acquisition nor working memory were affected by the inhibition of protein synthesis. The authors proposed that reference memory consolidation could lead to a transformation of the electrically induced early-LTP into a late LTP. Moreover, another relevant result was the fact that pseudo-trained animals showed depotentiation of the induced early-LTP. Thus, the authors showed that dentate gyrus early LTP can be reinforced to late-LTP by reference memory learning through a new protein synthesis-dependent mechanism. Using this same paradigm, the enhanced LTP and behavioural performance were subsequently shown to depend on mineralocorticoid receptors and D1/D5 receptors (Korz & Frey, 2007). Intracerebroventricular galanin administration to rats induces place learning deficits and has been proposed as an strong inhibitor of spatial memory consolidation (Kinney et al., 2003), and of LTP in CA3/CA1 and dentate gyrus synapses in slice electrophysiology (Badie-Mahdavi et al., 2005; Coumis & Davies, 2002). The administration of galanin to rats undergoing training in the Morris maze (four daily trials during two consecutive days) led to impairments in the reduction in escape latencies observed on the second day in the control group. The galanin reduced the phosphorylation of CREB and produced a reduction of LTP measured as the amplitude of the PS at least 60 minutes after the HFS (Kinney et al., 2009).

Genetic manipulations in mice displayed related deficiencies in LTP induction and maintenance in the dentate gyrus and spatial learning tests. Mice with the conditional deletion of the NT3 gene showed reduced neurogenesis, impaired LTP in the lateral pp to dentate gyrus and profound deficiencies in Morris maze training (Shimazu et al., 2006), whereas the overexpression of the NR2b subunit of the NMDAR induces enhanced LTP, learning and memory (Tang, et al., 1999; 2001). However, as was mentioned previously, the inhibition of LTP only impairs spatial learning in naive animals, but animals with previous exposure to both spatial and non-spatial tasks were not impaired by the LTP inhibition induced by NMDAR antagonists (Bannerman, et al., 1995; Saucier & Cain, 1995). Thus, spatial learning can occur in the absence of LTP when previous experience in the context of the learning has taken place. Niewoehneret al., (2007) showed a dependence of working memory ability on dentate NMDAR function. The authors generated mice exhibiting the complete loss of the NR1 subunit of the NMDAR restricted to dentate gyrus neurons and evaluated spatial working memory, reference memory and the associated synaptic plasticity using a radial maze (three arms baited from a six radial arm maze). The mice lacking the NR1 subunit showed intact spatial reference memory but impaired working memory, and concomitantly exhibited impaired LTP induction for pp stimulation, but preserved LTP at Schaffer collaterals-CA1 synapses. The authors previously evaluated the consequences of the ablation of the GluR-A subunit of AMPA receptors in mice and found that it disrupts the ability to express hippocampal LTP on spatial working memory, which was impaired, whereas spatial reference memory remained unaffected (Schmitt et al., 2003; Zamanillo et al., 1999). Also, mutant mice expressing a low proportion (10%) of coincidence-detection impaired NMDARs caused by an insensitivity to Mg^{2+} and impermeability to calcium Ca^{2+} (Burnashev et al., 1992), showed normal early CA1 LTP but impaired dentate gyrus LTP, reduced spike populations in the dentate gyrus and impaired spatial learning and spatial recognition in Morris maze, whereas novel object recognition was unaltered (Chen et al., 2009).

6.2. CA3 LTP and Spatial Learning

LTP and LTD of the associative/commissural synapse onto CA3 were evaluated in aged rats following their classification as good learners and bad learners in a spatial hippocampal-dependent learning task. Aged rats, both memory impaired and good learners, showed reduced NMDAR-dependent LTD and intact NMDAR-dependent LTP; however, metabotropic glutamate receptor-dependent LTD was unaltered in aged efficient rats but was absent in deficient rats. Moreover, it was observed that NMDAR-dependent forms of plasticity did not correlate with performance of the rats at any age, whereas the mGluR-dependent forms of plasticity were correlated with performance. Thus, successful aging was related to preserved mGluR dependent LTD in the commissural/CA3 synapses (Yang et al., 2013). A difference of Schaffer collaterals-CA1 synapses were has been observed age impaired NMDAR-dependent synaptic plasticity (Rosenzweig & Barnes, 2003), and increased VGCC-dependent LTP has specifically been uncovered in age unimpaired individuals (Boric et al., 2008).

Different works have revealed a relationship between spatial learning experiences and the facilitated induction of LTP or LTD from short forms of synaptic plasticity depending of the stimulation conditions and the behavioural experiences involving some learning (Kemp &

Manahan-Vaughan, 2007). Manahan-Vaughn and co-workers showed that the exploration of novel environments leads to the strengthening of weak plasticity inducing LTP both on mf-CA3 synapses and in commissural-CA3 synapses. However, LTD strengthening occurs with differential characteristics at each synapse. Mossy fibres-CA3 synaptic LTP is facilitated by exposure to novel landmarks, whereas LTD at commissural-CA3 is facilitated by small spatial cues (Hagena & Manahan-Vaughan, 2011, 2012).

Huang et al., tested the effect of ablations of the Cβ1 catalytic sub-unit or the regulatory R1β subunit OF PKA in mice, on the expression of LTP and place learning. The ablations induced the complete elimination of LTP at mossy fibre-CA3 synapses without causing alterations in the reaction to novelty, spatial learning or contextual conditioning (Huang et al., 1995). Furthermore, mice lacking mGluR5 showed reduced CA1 LTP (NMDAR-dependent) and the impaired acquisition of learning in the Morris maze tasks (as was previously mentioned), whereas NMDAR-independent mf-CA3 LTP remained intact (Lu, et al., 1997). Also, mice with ablations of NMDAR specifically at CA3 pyramidal cells were observed to have normal acquisition and retrieval of spatial reference information in the Morris water maze; however, deficiencies were present when the mice were exposed only to a fraction of the spatial information previously acquired during a probe trial, in which the mice showed reduced searching in the previous platform position relative to control mice, which searched in the platform position as well as in the condition of complete spatial cues. These findings support a role for CA3 in memory pattern retrieval and suggest that mutant mice cannot establish the full pattern previously activated under partial spatial information exposure, which requires CA3 NMDAR LTP. In the mutant mice, CA1 place cells showed normal activity in the original environment but reduced activity under the limited spatial cues condition (Nakazawa et al., 2002), this is in according with the proposed role of CA3 in pattern completion.

6.3. CA1 LTP and Spatial Learning

Environmental enrichment (EE) has profound effects on behavioural performance in rats of adult ages. In fact, it was Donald Hebb who noted that rats reared as pets performed better than rats reared in standard laboratory conditions (Hebb, 1949). Subsequently, a considerable research effort was aimed at assessing the effects of EE on cognition. One such study observed that exposure to enrichment for one night caused an increase in synaptic strength and cellular excitability in the dentate gyrus (Irvine et al., 2006), whereas in CA1 a dual effect was observed in which increased fEPSP occurred after high intensity stimulation but a decrease was observed at low intensities of stimulation (Irvine & Abraham, 2005). Further research revealed that periods of EE longer than months improve performance in hippocampal dependent tasks, including the Morris maze (Kempermann et al., 2002; Pham et al., 1999). In addition, it was observed that EE in rats from weaning to two years of age produced better performance compared with short-term exposure in aged rats (Kobayashi et al., 2002). Three months of exposure to EE induced an improvement in the Morris maze place-learning test, which was evident in a reduced path length through all training sessions; however, in the last of the six days of training no differences persisted since both groups reached their maximal performance. Brain slices were taken from the rats and LTP and LTD were induced in the CA1 region (radiatum and oriens strata). No changes were observed in basal strength of the fEPSP, in excitability of the neurons, or in paired pulse facilitation. This was interpreted as the absence of changes in the presynaptic short-term plasticity. Also, LTP was induced and no differences were observed in the strength and persistence of the HFS induced LTP in any strata. The only observed difference was a higher resistance to LFS induced reversal for the oriens LTP. Both enriched rats and control showed displayed depotentiation after the LFS, however the potentiation in the enriched group showed a recovery after LFS, whereas the control group slices remained depotentiated at least up to 40 minutes after (Eckert et al., 2010). In other work, it was observed that unimpaired aged Long-Evans rats showed a general reduction in NMDAR-dependent LTD and increased mGluR-dependent LTD that was possibly compensatory. This finding was interpreted as an age-dependent switch with learning performance and NMDAR-dependent forms of plasticity correlated during young age, whereas in aged rats a correlation was observed between learning performance and non-NMDAR forms of plasticity (Boric, et al., 2008; H. K. Lee, Min, Gallagher, & Kirkwood, 2005). The proposed age-dependent switch would require the preservation of mechanisms of the CA3, and it was also evident that different mechanisms of aging could exist in different regions of the hippocampus (Yang, et al., 2013).

Other results revealed that CA1 LTP was impaired when it was evoked by HFS in slices from rats submitted to two hours of stressful noise. A different group of animals was submitted to noise for 30-60 minutes before receiving training in the Morris maze during sixteen collapsed trials (one day of training). The rats showed a similar learning rate as the controls, but the retention tests conducted 24 hours after showed the reduced recall of the platform position for the stressed rats. Stressed rats also showed instability in the place fields of CA1 neurons (Kim et al., 2007).

A relationship between impairment in spatial ability and LTP alterations has been observed in other models involving mutations of additional components of the glutamatergic system, such as the glutamate transporter. Balschunet al., (2010) observed a reduction in the magnitude of CA1 LTP in heterozygous VGLUT1 deficient mice in which occurs a reduction in VGLUT1 transporter of 40 %. Deficient mice had unaltered reference spatial memory and were able to realize the reversal learning in the Morris maze; these mice only showed a higher time near the previous platform position from the first reversal trials. Also, mice with a deletion of NMDAR1 restricted to CA1 pyramidal neurons showed lack of synaptic currents and NMDAR-mediated LTP at CA1. Furthermore, place learning in the Morris maze hidden platform version was impaired, whereas a cued version of the task was unimpaired in these mice, supporting a relevant role of CA1 NMDAR-dependent LTP in the learning of spatial information (Tsien et al., 1996). In other mutant mice expressing an inhibitory form of the regulatory sub-unit of PKA, late LTP and PKA activity were significantly decreased in CA1 with concomitant behavioural deficits in place learning and long-term contextual fear conditioning, similar to the deficits induced by the inhibition of protein synthesis (Abel et al., 1997). Transgenic over-expression of the NR2B subunit containing NMDAR in rats caused an increase in LTP at CA1 associated with enhanced memory performance in the spatial water maze, novel object recognition, and the delayed not-matching working memory test (Wang et al., 2009).

7. LTD AND SPATIAL LEARNING

NMDA-dependent LTD and LTP have been proposed as substrates for learning and memory, principally through studies that manipulate NMDA receptors using agonists and antagonists as well as by transgenic studies; however, because these strategies affect both LTD and LTP, it has been difficult to determine which role corresponds to each form of synaptic plasticity. It was observed that GluN2A containing NMDAR preferentially contributes to LTP induction, whereas GluN2B containing NMDAR preferentially contributes to LTD (Fox et al., 2006). In freely moving adult rats, it was shown that there is a differential participation of the GluN2A sub-unit preferential antagonist NVP-AAM077 and the GluN2B sub-unit preferential antagonist Ro 25-6981 in LTP and LTD, respectively. NVP blocks LTP induction in CA1, whereas Ro 25-6981 blocked the LTD expression. The rats were trained on a Morris maze task for two days, with eight trials on the first day and a probe trial on the second day. The antagonists were applied (ip) before the start of the first training day; saline, NVP and Ro 25-6981 groups reduced their escape latencies in the five-eight trials compared with the first four trials (the data were collapsed into two blocks of four trials and compared); however, in the probe test 24 h later, the Ro 25-6981 group did not show preference for the platform quadrant compared with the opposite. Additionally, the Ro 25-6981 group had a small amount of time in the platform quadrant compared with the saline and NVP groups, a small number of crossings on the platform position and a higher latency to reaching the platform position in the probe trial. Thus, whereas NMDA-dependent LTP block had no effect on spatial learning and memory, the participation of LTD in place memory, but not in place learning, was supported by the studio. Additionally, a different blocker of LTD was used, the Tat-GluA23Y peptide, which avoids LTD expression by impairing regulated AMPA endocytosis (Ahmadian et al., 2004), and similar behavioural impairments were observed. Finally, the authors showed that the LTD block had an effect on the behaviour only when it was applied before the consolidation took place; when the drugs were administered 24 h after training, no effect was observed on place learning. These results support the participation of CA1 LTD on place learning consolidation (Ge et al., 2010).

It was shown that spatial learning training in the Morris maze facilitates the induction of LTD at CA1, after LFS, which failed to induce LTD previously the training. Selective antagonists for GluN2B containing NMDA receptors, avoided the Morris learning induced LTD, through the inhibition of AMPA receptors endocytosis, this last was tested using a systemic injection of Tat-GluA23Y peptide which avoid the endocytosis of AMPA receptors (Fox et al., 2007) and also blocks LTD Morris-induced learning. Both GluN2B antagonist and Tat-GluA23Y impaired reversal learning when applied systemic or intra-hippocampally. Additionally, acute stress that was induced by exposition to an elevated platform induced the facilitation of LTD that was mediated by GluN2B and AMPA receptor endocytosis and also induced a modest beneficial effect on spatial learning reversal (Dong et al., 2013).

Spatial reversal learning is evaluated after the initial training in the Morris maze, changing the position of the platform in the maze. LTD has been related to spatial reversal learning in several studies. Administration of endogenous D-serine, whose binding to the glycine site on the NR1 subunit is required by the activation of NMDA receptors (Johnson & Ascher, 1987), induces an increase in GluN2B-dependent LTD and improves reversal learning, without affecting the spatial learning normal acquisition, in the water maze (Duffy et al., 2008). Conversely, transgenic mice that lack NMDAR-dependent LTP showed delayed acquisition of reversal learning and unimpaired spatial learning ability in the same task (Nicholls et al., 2008). Additionally, a relation between LTD and long-term contextual fear memory was shown in Bax knock-out mice with deleted expression of Bax in pyramidal neurons of the CA1 region, a mutation that eliminated the expression of NMDA-dependent LTD without altering LTP. Additionally, the mice were efficient in the performance of innate fear, cued fear memory and short-term contextual memory, but they were impaired in long-term contextual fear, which implies LTD expression in consolidation but not in acquisition of this type of memory (Liu et al., 2014).

Another mutant mice knockout for P13K$_{\gamma}$ (phosphoinositide-3-kinase) showed selective impairment in CA1 NMDAR-dependent LTD and deficiency in spatial reversal learning in the Morris water maze tasks (Kim et al., 2011). However, a mutant that expressed increased expression of P13K$_{\gamma}$ also impaired CA1 NMDA-dependent LTD without altering NMDAR-dependent LTP and also caused impairment in place learning ability in the Morris water maze, whereas the contextual fear memory was not affected (Choi et al., 2014). Additionally, increased LTD has been related to deficiencies in place learning. Transgenic mice with increased activity of Rap2 protein, which constitutive activity-induced loss of surface AMPA receptors, shortening of dendrites and axons and loss of synapses (Fu et al., 2007), induced place learning deficiencies in the Morris maze and impaired extinction in contextual fear tests as well as having increased LTD evoked by 3 Hz/5 min stimulation on the slice. No effects were observed in LTP or depotentiation (Ryu et al., 2008).

Although the study of LTD and behavioural performance involves difficulty in the reliable induction of LTD in adult awake animals (Goh & Manahan-Vaughan, 2013b; Staubli & Scafidi, 1997), it was consistently observed that the coupling of afferent stimulation both through test-pulses or weak synaptic plasticity protocols with spatial learning events (exposure to novelty, exploration events, trials of training in place learning tasks) facilitates the expression of LTD (Kemp & Manahan-Vaughan, 2004; Kemp et al., 2013; Manahan-Vaughan & Braunewell, 1999). Goh and Manahan-Vaughan investigated the effect of object recognition memory in mice on learning-related plasticity. Mice were exposed to one arena containing two different objects and simultaneously were stimulated with paired pulse or HFS. Exposure to the arena with objects in the learning phase and recognition test induced LTD with a duration of at least 24 h. The result that both the training phase and recognition phase (with one novel object replacing a known object) facilitated LTD at CA1 conduced the authors to ask if the hippocampus treated the two sessions as novel events in view of the novel object introduced in the arena. To test this assumption, the authors contrasted the results with configural changes of known objects and observed that LTD facilitation occurred during the acquisition phase and in the novel configuration of new objects, but not during re-exposure to a similar arena (the same objects in the same places). LTP induced by HFS was curtailed by object recognition learning and recognition (re-exposure); however, during re-exposure to the same objects in the same places, the LTP was not inhibited and had a similar magnitude to that observed in non-trained stimulated animals. This work showed that intrinsic endogen synaptic depression occurs when the mice are exposed to a novel environment where objects are present (Goh & Manahan-Vaughan, 2013a). Thus, CA1 LTD appears to be reactive to novelty detection (new object-position and new position of known objects). Similar changes in synaptic plasticity related to spatial novelty had been reported for dentate gyrus, were LTP is induced through changes in an empty space (Straube et al., 2003a; Straube et al., 2003b). Kemp, et al., (2013) showed that exposure to a novel configuration of objects that induces enhanced LTD in hippocampal CA1 also triggers CA1 c-fos activation, and similarly, a blockade of c-fos expression and administration of actinomycin-D eliminated the learning-facilitated LTD expression in this hippocampal area.

The effect of exposure to a new environment on field potentials evoked in the CA1 area by stimulation of commissural/SC pathways to CA1 was assessed in Sprague-Dawley rats, and no effects were observed either for the exploration (novel objects) or re-exploration (familiar objects) in the evoked potentials. Additionally, it was observed that standard LFS was unable to induce LTD; however, paired LFS and the exploration of novel objects induced reliable LTD with a duration of at least 24 h. When LFS was paired with re-exposure to objects (familiar objects), no facilitation of LTD induction was observed. LTP induced by HFS (four trains of 30 pulses at 100 Hz, a strong protocol with interval inter train of 5 minutes) paired with novelty exposure or re-exposure to familiar objects was not altered. In addition, early LTP induced by weak stimulation (two trains of 30 pulses at 100 Hz, with inter train interval of 5 min) was paired with novelty exposition and re-exposure to familiar objects, and no effect was observed. Together, these results indicate that only CA1 LTD was facilitated by exposure to novelty. Because CA1 LTD has NMDA dependence, especially through the GluN2B-containing subunit, the antagonist Ro25-6981, which is specific to NMDAR, was administered with the previous stimulation protocols. The facilitation of LTD by novelty exposure was eliminated by the antagonist and by the administration of the peptide Tat-GluA23Y, which (as mentioned previously) impairs the internalization of AMPA receptors. These results support a relevant role of NMDA-dependent LTD in novel object exploration and the learning implied by such a role (Dong et al., 2012).

As was mentioned previously, LTD has been implied in spatial reversal learning and behavioural flexibility; in addition, it has been suggested to have a role of LTD in the depotentiation of synapses that were previously involved in the storage of memories, to permit the storage of new information (Nicholls, et al., 2008). Millset al., (2014) showed a vinculum between the cadherin/beta-catenin adhesion complex, LTD and cognitive flexibility. Cadherin is a key mediator of the bidirectional changes in synaptic strength and stability because the recruitment of cadherin to synapses is required for the maintenance of LTP and for memory consolidation (Bozdagi et al., 2000). Activity patterns that conduce to LTD cause cadherin internalization, disrupting beta-cathenin/cadherin interactions under in vitro conditions (Tai et al., 2007). Millset al., (2014) generated transgenic mice that presented stabilized beta-cathenin and abolished LTD, without alterations in basal synaptic transmission or LTP at CA1. These mice showed impaired spatial reversal learning in the Morris maze in association with the perseveration of searching in the former platform position and deficient performance in a delayed non-match to the place task in a Y maze, which was evident in the low percent of correct choices in the last days of training (6-10 days). Thus, these mice had impaired cognitive flexibility that was probably related to increased perseveration of obsolete spatial information. The suppression of obsolete information and acquisition of new information are implied in behavioural flexibility and adaptation to a changing environment. It has been shown that obsolete memory suppression requires the modification of neuronal activity-dependent processes (Myers & Davis, 2007).

However, other results are conflicting with respect to the role of LTD in behavioural flexibility. Mice that over-expressed adenylyl cyclase type 1 (AC) and then increased cAMP-calcium signalling showed impaired LTD expression but unaltered LTP at SC-CA1 synapses.

In spite of the impaired LTD, these mice showed normal depotentiation of previously generated LTP. Behavioural testing showed an improvement (faster acquisition) in the Morris maze task during the six days of training (one daily trial), and a similar performance to the wild type during a probe trial on the seventh day of training. Reversal learning was evaluated for another six days, and the over-expressing AC mice acquired faster the new position of the platform, while again no differences were observed during the probe trials. Thus, these mice had impaired SC-CA1 LTD and improved spatial learning and reversal learning but had similar memory and extinction of the information (Zhang & Wang, 2013). These results imply that there is a principal role of LTP and depotentiation in spatial learning and reversal learning, in the absence of LTD.

Another report on transgenic rats with increased expression of NR2B sub-units showed unchanged CA1 LTD, in opposition to the results on the transgenic mice, in which a crucial role of the NMDA-containing NR2B subunit in LTD expression was shown (Wang et al., 2009). Finally, a role of LTD in the stress-dependent impairment of learning has been observed in some studies. Acute stress was able to induce the facilitation of LTD induction at the CA1 *radiatum stratum* using a similar weak stimulation protocol, as described for novelty and exploration facilitation of LTD (Xu et al., 1997). Stress-facilitated LTD was dependent on NR2B-containing NMDA receptors because LTD induction was blocked by the antagonist Ro without altering the LTP induction, in rats, in vivo. The rats were trained on the Morris maze task using eight trials of training in one day, and their memory was tested for the platform location 24 h later. Acute stress caused by exposure to 30 min on an elevated maze before the probe trial caused a lack of spatial memory, which was blocked by the administration of Ro 30 min before the acute stress exposure. The peptide Tat-GluR23Y was administered to block LTD before the exposure to the acute stress, and it was observed that this peptide prevented memory impairment induced by stress. Finally, the authors blocked the glutamate transporter to induce a facilitation of LTD induction due to a different cause (not stress) and observed that this facilitation of LTD induction conduced spatial memory impairment similar to that produced by acute stress exposure. Thus, CA1 LTD promotion through NR2B-containing NMDA receptors appears to be a mechanism for spatial memory erasure.

Conclusion

The synaptic plasticity is intimately related to spatial learning. The evidence here revised show a strong relation between LTP facilitation and exploration, and between LTD and novelty coding, spatial reversal learning and behavioural flexibility as well as in the depotentiation of synapses that were previously involved in the storage of memories, to permit the storage of new information. However in relation to spatial learning the evidence is complex and depends on induction protocols and experimental strategies used in the evaluation of spatial cognition. CA1 NMDA dependent LTP appear to play a role in spatial learning abilities, whereas dentate gyrus NMDA dependent LTP would to have a minor role in spatial learning. NMDA dependent LTP appear to be involved principally in working memory processes, whereas spatial learning can be realized without NMDA participation. Also dissociations between short term memory and long term memory of spatial information appear exists. However, evidence showing punctual modifications of hippocampal sub-regions and spatial learning specific processes is scarce. It is very urgent to realize efforts to dissect factors as learning process (short-term memory versus long term memory; reference vs. working memory; acquisition, consolidation, recovery of information; etc.) and nature of evoked LTP (composite vs. NMDA-dependent or NMDA-independent), in experimental designs attempted to verify if the functions of hippocampal sub-regions are linked with specific LTP and LTD modifications. As was evident in the studies revised in this chapter, the evidence reflects a complex picture under construction despite of the strong effort realized in the past years.

REFERENCES

Abraham, W. C. & Goddard, G. V. (1983) Asymmetric relationships between homosynaptic long-term potentiation and heterosynaptic long-term depression. *Nature,* 305, 717-719.

Acsady, L., Kamondi, A., Sik, A., Freund, T. & Buzsaki, G. (1998) GABAergic cells are the major postsynaptic targets of mossy fibers in the rat hippocampus. *J. Neurosci.,* 18, 3386-3403.

Ahmadian, G., Ju, W., Liu, L., Wyszynski, M., Lee, S. H., Dunah, A. W., Taghibiglou, C., Wang, Y., Lu, J., Wong, T. P., Sheng, M. & Wang, Y. T. (2004) Tyrosine phosphorylation of GluR2 is required for insulin-stimulated AMPA receptor endocytosis and LTD. *EMBO J.,* 23, 1040-1050.

Amaral, D. G. & Witter, M. P. (1989) The three-dimensional organization of the hippocampal formation: a review of anatomical data. *Neuroscience,* 31, 571-591.

Andersen, P., Moser, E., Moser, M. B. & Trommald, M. (1996) Cellular correlates to spatial learning in the rat hippocampus. *J. Physiol. Paris,* 90, 349.

Ayala, J. E., Chen, Y., Banko, J. L., Sheffler, D. J., Williams, R., Telk, A. N., Watson, N. L., Xiang, Z., Zhang, Y., Jones, P. J., Lindsley, C. W., Olive, M. F. & Conn, P. J. (2009) mGluR5 positive allosteric modulators facilitate both hippocampal LTP and LTD and enhance spatial learning. *Neuropsychopharmacology,* 34, 2057-2071.

Bach, M. E., Barad, M., Son, H., Zhuo, M., Lu, Y. F., Shih, R.,et al., Mansuy, I., Hawkins, R. D. & Kandel, E. R. (1999) Age-related defects in spatial memory are correlated with defects in the late phase of hippocampal long-term potentiation in vitro and are attenuated by drugs that enhance the cAMP signaling pathway. *Proc. Natl. Acad. Sci. U S A*, 96, 5280-5285.

Bach, M. E., Hawkins, R. D., Osman, M., Kandel, E. R. & Mayford, M. (1995) Impairment of spatial but not contextual memory in CaMKII mutant mice with a selective loss of hippocampal LTP in the range of the theta frequency. *Cell,* 81, 905-915.

Badie-Mahdavi, H., Lu, X., Behrens, M. M. & Bartfai, T. (2005) Role of galanin receptor 1 and galanin receptor 2 activation in synaptic plasticity associated with 3',5'-cyclic AMP response element-binding protein phosphorylation in the dentate gyrus: studies with a galanin receptor 2 agonist and galanin receptor 1 knockout mice. *Neuroscience,* 133, 591-604.

Balschun, D., Manahan-Vaughan, D., Wagner, T., Behnisch, T., Reymann, K. G. & Wetzel, W. (1999) A specific role for group I mGluRs in hippocampal LTP and hippocampus-dependent spatial learning. *Learn Mem,* 6, 138-152.

Balschun, D., Moechars, D., Callaerts-Vegh, Z., Vermaercke, B., Van Acker, N., Andries, L. & D'Hooge, R. (2010) Vesicular glutamate transporter VGLUT1 has a role in hippocampal long-term potentiation and spatial reversal learning. *Cereb Cortex,* 20, 684-693.

Bannerman, D. M., Good, M. A., Butcher, S. P., Ramsay, M. & Morris, R. G. (1995) Distinct components of spatial learning revealed by prior training and NMDA receptor blockade. *Nature,* 378, 182-186.

Barnes, C. A. (1979) Memory deficits associated with senescence: a neurophysiological and behavioral study in the rat. *J. Comp. Physiol. Psychol.,* 93, 74-104.

Barria, A., & Malinow, R. (2005) NMDA receptor subunit composition controls synaptic plasticity by regulating binding to CaMKII. *Neuron,* 48, 289-301.

Bashir, Z. I., Jane, D. E., Sunter, D. C., Watkins, J. C. & Collingridge, G. L. (1993) Metabotropic glutamate receptors contribute to the induction of long-term depression in the CA1 region of the hippocampus. *Eur. J. Pharmacol.*, 239, 265-266.

Bast, T., da Silva, B. M. & Morris, R. G. (2005) Distinct contributions of hippocampal NMDA and AMPA receptors to encoding and retrieval of one-trial place memory. *J. Neurosci.,* 25, 5845-5856.

Bast, T., Wilson, I. A., Witter, M. P. & Morris, R. G. (2009) From rapid place learning to behavioral performance: a key role for the intermediate hippocampus. *PLoS Biol.,* 7, e1000089.

Bayazitov, I. T., Richardson, R. J., Fricke, R. G. & Zakharenko, S. S. (2007) Slow presynaptic and fast postsynaptic components of compound long-term potentiation. *J. Neurosci.,* 27, 11510-11521.

Bear, M. F. & Malenka, R. C. (1994) Synaptic plasticity: LTP and LTD. *Curr. Opin. Neurobiol.,* 4, 389-399.

Bear, M. F., Cooper, L. N. & Ebner, F. F. (1987) A physiological basis for a theory of synapse modification. *Science,* 237, 42-48.

Bennett, M. R. (2000) The concept of long term potentiation of transmission at synapses. *Prog. Neurobiol.,* 60, 109-137.

Bikbaev, A., Neyman, S., Ngomba, R. T., Conn, P. J., Nicoletti, F. & Manahan-Vaughan, D. (2008) MGluR5 mediates the interaction between late-LTP, network activity, and learning. *PLoS One,* 3, e2155.

Bliss, T. V. & Collingridge, G. L. (1993) A synaptic model of memory: long-term potentiation in the hippocampus. *Nature*, 361, 31-39.

Bliss, T. V. & Gardner-Medwin, A. R. (1973) Long-lasting potentiation of synaptic transmission in the dentate area of the unanaestetized rabbit following stimulation of the perforant path. *J. Physiol.,* 232, 357-374.

Bliss, T. V. & Lomo, T. (1973) Long-lasting potentiation of synaptic transmission in the dentate area of the anaesthetized rabbit following stimulation of the perforant path. *J. Physiol.,* 232, 331-356.

Bliss, T. V., Errington, M. L. & Lynch, M. A. (1990) Long-term potentiation in the dentate gyrus in vivo is associated with a sustained increase in extracellular glutamate. *Adv. Exp. Med. Biol.,* 268, 269-278.

Blundon, J. A. & Zakharenko, S. S. (2008) Dissecting the components of long-term potentiation. Neuroscientist, 14, 598-608.

Boric, K., Munoz, P., Gallagher, M. & Kirkwood, A. (2008) Potential adaptive function for altered long-term potentiation mechanisms in aging hippocampus. *J. Neurosci.,* 28, 8034-8039.

Borroni, A. M., Fichtenholtz, H., Woodside, B. L. & Teyler, T. J. (2000) Role of voltage-dependent calcium channel long-term potentiation (LTP) and NMDA LTP in spatial memory. *J. Neurosci.,* 20, 9272-9276.

Bozdagi, O., Shan, W., Tanaka, H., Benson, D. L. & Huntley, G. W. (2000) Increasing numbers of synaptic puncta during late-phase LTP: N-cadherin is synthesized, recruited to synaptic sites, and required for potentiation. *Neuron,* 28, 245-259.

Brun, V. H., Ytterbo, K., Morris, R. G., Moser, M. B. & Moser, E. I. (2001) Retrograde amnesia for spatial memory induced by NMDA receptor-mediated long-term potentiation. *J. Neurosci.,* 21, 356-362.

Burnashev, N., Schoepfer, R., Monyer, H., Ruppersberg, J. P., Gunther, W., Seeburg, P. H. & Sakmann, B. (1992) Control by asparagine residues of calcium permeability and magnesium blockade in the NMDA receptor. *Science,* 257, 1415-1419.

Cain, D. P., Saucier, D., Hall, J., Hargreaves, E. L. & Boon, F. (1996). Detailed behavioral analysis of water maze acquisition under APV or CNQX: contribution of sensorimotor disturbances to drug-induced acquisition deficits. *Behav. Neurosci.,* 110, 86-102.

Castillo, P. E. (2012) Presynaptic LTP and LTD of excitatory and inhibitory synapses. Cold. *Spring Harb. Perspect Biol.,* 4(2).

Cavus, I. & Teyler, T. (1996) Two forms of long-term potentiation in area CA1 activate different signal transduction cascades. *J. Neurophysiol.*, 76, 3038-3047.

Chen, P. E., Errington, M. L., Kneussel, M., Chen, G., Annala, A. J., Rudhard, Y. H., Rast, G. F., Specht, C. G., Tigaret, C. M., Nassar, M. A., Morris, R. G., Bliss, T. V. & Schoepfer, R. (2009) Behavioral deficits and subregion-specific suppression of LTP in mice expressing a population of mutant NMDA receptors throughout the hippocampus. *Learn. Mem.,* 16, 635-644.

Choi, J. H., Park, P., Baek, G. C., Sim, S. E., Kang, S. J., Lee, Y., et al. Ahn, S. H., Lim, C. S., Lee, Y. S., Collingridge, G. L., Kaang, B. K. (2014) Effects of PI3Kgamma overexpression in the hippocampus on synaptic plasticity and spatial learning. *Mol. Brain,* 7, 78.

Churchwell, J. C. & Kesner, R. P. (2011) Hippocampal-prefrontal dynamics in spatial working memory: interactions and independent parallel processing. *Behav. Brain Res.* 225, 389-395.

Cohen, N. J. & Squire, L. R. (1980) Preserved learning and retention of pattern-analyzing skill in amnesia: dissociation of knowing how and knowing that. *Science,* 210, 207-210.

Contractor, A., Swanson, G. & Heinemann, S. F. (2001) Kainate receptors are involved in short- and long-term plasticity at mossy fiber synapses in the hippocampus. *Neuron,* 29, 209-216.

Coumis, U. & Davies, C. H. (2002) The effects of galanin on long-term synaptic plasticity in the CA1 area of rodent hippocampus. *Neuroscience, 112*(1), 173-182.

Debanne, D., Gahwiler, B. H. & Thompson, S. M. (1996) Cooperative interactions in the induction of long-term potentiation and depression of synaptic excitation between hippocampal CA3-CA1 cell pairs in vitro. *Proc. Natl. Acad. Sci. U S A,* 93, 11225-11230.

Delatour, B. & Witter, M. P. (2002) Projections from the parahippocampal region to the prefrontal cortex in the rat: evidence of multiple pathways. *Eur. J. Neurosci.,* 15, 1400-1407.

Diamond, A. (1990) The development and neural bases of higher cognitive functions. Introduction. *Ann N Y Acad. Sci.,* 608, xiii-lvi.

Dolphin, A. C., Errington, M. L. & Bliss, T. V. (1982) Long-term potentiation of the perforant path in vivo is associated with increased glutamate release. *Nature,* 297, 496-498.

Dong, Z., Bai, Y., Wu, X., Li, H., Gong, B., Howland, J. G., et al. Huang, Y., He, W., Li, T. & Wang, Y. T. (2013) Hippocampal long-term depression mediates spatial reversal learning in the Morris water maze. *Neuropharmacology,* 64, 65-73.

Dong, Z., Gong, B., Li, H., Bai, Y., Wu, X., Huang, Y., He, W., Li, T. & Wang, Y. T. (2012) Mechanisms of hippocampal long-term depression are required for memory enhancement by novelty exploration. *J. Neurosci.*, 32, 11980-11990.

Douglas, R. M. & Goddard, G. V. (1975) Long-term potentiation of the perforant path-granule cell synapse in the rat hippocampus. *Brain Res.*, 86, 205-215.

Doyere, V., Srebro, B. & Laroche, S. (1997) Heterosynaptic LTD and depotentiation in the medial perforant path of the dentate gyrus in the freely moving rat. *J. Neurophysiol.,* 77, 571-578.

Dragoi, G., Harris, K. D. & Buzsaki, G. (2003) Place representation within hippocampal networks is modified by long-term potentiation. *Neuron*, 39, 843-853.

Dudek, S. M. & Bear, M. F. (1992) Homosynaptic long-term depression in area CA1 of hippocampus and effects of N-methyl-D-aspartate receptor blockade. *Proc. Natl. Acad. Sci. U S A,* 89, 4363-4367.

Duffy, S., Labrie, V. & Roder, J. C. (2008) D-serine augments NMDA-NR2B receptor-dependent hippocampal long-term depression and spatial reversal learning. *Neuropsychopharmacology*, 33, 1004-1018.

Eckert, M. J., Bilkey, D. K. & Abraham, W. C. (2010) Altered plasticity in hippocampal CA1, but not dentate gyrus, following long-term environmental enrichment. *J. Neurophysiol.,* 103, 3320-3329.

Erickson, C. A., McNaughton, B. L. & Barnes, C. A. (1993) Comparison of long-term enhancement and short-term exploratory modulation of perforant path synaptic transmission. *Brain Res.,* 615, 275-280.

Fan, W., Ster, J. & Gerber, U. (2010) Activation conditions for the induction of metabotropic glutamate receptor-dependent long-term depression in hippocampal CA1 pyramidal cells. *J. Neurosci.*, 30, 1471-1475.

Fox, C. J., Russell, K. I., Wang, Y. T. & Christie, B. R. (2006) Contribution of NR2A and NR2B NMDA subunits to bidirectional synaptic plasticity in the hippocampus in vivo. *Hippocampus,* 16, 907-915.

Fox, C. J., Russell, K., Titterness, A. K., Wang, Y. T. & Christie, B. R. (2007) Tyrosine phosphorylation of the GluR2 subunit is required for long-term depression of synaptic efficacy in young animals in vivo. *Hippocampus,* 17, 600-605.

Frey, S., Bergado-Rosado, J., Seidenbecher, T., Pape, H. C. & Frey, J. U. (2001) Reinforcement of early long-term potentiation (early-LTP) in dentate gyrus by stimulation of the basolateral amygdala: heterosynaptic induction mechanisms of late-LTP. *J. Neurosci.,* 21, 3697-3703.

Frey, U., Krug, M., Reymann, K. G. & Matthies, H. (1988) Anisomycin, an inhibitor of protein synthesis, blocks late phases of LTP phenomena in the hippocampal CA1 region in vitro. *Brain Res.,* 452, 57-65.

Fu, Z., Lee, S. H., Simonetta, A., Hansen, J., Sheng, M. & Pak, D. T. (2007). Differential roles of Rap1 and Rap2 small GTPases in neurite retraction and synapse elimination in hippocampal spiny neurons. *J. Neurochem.,* 100, 118-131.

Fyhn, M., Molden, S., Witter, M. P., Moser, E. I. & Moser, M. B. (2004) Spatial representation in the entorhinal cortex. Science, 305, 1258-1264.

Gaffan, D. (1991) Spatial organization of episodic memory. *Hippocampus,* 1, 262-264.

Ge, Y., Dong, Z., Bagot, R. C., Howland, J. G., Phillips, A. G., Wong, T. P. & Wang, Y. T. (2010) Hippocampal long-term depression is required for the consolidation of spatial memory. *Proc. Natl. Acad. Sci. U S A,* 107, 16697-16702.

Giese, K. P., Fedorov, N. B., Filipkowski, R. K. & Silva, A. J. (1998) Autophosphorylation at Thr286 of the alpha calcium-calmodulin kinase II in LTP and learning. *Science*, 279, 870-873.

Gladding, C. M., Fitzjohn, S. M. & Molnar, E. (2009) Metabotropic glutamate receptor-mediated long-term depression: molecular mechanisms. *Pharmacol Rev.,* 61, 395-412.

Goh, J. J. & Manahan-Vaughan, D. (2013a) Spatial object recognition enables endogenous LTD that curtails LTP in the mouse hippocampus. *Cereb. Cortex*, 23, 1118-1125.

Goh, J. J. & Manahan-Vaughan, D. (2013b) Synaptic depression in the CA1 region of freely behaving mice is highly dependent on afferent stimulation parameters. *Front. Integr. Neurosci., 7*, 1.

Goldman-Rakic, P. S. (1995) Cellular basis of working memory. *Neuron,* 14, 477-485.

Green, E. J., McNaughton, B. L. & Barnes, C. A. (1990a) Exploration-dependent modulation of evoked responses in fascia dentata: dissociation of motor, EEG, and sensory factors and evidence for a synaptic efficacy change. *J Neurosci,* 10, 1455-1471.

Green, E. J., McNaughton, B. L. & Barnes, C. A. (1990b) Role of the medial septum and hippocampal theta rhythm in exploration-related synaptic efficacy changes in rat fascia dentata. *Brain Res*, 529, 102-108.

Grover, L. M. & Teyler, T. J. (1990a) Differential effects of NMDA receptor antagonist APV on tetanic stimulation induced and calcium induced potentiation. *Neurosci Lett.,* 113, 309-314.

Grover, L. M. & Teyler, T. J. (1990b) Two components of long-term potentiation induced by different patterns of afferent activation. *Nature,* 347, 477-479.

Gustafsson, B. & Wigstrom, H. (1990) Long-term potentiation in the hippocampal CA1 region: its induction and early temporal development. *Prog. Brain Res.,* 83, 223-232.

Gustafsson, B., Asztely, F., Hanse, E. & Wigstrom, H. (1989) Onset Characteristics of Long-Term Potentiation in the Guinea-Pig Hippocampal CA1 Region in Vitro. *Eur. J. Neurosci.,* 1, 382-394.

Hagena, H. & Manahan-Vaughan, D. (2011) Learning-facilitated synaptic plasticity at CA3 mossy fiber and commissural-associational synapses reveals different roles in information processing. *Cereb. Cortex,* 21, 2442-2449.

Hagena, H., & Manahan-Vaughan, D. (2012). Learning-facilitated long-term depression and long-term potentiation at mossy fiber-CA3 synapses requires activation of beta-adrenergic receptors. *Front Integr Neurosci, 6*, 23.

Halt, A. R., Dallapiazza, R. F., Zhou, Y., Stein, I. S., Qian, H., Juntti, S., et al. (2012). CaMKII binding to GluN2B is critical during memory consolidation. *EMBO J, 31*(5), 1203-1216.

Harris, E. W., & Cotman, C. W. (1986). Long-term potentiation of guinea pig mossy fiber responses is not blocked by N-methyl D-aspartate antagonists. *Neurosci Lett, 70*(1), 132-137.

Harris, K. M., & Teyler, T. J. (1984). Developmental onset of long-term potentiation in area CA1 of the rat hippocampus. *J Physiol, 346*, 27-48.

Hebb, D. (1949). *The Organization of Behavior: A Neuropsychological Theory*. New York: Wiley.

Hess, G., & Gustafsson, B. (1990). Changes in field excitatory postsynaptic potential shape induced by tetanization in the CA1 region of the guinea-pig hippocampal slice. *Neuroscience, 37*(1), 61-69.

Hoh, T., Beiko, J., Boon, F., Weiss, S., & Cain, D. P. (1999). Complex behavioral strategy and reversal learning in the water maze without NMDA receptor-dependent long-term potentiation. *J Neurosci, 19*(10), RC2.

Huang, Y. Y., Kandel, E. R., Varshavsky, L., Brandon, E. P., Qi, M., Idzerda, R. L., et al. (1995). A genetic test of the effects of mutations in PKA on mossy fiber LTP and its relation to spatial and contextual learning. *Cell, 83*(7), 1211-1222.

Huang, Y. Y., Li, X. C., & Kandel, E. R. (1994). cAMP contributes to mossy fiber LTP by initiating both a covalently mediated early phase and macromolecular synthesis-dependent late phase. *Cell, 79*(1), 69-79.

Irvine, G. I., & Abraham, W. C. (2005). Enriched environment exposure alters the input-output dynamics of synaptic transmission in area CA1 of freely moving rats. *Neurosci Lett, 391*(1-2), 32-37.

Irvine, G. I., Logan, B., Eckert, M., & Abraham, W. C. (2006). Enriched environment exposure regulates excitability, synaptic transmission, and LTP in the dentate gyrus of freely moving rats. *Hippocampus, 16*(2), 149-160.

Johnson, J. W., & Ascher, P. (1987). Glycine potentiates the NMDA response in cultured mouse brain neurons. *Nature, 325*(6104), 529-531.

Johnston, D., Williams, S., Jaffe, D., & Gray, R. (1992). NMDA-receptor-independent long-term potentiation. *Annu Rev Physiol, 54*, 489-505.

Jones, M. W., Errington, M. L., French, P. J., Fine, A., Bliss, T. V., Garel, S., et al. (2001). A requirement for the immediate early gene Zif268 in the expression of late LTP and long-term memories. *Nat Neurosci, 4*(3), 289-296.

Kakegawa, W., Tsuzuki, K., Yoshida, Y., Kameyama, K., & Ozawa, S. (2004). Input- and subunit-specific AMPA receptor trafficking underlying long-term potentiation at hippocampal CA3 synapses. *Eur J Neurosci, 20*(1), 101-110.

Kemp, A., & Manahan-Vaughan, D. (2004). Hippocampal long-term depression and long-term potentiation encode different aspects of novelty acquisition. *Proc Natl Acad Sci U S A, 101*(21), 8192-8197.

Kemp, A., & Manahan-Vaughan, D. (2005). The 5-hydroxytryptamine4 receptor exhibits frequency-dependent properties in synaptic plasticity and behavioural metaplasticity in the hippocampal CA1 region in vivo. *Cereb Cortex, 15*(7), 1037-1043.

Kemp, A., & Manahan-Vaughan, D. (2007). Hippocampal long-term depression: master or minion in declarative memory processes? *Trends Neurosci, 30*(3), 111-118.

Kemp, A., & Manahan-Vaughan, D. (2008). The hippocampal CA1 region and dentate gyrus differentiate between environmental and spatial feature encoding through long-term depression. *Cereb Cortex, 18*(4), 968-977.

Kemp, A., Tischmeyer, W., & Manahan-Vaughan, D. (2013). Learning-facilitated long-term depression requires activation of the immediate early gene, c-fos, and is transcription dependent. *Behav Brain Res, 254*, 83-91.

Kempermann, G., Gast, D., & Gage, F. H. (2002). Neuroplasticity in old age: sustained fivefold induction of hippocampal neurogenesis by long-term environmental enrichment. *Ann Neurol, 52*(2), 135-143.

Kenney, J., & Manahan-Vaughan, D. (2013a). Learning-facilitated synaptic plasticity occurs in the intermediate hippocampus in association with spatial learning. *Front Synaptic Neurosci, 5*, 10.

Kenney, J., & Manahan-Vaughan, D. (2013b). NMDA receptor-dependent synaptic plasticity in dorsal and intermediate hippocampus exhibits distinct frequency-dependent profiles. *Neuropharmacology, 74*, 108-118.

Kesner, R. P. (2013). A process analysis of the CA3 subregion of the hippocampus. *Front Cell Neurosci, 7*, 78.

Kesner, R. P., Hunsaker, M. R., & Warthen, M. W. (2008). The CA3 subregion of the hippocampus is critical for episodic memory processing by means of relational encoding in rats. *Behav Neurosci, 122*(6), 1217-1225.

Kim, J. I., Lee, H. R., Sim, S. E., Baek, J., Yu, N. K., Choi, J. H., et al. (2011). PI3Kgamma is required for NMDA receptor-dependent long-term depression and behavioral flexibility. *Nat Neurosci, 14*(11), 1447-1454.

Kim, J. J., Lee, H. J., Welday, A. C., Song, E., Cho, J., Sharp, P. E., et al. (2007). Stress-induced alterations in hippocampal plasticity, place cells, and spatial memory. *Proc Natl Acad Sci U S A, 104*(46), 18297-18302.

Kinney, J. W., Sanchez-Alavez, M., Barr, A. M., Criado, J. R., Crawley, J. N., Behrens, M. M., et al. (2009). Impairment of memory consolidation by galanin correlates with in vivo inhibition of both LTP and CREB phosphorylation. *Neurobiol Learn Mem, 92*(3), 429-438.

Kinney, J. W., Starosta, G., & Crawley, J. N. (2003). Central galanin administration blocks consolidation of spatial learning. *Neurobiol Learn Mem, 80*(1), 42-54.

Kobayashi, K., Manabe, T., & Takahashi, T. (1996). Presynaptic long-term depression at the hippocampal mossy fiber-CA3 synapse. *Science, 273*(5275), 648-650.

Kobayashi, S., Ohashi, Y., & Ando, S. (2002). Effects of enriched environments with different durations and starting times on learning capacity during aging in rats assessed by a refined procedure of the Hebb-Williams maze task. *J Neurosci Res, 70*(3), 340-346.

Kohonen, T. (Ed.) (1984). *Self-Organization and Associative Memory*. New York, NY: Springer-Verlag.

Korz, V., & Frey, J. U. (2007). Hormonal and monoamine signaling during reinforcement of hippocampal long-term potentiation and memory retrieval. *Learn Mem, 14*(3), 160-166.

Krug, M., Lossner, B., & Ott, T. (1984). Anisomycin blocks the late phase of long-term potentiation in the dentate gyrus of freely moving rats. *Brain Res Bull, 13*(1), 39-42.

Lee, H. K., Kameyama, K., Huganir, R. L., & Bear, M. F. (1998). NMDA induces long-term synaptic depression and dephosphorylation of the GluR1 subunit of AMPA receptors in hippocampus. *Neuron, 21*(5), 1151-1162.

Lee, H. K., Min, S. S., Gallagher, M., & Kirkwood, A. (2005). NMDA receptor-independent long-term depression correlates with successful aging in rats. *Nat Neurosci, 8*(12), 1657-1659.

Lee, I., & Kesner, R. P. (2003). Differential roles of dorsal hippocampal subregions in spatial working memory with short versus intermediate delay. *Behav Neurosci, 117*(5), 1044-1053.

Lemon, N., & Manahan-Vaughan, D. (2006). Dopamine D1/D5 receptors gate the acquisition of novel information through hippocampal long-term potentiation and long-term depression. *J Neurosci, 26*(29), 7723-7729.

Li, S., Cullen, W. K., Anwyl, R., & Rowan, M. J. (2003). Dopamine-dependent facilitation of LTP induction in hippocampal CA1 by exposure to spatial novelty. *Nat Neurosci, 6*(5), 526-531.

Lisman, J. E., & Otmakhova, N. A. (2001). Storage, recall, and novelty detection of sequences by the hippocampus: elaborating on the SOCRATIC model to account for normal and aberrant effects of dopamine. *Hippocampus, 11*(5), 551-568.

Liu, X., Gu, Q. H., Duan, K., & Li, Z. (2014). NMDA receptor-dependent LTD is required for consolidation but not acquisition of fear memory. *J Neurosci, 34*(26), 8741-8748.

Lomo, T. (1971a). Patterns of activation in a monosynaptic cortical pathway: the perforant path input to the dentate area of the hippocampal formation. *Exp Brain Res, 12*(1), 18-45.

Lomo, T. (1971b). Potentiation of monosynaptic EPSPs in the perforant path-dentate granule cell synapse. *Exp Brain Res, 12*(1), 46-63.

Lomo, T. (2003). The discovery of long-term potentiation. *Philos Trans R Soc Lond B Biol Sci, 358*(1432), 617-620.

Lu, Y. M., Jia, Z., Janus, C., Henderson, J. T., Gerlai, R., Wojtowicz, J. M., et al. (1997). Mice lacking metabotropic glutamate receptor 5 show impaired learning and reduced CA1 long-term potentiation (LTP) but normal CA3 LTP. *J Neurosci, 17*(13), 5196-5205.

Lynch, G. S., Dunwiddie, T., & Gribkoff, V. (1977). Heterosynaptic depression: a postsynaptic correlate of long-term potentiation. *Nature, 266*(5604), 737-739.

Lynch, M. A. (2004). Long-term potentiation and memory. *Physiol Rev, 84*(1), 87-136.

Lynch, M. A., Errington, M. L., Clements, M. P., Bliss, T. V., Redini-Del Negro, C., & Laroche, S. (1990). Increases in glutamate release and phosphoinositide metabolism associated with long-term potentiation and classical conditioning. *Prog Brain Res, 83*, 251-256.

Mackes, J. L., & Willner, J. (2006). NMDA antagonist MK-801 impairs acquisition of place strategies, but not their use. *Behav Brain Res, 175*(1), 112-118.

Manahan-Vaughan, D. (1997). Group 1 and 2 metabotropic glutamate receptors play differential roles in hippocampal long-term depression and long-term potentiation in freely moving rats. *J Neurosci, 17*(9), 3303-3311.

Manahan-Vaughan, D., & Braunewell, K. H. (1999). Novelty acquisition is associated with induction of hippocampal long-term depression. *Proc Natl Acad Sci U S A, 96*(15), 8739-8744.

Manahan-Vaughan, D., Braunewell, K. H., & Reymann, K. G. (1998). Subtype-specific involvement of metabotropic glutamate receptors in two forms of long-term potentiation in the dentate gyrus of freely moving rats. *Neuroscience, 86*(3), 709-721.

McNaughton, B. L., Barnes, C. A., Rao, G., Baldwin, J., & Rasmussen, M. (1986). Long-term enhancement of hippocampal synaptic transmission and the acquisition of spatial information. *J Neurosci, 6*(2), 563-571.

McNaughton, B. L., Douglas, R. M., & Goddard, G. V. (1978). Synaptic enhancement in fascia dentata: cooperativity among coactive afferents. *Brain Res, 157*(2), 277-293.

Mills, F., Bartlett, T. E., Dissing-Olesen, L., Wisniewska, M. B., Kuznicki, J., Macvicar, B. A., et al. (2014). Cognitive flexibility and long-term depression (LTD) are impaired following beta-catenin stabilization in vivo. *Proc Natl Acad Sci U S A, 111*(23), 8631-8636.

Montgomery, J. M., & Madison, D. V. (2002). State-dependent heterogeneity in synaptic depression between pyramidal cell pairs. *Neuron, 33*(5), 765-777.

Moosmang, S., Haider, N., Klugbauer, N., Adelsberger, H., Langwieser, N., Muller, J., et al. (2005). Role of hippocampal Cav1.2 Ca^{2+} channels in NMDA receptor-independent synaptic plasticity and spatial memory. *J Neurosci, 25*(43), 9883-9892.

Morgan, S. L., & Teyler, T. J. (2001). Electrical stimuli patterned after the theta-rhythm induce multiple forms of LTP. *J Neurophysiol, 86*(3), 1289-1296.

Morris, R. G., & Frey, U. (1997). Hippocampal synaptic plasticity: role in spatial learning or the automatic recording of attended experience? *Philos Trans R Soc Lond B Biol Sci, 352*(1360), 1489-1503.

Morris, R. G., Anderson, E., Lynch, G. S., & Baudry, M. (1986). Selective impairment of learning and blockade of long-term potentiation by an N-methyl-D-aspartate receptor antagonist, AP5. *Nature, 319*(6056), 774-776.

Moser, E. I. (1995). Learning-related changes in hippocampal field potentials. *Behav Brain Res, 71*(1-2), 11-18.

Moser, E. I. (1996). Altered inhibition of dentate granule cells during spatial learning in an exploration task. *J Neurosci, 16*(3), 1247-1259.

Moser, E. I., & Moser, M. B. (1999). Is learning blocked by saturation of synaptic weights in the hippocampus? *Neurosci Biobehav Rev, 23*(5), 661-672.

Moser, E. I., Krobert, K. A., Moser, M. B., & Morris, R. G. (1998). Impaired spatial learning after saturation of long-term potentiation. *Science, 281*(5385), 2038-2042.

Myers, C. E., & Scharfman, H. E. (2011). Pattern separation in the dentate gyrus: a role for the CA3 backprojection. *Hippocampus, 21*(11), 1190-1215.

Myers, K. M., & Davis, M. (2007). Mechanisms of fear extinction. *Mol Psychiatry, 12*(2), 120-150.

Naie, K., & Manahan-Vaughan, D. (2005). Pharmacological antagonism of metabotropic glutamate receptor 1 regulates long-term potentiation and spatial reference memory in the dentate gyrus of freely moving rats via N-methyl-D-aspartate and metabotropic glutamate receptor-dependent mechanisms. *Eur J Neurosci, 21*(2), 411-421.

Nakazawa, K., Quirk, M. C., Chitwood, R. A., Watanabe, M., Yeckel, M. F., Sun, L. D., et al. (2002). Requirement for hippocampal CA3 NMDA receptors in associative memory recall. *Science, 297*(5579), 211-218.

Nicholls, R. E., Alarcon, J. M., Malleret, G., Carroll, R. C., Grody, M., Vronskaya, S., et al. (2008). Transgenic mice lacking NMDAR-dependent LTD exhibit deficits in behavioral flexibility. *Neuron, 58*(1), 104-117.

Nicoll, R. A., & Schmitz, D. (2005). Synaptic plasticity at hippocampal mossy fibre synapses. *Nat Rev Neurosci, 6*(11), 863-876.

Niewoehner, B., Single, F. N., Hvalby, O., Jensen, V., Meyer zum Alten Borgloh, S., Seeburg, P. H., et al. (2007). Impaired spatial working memory but spared spatial reference memory following functional loss of NMDA receptors in the dentate gyrus. *Eur J Neurosci, 25*(3), 837-846.

Nowak, L., Bregestovski, P., Ascher, P., Herbet, A., & Prochiantz, A. (1984). Magnesium gates glutamate-activated channels in mouse central neurones. *Nature, 307*(5950), 462-465.

O'Keefe, J., & Conway, D. H. (1978). Hippocampal place units in the freely moving rat: why they fire where they fire. *Exp Brain Res, 31*(4), 573-590.

Otnaess, M. K., Brun, V. H., Moser, M. B., & Moser, E. I. (1999). Pretraining prevents spatial learning impairment after saturation of hippocampal long-term potentiation. *J Neurosci, 19*(24), RC49.

Palmer, M. J., Irving, A. J., Seabrook, G. R., Jane, D. E., & Collingridge, G. L. (1997). The group I mGlu receptor agonist DHPG induces a novel form of LTD in the CA1 region of the hippocampus. *Neuropharmacology, 36*(11-12), 1517-1532.

Pham, T. M., Soderstrom, S., Winblad, B., & Mohammed, A. H. (1999). Effects of environmental enrichment on cognitive function and hippocampal NGF in the non-handled rats. *Behav Brain Res, 103*(1), 63-70.

Poschel, B., & Manahan-Vaughan, D. (2007). Persistent (>24h) long-term depression in the dentate gyrus of freely moving rats is not dependent on activation of NMDA receptors, L-type voltage-gated calcium channels or protein synthesis. *Neuropharmacology, 52*(1), 46-54.

Poschel, B., & Stanton, P. K. (2007). Comparison of cellular mechanisms of long-term depression of synaptic strength at perforant path-granule cell and Schaffer collateral-CA1 synapses. *Prog Brain Res, 163*, 473-500.

Racine, R. J., Milgram, N. W., & Hafner, S. (1983). Long-term potentiation phenomena in the rat limbic forebrain. *Brain Res, 260*(2), 217-231.

Rolls, E. T. (2013). The mechanisms for pattern completion and pattern separation in the hippocampus. *Front Syst Neurosci, 7*, 74.

Rolls, E. T., & Kesner, R. P. (2006). A computational theory of hippocampal function, and empirical tests of the theory. *Prog Neurobiol, 79*(1), 1-48.

Rolls, E. T., Stringer, S. M., & Elliot, T. (2006). Entorhinal cortex grid cells can map to hippocampal place cells by competitive learning. *Network, 17*(4), 447-465.

Rosenzweig, E. S., & Barnes, C. A. (2003). Impact of aging on hippocampal function: plasticity, network dynamics, and cognition. *Prog Neurobiol, 69*(3), 143-179.

Roth-Alpermann, C., Morris, R. G., Korte, M., & Bonhoeffer, T. (2006). Homeostatic shutdown of long-term potentiation in the adult hippocampus. *Proc Natl Acad Sci U S A, 103*(29), 11039-11044.

Ryu, J., Futai, K., Feliu, M., Weinberg, R., & Sheng, M. (2008). Constitutively active Rap2 transgenic mice display fewer dendritic spines, reduced extracellular signal-regulated kinase signaling, enhanced long-term depression, and impaired spatial learning and fear extinction. *J Neurosci, 28*(33), 8178-8188.

Sacchetti, B., Lorenzini, C. A., Baldi, E., Bucherelli, C., Roberto, M., Tassoni, G., et al. (2001). Long-lasting hippocampal potentiation and contextual memory consolidation. *Eur J Neurosci, 13*(12), 2291-2298.

Saucier, D., & Cain, D. P. (1995). Spatial learning without NMDA receptor-dependent long-term potentiation. *Nature, 378*(6553), 186-189.

Saucier, D., Hargreaves, E. L., Boon, F., Vanderwolf, C. H., & Cain, D. P. (1996). Detailed behavioral analysis of water maze acquisition under systemic NMDA or muscarinic antagonism: nonspatial pretraining eliminates spatial learning deficits. *Behav Neurosci, 110*(1), 103-116.

Schmitt, W. B., Deacon, R. M., Seeburg, P. H., Rawlins, J. N., & Bannerman, D. M. (2003). A within-subjects, within-task demonstration of intact spatial reference memory and impaired spatial working memory in glutamate receptor-A-deficient mice. *J Neurosci, 23*(9), 3953-3959.

Schulz, K., & Korz, V. (2010). Emotional and cognitive information processing: relations to behavioral performance and hippocampal long-term potentiation in vivo during a spatial water maze training in rats. *Learn Mem, 17*(11), 552-560.

Sharp, P. E., McNaughton, B. L., & Barnes, C. A. (1985). Enhancement of hippocampal field potentials in rats exposed to a novel, complex environment. *Brain Res, 339*(2), 361-365.

Shimazu, K., Zhao, M., Sakata, K., Akbarian, S., Bates, B., Jaenisch, R., et al. (2006). NT-3 facilitates hippocampal plasticity and learning and memory by regulating neurogenesis. *Learn Mem, 13*(3), 307-315.

Staubli, U., & Scafidi, J. (1997). Studies on long-term depression in area CA1 of the anesthetized and freely moving rat. *J Neurosci, 17*(12), 4820-4828.

Steele, R. J., & Morris, R. G. (1999). Delay-dependent impairment of a matching-to-place task with chronic and intrahippocampal infusion of the NMDA-antagonist D-AP5. *Hippocampus, 9*(2), 118-136.

Stein, I. S., Donaldson, M. S., & Hell, J. W. (2014). CaMKII binding to GluN2B is important for massed spatial learning in the Morris water maze. *F1000Res, 3*, 193.

Straube, T., Korz, V., & Frey, J. U. (2003). Bidirectional modulation of long-term potentiation by novelty-exploration in rat dentate gyrus. *Neurosci Lett, 344*(1), 5-8.

Straube, T., Korz, V., Balschun, D., & Frey, J. U. (2003). Requirement of beta-adrenergic receptor activation and protein synthesis for LTP-reinforcement by novelty in rat dentate gyrus. *J Physiol, 552*(Pt 3), 953-960.

Tai, C. Y., Mysore, S. P., Chiu, C., & Schuman, E. M. (2007). Activity-regulated N-cadherin endocytosis. *Neuron, 54*(5), 771-785.

Tang, Y. P., Shimizu, E., Dube, G. R., Rampon, C., Kerchner, G. A., Zhuo, M., et al. (1999). Genetic enhancement of learning and memory in mice. *Nature, 401*(6748), 63-69.

Tang, Y. P., Wang, H., Feng, R., Kyin, M., & Tsien, J. Z. (2001). Differential effects of enrichment on learning and memory function in NR2B transgenic mice. *Neuropharmacology, 41*(6), 779-790.

Teskey, G. C., & Valentine, P. A. (1998). Post-activation potentiation in the neocortex of awake freely moving rats. *Neurosci Biobehav Rev, 22*(2), 195-207.

Tsien, J. Z., Huerta, P. T., & Tonegawa, S. (1996). The essential role of hippocampal CA1 NMDA receptor-dependent synaptic plasticity in spatial memory. *Cell, 87*(7), 1327-1338.

Uekita, T., Okaichi, Y., & Okaichi, H. (2006). Dissociation of the roles of NMDA receptor and hippocampus in rats' spatial learning: the effects of environmental familiarity and task familiarity. *Rev Neurosci, 17*(1-2), 163-173.

Uzakov, S., Frey, J. U., & Korz, V. (2005). Reinforcement of rat hippocampal LTP by holeboard training. *Learn Mem, 12*(2), 165-171.

Wang, D., Cui, Z., Zeng, Q., Kuang, H., Wang, L. P., Tsien, J. Z., et al. (2009). Genetic enhancement of memory and long-term potentiation but not CA1 long-term depression in NR2B transgenic rats. *PLoS One, 4*(10), e7486.

Wang, G. W., & Cai, J. X. (2006). Disconnection of the hippocampal-prefrontal cortical circuits impairs spatial working memory performance in rats. *Behav Brain Res, 175*(2), 329-336.

Whishaw, I. Q., & Jarrard, L. E. (1996). Evidence for extrahippocampal involvement in place learning and hippocampal involvement in path integration. *Hippocampus, 6*(5), 513-524.

Whishaw, I. Q., Cassel, J. C., & Jarrad, L. E. (1995). Rats with fimbria-fornix lesions display a place response in a swimming pool: a dissociation between getting there and knowing where. *J Neurosci, 15*(8), 5779-5788.

Whitlock, J. R., Heynen, A. J., Shuler, M. G., & Bear, M. F. (2006). Learning induces long-term potentiation in the hippocampus. *Science, 313*(5790), 1093-1097.

Wigstrom, H., & Gustafsson, B. (1986). Postsynaptic control of hippocampal long-term potentiation. *J Physiol (Paris), 81*(4), 228-236.

Williams, J. H., Errington, M. L., Lynch, M. A., & Bliss, T. V. (1989). Arachidonic acid induces a long-term activity-dependent enhancement of synaptic transmission in the hippocampus. *Nature, 341*(6244), 739-742.

Wilson, D. A. (1984). A comparison of the postnatal development of post-activation potentiation in the neocortex and dentate gyrus of the rat. *Brain Res, 318*(1), 61-68.

Wilson, I. A., Ikonen, S., Gallagher, M., Eichenbaum, H., & Tanila, H. (2005). Age-associated alterations of hippocampal place cells are subregion specific. *J Neurosci, 25*(29), 6877-6886.

Wilson, M. A., & McNaughton, B. L. (1993). Dynamics of the hippocampal ensemble code for space. *Science, 261*(5124), 1055-1058.

Witter, M. P. (1993). Organization of the entorhinal-hippocampal system: a review of current anatomical data. *Hippocampus, 3 Spec No*, 33-44.

Xu, L., Anwyl, R., & Rowan, M. J. (1997). Behavioural stress facilitates the induction of long-term depression in the hippocampus. *Nature, 387*(6632), 497-500.

Xu, L., Anwyl, R., & Rowan, M. J. (1998). Spatial exploration induces a persistent reversal of long-term potentiation in rat hippocampus. *Nature, 394*(6696), 891-894.

Yang, S., Megill, A., Ardiles, A. O., Ransom, S., Tran, T., Koh, M. T., et al. (2013). Integrity of mGluR-LTD in the associative/commissural inputs to CA3 correlates with successful aging in rats. *J Neurosci, 33*(31), 12670-12678.

Zakharenko, S. S., Patterson, S. L., Dragatsis, I., Zeitlin, S. O., Siegelbaum, S. A., Kandel, E. R., et al. (2003). Presynaptic BDNF required for a presynaptic but not postsynaptic component of LTP at hippocampal CA1-CA3 synapses. *Neuron, 39*(6), 975-990.

Zakharenko, S. S., Zablow, L., & Siegelbaum, S. A. (2001). Visualization of changes in presynaptic function during long-term synaptic plasticity. *Nat Neurosci, 4*(7), 711-717.

Zalutsky, R. A., & Nicoll, R. A. (1990). Comparison of two forms of long-term potentiation in single hippocampal neurons. *Science, 248*(4963), 1619-1624.

Zamanillo, D., Sprengel, R., Hvalby, O., Jensen, V., Burnashev, N., Rozov, A., et al. (1999). Importance of AMPA receptors for hippocampal synaptic plasticity but not for spatial learning. *Science, 284*(5421), 1805-1811.

Zhang, J., Wang, C., Deng, T., Xue, Z., Chen, X., Chang, L., et al. (2013). The preventive effect of NR2B and NR2D-containing NMDAR antagonists on Abeta-induced LTP disruption in the dentate gyrus of rats. *Metab Brain Dis, 28*(4), 697-704.

Zhang, M., & Wang, H. (2013). Mice overexpressing type 1 adenylyl cyclase show enhanced spatial memory flexibility in the absence of intact synaptic long-term depression. *Learn Mem, 20*(7), 352-357.

Zhang, X. H., Liu, S. S., Yi, F., Zhuo, M., & Li, B. M. (2013). Delay-dependent impairment of spatial working memory with inhibition of NR2B-containing NMDA receptors in hippocampal CA1 region of rats. *Mol Brain, 6*, 13.

Zhao, M. G., Toyoda, H., Lee, Y. S., Wu, L. J., Ko, S. W., Zhang, X. H., et al. (2005). Roles of NMDA NR2B subtype receptor in prefrontal long-term potentiation and contextual fear memory. *Neuron, 47*(6), 859-872.

In: Synaptic Fundamentals of Memory Performance
Editor: Ignacio González-Burgos
ISBN: 978-1-63483-279-3

Chapter 5

CONSOLIDATION, RETRIEVAL, AND EXTINCTION: DISSIMILAR MOLECULAR REQUIREMENTS

Sofía González-Salinas, Gina Lorena Quirarte, Andrea Cristina Medina and Roberto Agustín Prado-Alcalá*

Laboratorio de Aprendizaje y Memoria, Departamento de Neurobiología Conductual y Cognitiva, Instituto de Neurobiología, Universidad Nacional Autónoma de México, Campus Juriquilla, Querétaro, México

ABSTRACT

Memory is an essential process that allows animals to adapt to their environment. This process has several stages in which learned information is acquired, stored, retrieved, and it is susceptible to extinction. In this chapter, we will mention the principal concepts used in the field of memory, and we will talk about the neurobiological features common to the different stages of memory, and about characteristics that differentiate them. In spite of the attributes that have been proposed to characterize each of the memory stages, it seems that the relative importance of particular mechanisms correlates with the strength of learning. A growing body of evidence shows that typical treatments that impede memory consolidation of learning mediated by low or moderate degrees of training, become innocuous when learning results from high degrees of training. These dissimilar training-dependent effects illustrate how far we still are from understanding the rules that govern consolidation, retrieval, and extinction of learned behaviors.

Keywords: memory, stress, hormones, neurotransmitters, molecular biology

* Send correspondence to: Roberto Agustín Prado-Alcalá, PhD; Laboratorio de Aprendizaje y Memoria, Departamento de Neurobiología Conductual y Cognitiva, Instituto de Neurobiología, Universidad Nacional Autónoma de México, Campus Juriquilla, Querétaro 76230, Qro. México. Email: prado@unam.mx.

1. Introduction

Daily experiences can modify behavior in a more or less permanent way, as evidenced by the learning of information derived from such experiences. In order for this information to persist and be available for future use, it must be stored in what is known as long-term memory (Kandel et al., 2000). Learning and memory are processes that come about in a natural way in humans and other animals that possess the adequate neurobiological machinery (McGaugh, 1973).

2. Categories of Memory

Initially based on records from patients with brain damage and subsequently on experimental data provided by animal models, memory has been classified in a number of ways; one is based on the kind of information that is stored, i.e., declarative and procedural (Squire, 1986). Thus, the contents of declarative memory include facts and concepts (semantic memory) or events and personal experiences (episodic memory), such as the names of Latin American countries and their capital cities or recalling things we did during last year´s trip to the mountains. On the other hand, procedural (or implicit) memory refers to skills and the storage of classical and instrumental learning. Riding a bicycle or playing a piano is an example of behaviors that depend on procedural memory.

Another widely used classification of memory is based on its duration. Short-term memory (STM) may last seconds or just a few hours, whereas long-term memory (LTM) may last for hours, months, years, and even for a lifetime (McGaugh, 2000). LTM, in turn, has several stages: acquisition (or learning), consolidation, and retrieval. A closely related process is extinction, by which the performance of a learned behavior can be diminished. All of these processes have distinct behavioral, biochemical, and molecular signatures, although they may share some of them, as described below.

During acquisition or learning, new information is generally obtained from an experience in a particular context and is initially stored in STM; in the course of consolidation this information is transferred to LTM. The only objective manner by which memory can be shown to exist is through retrieval, expressed as changes in behavior after learning has occurred. Retrieval is an important process because, depending on the consequences of the behavior, it can lead to strengthening or to weakening of the learned response. In the latter case, if behavior is performed in the absence of the stimulus that was associated with the response (for example, food, foot-shock, social approval), then extinction ensues, i.e., the intensity or frequency of the response will diminish and may, eventually, disappear for a period of time. Extinction is considered a new learning, in which animals learn not to respond when there are no important consequences; this process sets in motion some of the machinery of consolidation to form a new memory (Szapiro et al., 2002), although not all of the molecular details are shared by these processes (Tronson et al., 2012).

3. Rodents As Good Models to Study Emotional Memories

Rodents, especially mice and rats, are the animals used most frequently to study the biochemical and cellular basis of the different memory stages (Abel & Lattal, 2001). These rodents offer several advantages for such studies: they can learn relatively simple behavioral tasks in a short period of time (Buccafusco, 2009), and most of the cerebral regions involved in these tasks have a structural equivalent in the human brain (Bayer et al., 1993); also, about 79% of the genes related to neurological functions show a conserved expression pattern in mice and humans (Zeng et al., 2012).

Techniques used in rodents for the study of memory processes include manipulations of the brain through lesions, administration of drugs, electrical recordings, and molecular analyses. Behavioral tasks used most frequently in this field include spatial navigation (e.g., T-maze, Barnes maze, and Morris water maze), and emotional tasks (e. g., inhibitory and active avoidance, contextual and cued fear conditioning, and conditioned taste aversion); for a description of the procedural details of some of the tasks see Buccafusco (2009).

In this chapter, we will focus on tasks that have an emotional aversive component. We will also discuss how memory stages are modulated by hormones and neurotransmitters released after stressful experiences. The study of emotional memories has received a great deal of attention, because it may shed light on psychological disorders that are produced by traumatic events and are characterized by repetitious, disturbing memories that are very hard to eradicate. One such disorder is post-traumatic stress disorder (PTSD). Contextual fear conditioning seems to be a good model for the study of this pathology because, as in the case of PTSD, it is produced by pairing an emotionally neutral context (environment) with an aversive, negative experience (Milad & Quirk, 2012). A typical experiment involves placing a mouse or a rat inside a small chamber with a grid floor, and then it receives one or several foot-shocks. When the animal is later returned to the chamber, a freezing behavior that may last for several months is observed (Rau & Fanselow, 2009). Inhibitory and active avoidance tasks are also good models of PTSD, due to the relatively long-lasting aversive memory they produce (Edo Izquierdo et al., 1994; Roldán-Roldán et al., 2001; Zoladz et al., 2010). In the former, the animal learns not to return to a place where it was punished previously; in the latter, the animal learns to perform a response to get away from a place where it was previously punished.

4. The ABC of Stress

An important reason for studying emotional memories is that they may lead us to understand the role of molecules released during a stressful situation, to determine how molecular mechanisms required for the formation of that memory are initiated, and to begin to identify the brain regions involved. A stressor can be defined as any circumstance, object, or experience that exerts a real or potential negative effect on the integrity of an individual; the stressor induces rapid bodily changes in the organism that allows it to cope with the current situation, as well as delayed changes that will be useful in the future (Jöels & Baram, 2009).

In general, physical stressors, such as blood loss, respiratory stress, cold, and pain, recruit the activity of the brain stem and the hypothalamus (Ulrich-Lai & Herman, 2009), whereas psychological stressors, such as the presence of a predator, or the exposure to a context that was associated with an aversive experience, engage cerebral structures related to emotions (amygdala, prefrontal cortex, hippocampus, insular cortex), decision making (prefrontal cortex, striatum), and memory (hippocampus, amygdala, prefrontal cortex, striatum, insular cortex) (Sanders et al., 2003; Phelps & LeDoux, 2005; Miranda et al., 2008; Sierra-Mercado et al., 2011; Flores & Disterhoft, 2013; Lozano et al., 2013).

Stress molecules are released from the adrenal gland; the hormones epinephrine and norepinephrine are secreted by the adrenal medulla, while corticosteroids are released from the adrenal cortex (Rodrigues et al., 2009; Riedemann et al., 2010). Epinephrine does not cross the blood-brain barrier, but it can activate vagal afferent fibers that will induce the release of norepinephrine in brain regions such as the amygdala (Roozendaal et al., 2009).

There are two types of corticosteroids: glucocorticoids (corticosterone and cortisol) and mineralocorticoids (aldosterone and deoxycorticosterone) (Arlt & Stewart, 2005). corticosterone is the glucocorticoid present in rodents, while in humans cortisol predominates, but a small amount of corticosterone (10-20 fold lower levels compared to cortisol) is also found in humans (Steckler et al., 2005).

When released from the adrenal cortex, corticosterone is transported to the brain by way of p-glycoprotein (Karssen et al., 2001). Once it has crossed the blood-brain barrier, corticosterone may activate two types of receptors, namely, the high affinity mineralocorticoid receptors and the glucocorticoid receptors with 10-fold lower affinity (Reul & de Kloet, 1985).

5. Acquisition and Consolidation Are Interwoven through Enzymatic Activity, Neurotransmitter Systems, and Hormones

It is beyond the scope of this chapter to review exhaustively the known molecules that participate in learning and memory processes, so we will offer only a brief overview of some of the most-studied messengers.

The information derived from a learning experience (visual, tactile, auditory, contextual, noxious stimulation, etc.), produces fast cellular events which are initiated at the neuronal membrane; this information is then transferred, through different biochemical codes, to distinct neuronal compartments in specific brain regions. Figure 1 depicts the cellular events involved in memory that are triggered by the activation of neuronal membrane receptors, and Table I summarizes the molecular events that participate in the different stages of memory and extinction. The main mechanism that allows for propagation of information along neuronal pathways is the release of neurotransmitters. Neurotransmitters are molecules released from the presynaptic neuron subsequent to an electrochemical event; these molecules will activate receptors located in the postsynaptic neuron, but sometimes they can act at the presynapse itself (Figure 1:1).

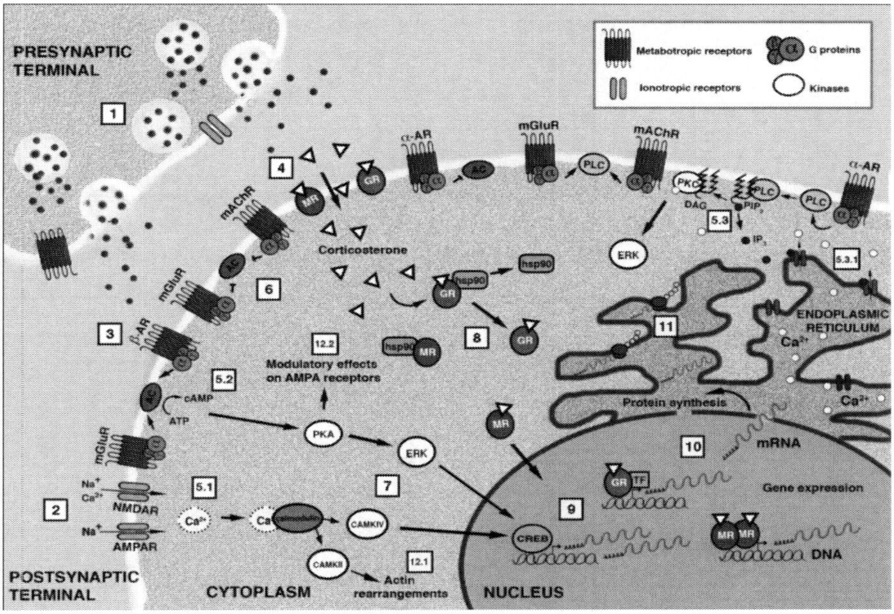

Figure 1. Trans-synaptic localization of the molecular events participating in memory. Neurotransmitters are released from the presynaptic terminal (1) and bind to the appropriate ionotropic (2) or metabotropic (3) receptors localized in the postsynaptic terminal. Corticosterone can freely diffuse through the membrane and also can activate membrane receptors (4). The activation of the membrane receptors transduces their signal by means of second messengers such as calcium (5.1), cAMP (5.2), DAG and IP_3 (5.3). IP_3 will later activate receptors localized in the endoplasmic reticulum that will release calcium into the cytoplasm (5.3.1). G proteins, which are coupled to metabotropic receptors, will interact with membrane enzymes like adenylate cyclase (AC) and phospholipase C (PLC) (6). The second messengers will activate a variety of kinases such as PKA, PKC, ERK, CAMKII, and CAMKIV (7). Cytosolic glucocorticoid (GR) and mineralocorticoid (MR) receptors are kept inactive by the heat shock protein 90 (hsp90) until corticosterone binds to them, allowing them to translocate to the nucleus (8). Transcription factors (TF) will induce the expression of diverse genes (9); the corresponding mRNAs (10) will be sent to the endoplasmic reticulum to be translated into proteins (11). The intracellular activity initiated by the presynaptic neurotransmitters will produce actin rearrangements (12.1) and modulation of membrane receptors like the AMPAR (12.2).

As stated above, once learning has occurred, this new information can be stored in the short-lived, labile STM store. To become stable, the information derived from the learning experience must be transferred to a longer-lasting store, the LTM store. This transfer of information takes place through memory consolidation, a time-dependent process that may be affected by different pharmacological and physical interventions (Dudai, 2004). According to McGaugh (2000), memory consolidation may have an adaptive role because, in spite of its limited duration, the neurophysiological processes activated by an experience can modulate the intensity with which an event can be recalled. Sometimes it is difficult to differentiate between elements that participate exclusively in acquisition from those in consolidation, because some are required for both processes (Mayford et al., 1996; Galindo et al., 2008) and because of methodological issues (Abel & Lattal, 2001). For this reason we will discuss learning and consolidation in the same section, and we suggest readers to refer directly to the references given above for a close view of these issues.

Table 1. Molecular requirements for memory

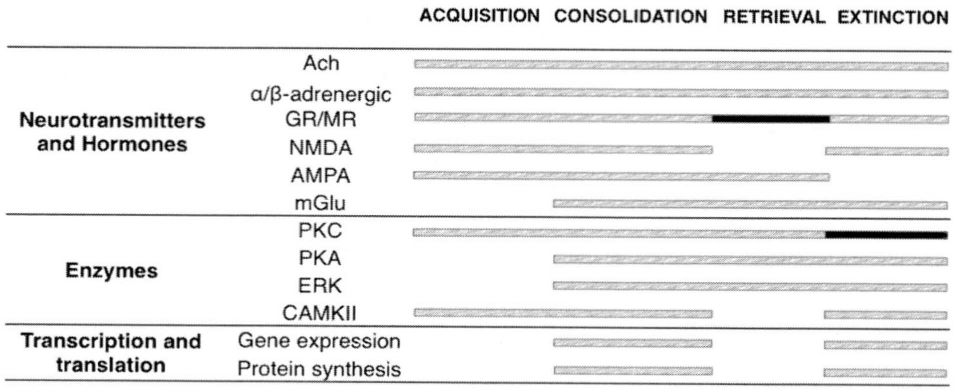

The gray lines depict the elements required for acquisition, consolidation, retrieval, and/or extinction. The gaps mean that those elements are not needed for acquisition retrieval or extinction; the black segments show the elements that are required, but have a negative effect on retrieval or extinction.

5.1. Neurotransmitters

The effect of neurotransmitters propagates by activating membrane receptors. In the cellular membrane there are ionotropic and metabotropic receptors; the former are channels composed by multiple subunits that allow the entry of ions, such as Na+, K+, Ca^{2+}, and Cl^{-}, and produce, within a matter of milliseconds, ionic currents that end when the neurotransmitters are uncoupled from their receptors (Figure 1: 2). Metabotropic receptors are proteins that have seven transmembrane domains; they have a slower but longer-lasting effect that involves the activity of G proteins that will engage the activity of several enzymes located inside the neuron (Figure 1: 3, 6). Ionotropic and metabotropic receptors trigger signaling cascades that will reach the neuronal nucleus, producing long-term changes such as cytoarchitectonic remodeling and receptor relocalization.

There is an extensive literature regarding the involvement of neurotransmitters in memory processes, including acetylcholine (Gold, 2003), dopamine (El-Ghundi et al., 2011), noradrenaline (Kobayashi & Yasoshima, 2001); serotonin (Meneses & Liv-Salmeron, 2012), and gamma-aminobutyric acid (GABA) (Makkar et al., 2010) systems. Plastic changes in neurons will be produced by only those neurotransmitters that are released in sites with an appropriate number of receptors with sufficient affinity for them (Jöels & Baram, 2009). We shall get back to this issue later in the chapter focusing in the glutamate, cholinergic and noradrenergic systems.

Immediately after a stressful situation, the levels of dopamine, serotonin, noradrenalin, and other neurotransmitters increase in various cerebral regions, including the hippocampus, amygdala, and prefrontal cortex (Quirarte et al., 1998; Goto et al., 2007; Linthorst & Reul, 2008).

Lesions of noradrenergic tracts have been shown to produce learning impairments in different tasks (Everitt et al., 1983; Cole & Robbins, 1987). Subsequent studies showed that intra-amygdala injection of noradrenaline facilitates memory consolidation and that α- and β-adrenoceptor antagonists produce impairment of consolidation (Ferry et al., 1999; Hatfield & McGaugh, 1999). In a similar way, studies addressing the participation of acetylcholine in memory have shown that this neurotransmitter is required for acquisition, consolidation, and retrieval (Prado-Alcalá et al., 1985; McIntyre et al., 1998; Szapiro et al., 2000; Wallenstein & Vago, 2001; Rogers & Kesner, 2003; Barros et al., 2004).

During learning, it seems that glutamate acts mainly through its ionotropic NMDA and AMPA receptors, and that during consolidation the metabotropic mGlu receptors become in charge of information processing, while NMDA and AMPA receptors appear to have a less important role in the formation of LTM (Atkins et al., 1998; Riedel et al., 2003). Thus, the noradrenergic, cholinergic, and glutamatergic systems are all required for learning and memory consolidation.

5.2. Stress Hormones

Stress molecules can enhance learning, and sometimes the effects are observed on consolidation after a memory test. The delivery of a small number of tail-shocks 1 day before eye-blink conditioning did not affect learning, while enhanced stress induced by a higher number of tail-shocks improved acquisition (Beylin & Shors, 1998). Importantly, Beylin & Shors (2003) showed that this facilitated eye-blink conditioned learning depended on the presence of intact adrenal glands, particularly on corticosterone. Other studies have shown that the administration of a foot-shock two days before fear conditioning did not affect learning; however, when the same animals were evaluated 24 hours later, they showed memory facilitation (Cordero et al., 2003). These results show that the effects of stress on acquisition depend on the number of presentations of the stressor prior to learning, and particularly on corticosterone, as in the case of eye-blink conditioning mentioned above, and that stress does not always produce immediate effects on behavior, as it can have delayed effects on memory stabilization.

Corticosterone is also importantly involved in consolidation of emotionally arousing experiences. It has been shown that blockade of corticosterone receptors or of corticosterone biosynthesis impairs consolidation, and that activation of corticosterone receptors facilitates memory consolidation of mildly stressful and appetitive experiences (Roozendaal & McGaugh, 1997; Sandi et al., 1997; Miranda et al., 2008; Barsegyan et al., 2010).

Brain regions with a low density of glucocorticoid receptors also modulate memory consolidation. For example, we have shown that in the dorsal striatum administration of corticosterone enhances consolidation (Medina et al., 2007). The effect of corticosterone depends upon the type of memory being studied; procedural memory is improved but spatial memory is not, thus supporting the known role of the dorsal striatum in procedural memories (Quirarte et al., 2009). However, because of its connections with the hippocampus, infusion of corticosterone specifically into the dorso-medial portion of the striatum can facilitate spatial memory but not procedural memory, showing that pharmacological studies addressing smaller sub-regions can reveal a multimodal role of certain brain regions (Lozano et al., 2013).

5.3. Second Messengers and Enzymes

During acquisition (learning), activation of the different types of membrane receptors promotes the action of second messengers like Ca^{2+}, cyclic adenosine monophosphate (cAMP), diacylglycerol (DAG), and inositol triphosphate (Figure 1: 5.1, 5.2, 5.3). When Ca^{2+} enters the cell it can adhere to calmodulin which, in turn, activates proteins such as calcium/calmodulin-dependent protein kinase II (CAMKII) and calcium/calmodulin-dependent protein kinase IV (CAMKIV) (Wang et al., 2006) (Figure 1: 7). Kinases are proteins that add phosphate groups to other proteins; this change will usually activate the tagged proteins.

Using pharmacogenetic tools, it was found that increased activity of CAMKII produces deterioration in acquisition and consolidation of water maze and fear conditioning tasks (Mayford et al., 1996; Bejar et al., 2002). Behavioral tests of transgenic mice that have reduced CAMKIV activity showed that this enzyme is not required during learning, but is needed to consolidate memories (Kang et al., 2001).

The aforementioned second messengers also promote the activation of the enzymes protein kinase C (PKC), protein kinase A (PKA), and mitogen activated protein kinases (MAPKs) (Figure 1: 7). PKC is needed for acquisition and consolidation, while PKA seems to be required only during consolidation (Paylor et al., 1991; Noguès et al., 1996; Abel et al., 1997; Schafe & Le Deux, 2000; Vianna et al., 2000). MAPKs, and specifically the extracellular signal-regulated kinase (ERK) sub-family, have been broadly studied in different paradigms and stages of memory. Many neurotransmitters and molecular cascades activate ERK; in turn, ERK acts on transcription factors that are also required to consolidate memories (Peng et al., 2010). Studies using pharmacological treatments have consistently shown that the phosphorylation of ERK is not needed during acquisition but is required to consolidate different memories, such as those formed by contextual and tone fear conditioning (Atkins et al., 1998; Schafe et al., 2000) and the water maze with hidden platform (Blum et al., 1999). Even though drugs blocking ERK phosphorylation do not seem to affect learning, the phosphorylation of ERK is increased as early as 5 minutes after the learning experience; ERK phosphorylation is most commonly detected at 1 hour after training, but the activation kinetics depends on the brain region and the behavioral paradigm under study (Atkins et al., 1998; Blum et al., 1999; Schafe et al., 2000). These studies suggest that ERK becomes active after learning and allows long-term storage of information. Participation of ERK is particularly important in memory consolidation, since it has a direct impact on the expression of genes, thus giving rise to long-term changes (Peng et al., 2010), such as the formation of new dendritic spines, which may represent a substrate for LTM (Sweatt, 2004).

6. Nuclear Activity and Memory Consolidation

The intracellular signals that are triggered during acquisition and later in consolidation must reach the nucleus of the neuron in order to promote stable changes that will result in long-term memory storage. The requirement of gene expression and *de novo* protein synthesis, deduced by using drugs that block these processes, are key features of consolidation that are not shared with learning. The production of proteins depends on two main processes: transcription, which is the synthesis of RNA from a DNA template, and translation, the assembly of a protein from messenger RNA (mRNA).

Inside the nucleus, transcription factors interact with specific regions of DNA and with the RNA polymerase to bring about the synthesis of mRNA from specific genes (Alberini, 2009) (Figure 1: 9, 10). One of the most studied transcription factors in memory is the cAMP-response element binding protein (CREB). CREB is constitutively expressed and becomes active after being phosphorylated by proteins like ERK and CAMKIV; this transcription factor has attracted attention in the field because it has been shown that the neurons that are recruited during learning to form the memory are those that express higher levels of CREB (Han et al., 2007). The mRNA synthesized in response to CREB or another transcription factors is later edited and sent to the cytoplasm (Figure 1: 9,10), where this nucleotide message is translated into *de novo* proteins that are necessary for remodeling synapses that participate in stabilizing memory (Kandel, 2001) (Figure 1: 11, 12.1, 12.2). These cellular changes that occur during consolidation are known as synaptic consolidation (Dudai, 2004).

Gene expression is necessary at different moments during the consolidation process; the administration of transcription inhibitors indicates that gene expression is necessary around the time of training and within 3-6 hours after learning in order for consolidation to proceed, and the same temporal window was found when a protein synthesis inhibitor (PSI) was studied (Igaz et al., 2002).

Furthermore, it has been found that after learning, there is an increase in the expression of genes involved in transcription and synaptic remodeling, such as *camk2a, camk2b, grm7, snca, stx1a, bdnf, lrp3,* and *chrm2*, and immediate early genes such as *zif268, arc, homer1a*, and *c-fos* (Igaz et al., 2004; O'Sullivan et al., 2007; Sakaguchi & Hayashi, 2012).

Importantly, it has been reported that changes in gene expression correlate negatively with the degree of learning. Several genes are expressed when animals perform at a 50% level in an operant task, whereas less expression is observed when they have reached a 100% response level (Rapanelli et al., 2009, 2010). Similarly, rats trained for only one session in the spatial version of the water maze show a higher expression of *arc, zif268,* and *c-fos* in the hippocampus as compared with rats trained for seven sessions (Guzowski et al., 2001). These results suggest that greater changes in gene expression are required when the subjects are in the process of learning a task than later, when they have acquired all the necessary skills to perform the task.

7. Molecules to Access Memory

One way to confirm that a memory has been successfully stored is to access the stored information, which is accomplished by way of a process called retrieval. During retrieval, the stored information related to an event, the current context, and the mood we are in influence the strength of the recollection (Tulving & Thomson, 1973). Retrieving a memory may lead to strengthening of that memory, to its modification by adding new information, or to extinction (Eisenberg et al., 2003; Rodriguez-Ortiz et al., 2005).

Recalling the name of an acquaintance, a telephone number, or an address happens in a matter of milliseconds or in just a few seconds; such an extraordinary capacity is the result of the workings of neuronal mechanisms that do their job within that same time interval. The activity of cholinergic, AMPA, and mGlu receptors is required to retrieve a memory; these same activities are required during consolidation (Prado-Alcalá et al., 1985; Szapiro et al., 2000; Barros et al., 2004). Opposite to what happens during consolidation, NMDA receptors may not participate actively in retrieval (Liang et al., 1996; Barros et al., 2000; Bast et al., 2005).

A stressful event before retrieval causes a retrieval deficit, showing that those molecules released during the stress play an active role in retrieving information (de Quervain et al., 1998). Activation of β-adrenergic receptors in the amygdala and the hippocampus is important in modulating the negative effects that glucocorticoids exert on retrieval (Roozendaal et al., 2004). As mentioned above, the effects of stress on memory formation depend on multiple factors such as the particular stress molecule and its concentration prior to retrieval.

Some authors propose that corticosterone exerts rapid effects on consolidation and retrieval by means of membrane receptors; this hormone also exerts late effects that depend on activation of intracellular receptors (Barsegyan et al., 2010; Chauveau et al., 2010) (Figure 1: 4). It is worth noting that stress may have opposite effects on retrieval and consolidation; whereas stress can facilitate consolidation, it may impair retrieval (Roozendaal, 2002).

The activity of the enzymes PKA, PKC, and ERK is required for memory retrieval as well as for consolidation, and it seems that CAMKII activity is needed only for consolidation (Szapiro et al., 2000; Vianna et al., 2000; Huang et al., 2010). These enzymes work on a time scale of minutes, as opposed to the activation of membrane receptors and channels which takes place in milliseconds or just a few seconds. Thus, enzymatic activity is unlikely to have an impact on memory retrieval, which may take just a few seconds, as mentioned by Cammarotaet al., (2004).

Consistent with the pharmacological studies described above, it has been observed that retrieval induces phosphorylation of the enzymes PKA, ERK, and MSK1; the latter is regulated by the MAPK pathway (Huang et al., 2010; Myskiw et al., 2010; Besnard et al., 2013). Interestingly, the study of Besnardet al., (2013) showed that the changes in phosphorylation after retrieval are smaller than those observed after training; this may be due to the context conditions that characterize each stage (training-foot-shock in context, retrieval-no foot-shock in context).

Although interfering with CAMKII activity does not affect retrieval (Szapiro et al., 2000), this enzyme becomes active after animals are subjected to a memory test (Myskiw et al., 2010). The increase in enzymatic activity of CAMKII after the animals were re-exposed to the learning environment will affect other processes that are engaged during retrieval that will be described later.

While the blockade of transcription and protein synthesis does not affect retrieval (Vianna et al., 2003), recalling an experience induces nuclear activity. This has been shown by increases in phosphorylation of the histone H3 (Besnard et al., 2013) which, together with other proteins and DNA, gives rise to chromatin. The activity of the transcription factor CREB, gene expression (e.g., *arc* and *zif268*), and protein synthesis (e.g., c-Fos, Zif268, and Arc) are also increased during retrieval (Hall et al., 2001a, 2001b; Gusev et al., 2005; Besnard et al., 2013).

8. Modifying Behavior through Extinction

The making of a memory is not finished after consolidation, because reactivation of a memory can open the gates to plasticity. It is thought that because of retrieval, the contents of a consolidated memory can be changed, and even erased, by a hypothetical process called reconsolidation (Nader & Einarsson, 2010). In addition, a consolidated, learned behavior performed in the absence of the unconditioned (or reinforcing) stimulus that was initially associated with that behavior may produce a new learning, called extinction, whereby its strength or frequency declines (Pavlov, 1927). Spontaneous recovery, renewal, reinstatement, and fast reacquisition are behavioral manipulations that indicate that extinction is a new learning that does not erase the original learning but, instead, impedes its expression (Quirk & Mueller, 2007).

The outcome that prevails during retrieval depends on the duration and number of re-exposures to the context where the learning took place. If the number of retrieval sessions is small or the re-exposure time is brief, then the original memory trace will predominate, and it may be susceptible to reconsolidation. Conversely, if the number of retrieval episodes is high or if the time of re-exposure to the context is also high, then the trace of extinction will predominate (Eisenberg et al., 2003; Pedreira & Maldonado, 2003; Suzuki et al., 2004; Mamiya et al., 2009).

Extinction takes place in three phases, just as in other forms of learning: acquisition, consolidation, and retrieval, and it entails the formation of a new memory whose main neural substrate includes the hippocampus, amygdala, and the prefrontal cortex (Quirk & Mueller, 2007). Some of the molecules required for extinction, such as the neurotransmitters glutamate, noradrenaline, and stress hormones, are also involved in consolidation of the original memory.

Blockade of the mGlu and NMDA receptors impedes extinction as well as consolidation (Falls et al., 1992; Lin et al., 2003; Kim et al., 2007; Sotres-Bayon et al., 2007). Unlike consolidation, extinction seems not to require AMPA receptors as their blockade in the amygdala does not interfere with memory of this type of learning (Falls et al., 1992; Lin et al., 2003).

Regarding acetylcholine, numerous reports indicate that extinction learning is highly dependent upon the activity of this neurotransmitter, as shown by the facilitation and impediment produced by cholinergic agonists and antagonists, respectively; these effects have been found after systemic and localized injections into particular brain structures, such as the amygdala, infralimbic cortex, and hippocampus (Prado-Alcalá et al., 1994; Roldán-Roldán et al., 2001; Boccia et al., 2009; Tronson et al., 2009; Santini et al., 2012).

As occurs during consolidation, noradrenaline, and corticosterone allow extinction to take place. The administration of noradrenaline into the amygdala facilitates extinction and the use of systemic or intra-amygdala glucocorticoids agonists also facilitated extinction (Yang et al., 2005; Berlau & McGaugh, 2006).

Gene expression and protein synthesis are also required for behavioral extinction. It seems that the temporal window for these cellular functions that occur during extinction is shorter than during consolidation since treatment with inhibitors of transcription and of protein synthesis interfere with the behavior when administered 15 minutes before, but not when administered 1 or 3 hours after the first extinction session (Vianna et al., 2003). This suggests that during extinction, there is a limited period of time to renew the information derived from the novel experience because neuronal changes happen rapidly. Increased expression of mRNAs for *arc* and *bdnf*, and in the protein levels of CFos, Zif268, and the $GABA_A$ receptor have been found in the amygdala after the beginning of extinction (Herry & Mons, 2004; Chhatwal et al., 2005, 2006; Mamiya et al., 2009).

Enzymatic activity of PKA, ERK, and CAMKII is necessary for extinction (Szapiro et al., 2003; Herry et al., 2006; Myskiw et al., 2010). Contrary to what is observed in acquisition, consolidation, and retrieval, the blockade of PKC facilitates extinction (Tronson et al., 2007).

8.1. The Protective Effect of Enhanced Training

Studies focused on measuring specific proteins, and those where the machinery of transcription and translation was affected have led to the proposal that protein synthesis is required to consolidate memories (Alberini, 2008; Gkogkas et al., 2010). Other studies have found several time-points (windows) sensitive to the disrupting effects of protein synthesis inhibitors (PSIs); for example, Igazet al., (2002) reported that the temporal window during which protein synthesis participates in consolidating inhibitory avoidance is the same as in transcription, i.e., around training and 3-6 hours after conditioning.

In recent years a discussion about the participation of protein synthesis in consolidation has emerged, where the side effects of most of the antibiotics used to inhibit protein synthesis being the main argument against protein synthesis being essential for consolidation (Martinez et al., 1981; Routtenberg & Rekart, 2005; Alberini, 2008; Gold, 2008). Side effects of PSIs include massive release of neurotransmitters, silencing of neuronal activity, increased activity of some kinases, and over-induction of gene expression (Edwards & Mahadevan, 1992; Rauch et al., 2006; Canal et al., 2007; Sharma et al., 2012).

Moreover, there are training conditions where *de novo* protein synthesis seems to be unnecessary for memory consolidation. We have found that administration of a PSI greatly interferes with the formation of long-term memory of inhibitory and active avoidance, but it becomes innocuous when animals are subjected to enhanced training (higher foot-shock intensity during training), i.e., when the task becomes more emotive (Díaz-Trujillo et al., 2009; González-Salinas et al., 2015). The same is true in the case of extinction of active avoidance trained with high-intensity foot-shocks (González-Salinas et al., 2015). Infusion of a PSI into the nucleus accumbens impedes memory consolidation of cued (tone) fear conditioning trained with a foot-shock of low intensity, but consolidation develops when a higher intensity is used (Kishioka et al., 2013).

Taken together, these studies suggest that *de novo* protein synthesis is not critically involved in the formation of lasting, long-term memories. It has been proposed that post-translational modifications of pre-existing proteins, through phosphorylation, glycosylation, proteolytic cleavage, and cellular translocation, are necessary and sufficient for consolidation, and that transcription and translation only intervene to replenish proteins used at the synapse (Routtenberg & Rekart, 2005).

With respect to the participation of neurotransmitters, a growing body of evidence also demonstrates that enhanced training prevents the amnesic effects of manipulating synaptic activity. Infusions of acetylcholine, GABA, and serotonin antagonists as well as sodium channel blockers into the striatum, substantia nigra, or hippocampus produce marked, long-term memory deficits, which are not observed when the experimental animals are subjected to increased aversive experiences, as in the following few examples (for a recent review see Prado-Alcalá et al., 2012).

Using systemic and intracerebral treatments, we found that drugs that interfere with the activity of acetylcholine and GABA produce significant deficits in consolidation. However, if the training is stronger, blockade of these neurotransmitters does not impede memory consolidation (Giordano & Prado-Alcalá, 1986; Durán-Arévalo et al., 1990; Cobos-Zapiaín et al., 1996). We also found that when p-chloroamphetamine, a drug that destroys serotonergic neurons, is administered systemically prior to training, it produces acquisition and retention deficits in an active avoidance task trained with low-intensity foot-shocks, but no such effects are produced when the animals are trained with a relatively high-intensity foot-shock (Galindo et al., 2008). The same happens when rats are trained in inhibitory avoidance (Solana-Figueroa et al., 2002).

These results indicate that when there is an interference with the activity of a cerebral neurochemical system, memory consolidation of avoidance learning is disrupted. Under enhanced training conditions, however, the same interference is totally ineffective in modifying the consolidation process. Taken together, the data reviewed above strongly suggest that certain cerebral structures or neurochemical systems are necessary for consolidation; nevertheless, after enhanced training, the memory trace is not represented by the same particular set of structures or neurochemical systems. It is proposed that after an enhanced learning experience, the memory trace may be widely distributed in the brain, and it requires cellular mechanisms that are independent of *de novo* protein synthesis.

CONCLUSION

Memory comprises several stages: learning (acquisition), consolidation, and retrieval. Extinction is a form of learning whereby a conditioned behavior diminishes in frequency or strength when an unconditioned stimulus or a reinforcer does not follow it.

There are neuronal elements that participate in all stages of memory, some of which are the cholinergic and adrenergic systems, the glutamatergic AMPA receptors, and the enzyme PKC. Others, like the NMDA receptor and the enzyme CAMKII are mainly involved in acquisition and consolidation, while mGlu receptors and the enzymes PKA and ERK mediate consolidation and retrieval. There is still a scarcity of reports dealing with cellular and molecular aspects of extinction, but they point to the participation of the cholinergic, GABAergic, and adrenergic systems, the NMDA and mGlu receptors, and the enzymes PKA, PKC, CAMKII, and ERK in this type of learning.

Glucocorticoid hormones promote acquisition, consolidation, and extinction, although they interfere with retrieval. However, under certain circumstances it is possible that these hormones affect all the stages of memory, either positively or negatively, depending on the features of the stressor.

Administration of PSIs impedes memory consolidation and the development of extinction, but not acquisition or retrieval. There is evidence; however, indicating that the deficits produced by PSIs are due to their side effects, thus casting serious doubts about the validity of the hypothesis that protein synthesis is a requisite for memory consolidation. Along these lines, it has been reported that the amnestic effects produced by interference with the activity of some neurotransmitter systems and by PSIs are counteracted when the experimental subjects are subjected to an enhanced learning experience.

Taken together, the data we have reviewed indicates that the stages of memory share only some molecular mechanisms. Also, the data point to the conclusion that memory consolidation depends on some unknown process, and not on protein synthesis. Finally, the fact that amnestic treatments do not disturb memory of enhanced learning gives rise to the proposal that the memory derived from this kind of learning must follow rules and mechanisms that are different from those of regular learning.

ACKNOWLEDGMENTS

The authors thank N. Serafín for her excellent technical assistance, F. G. Vázquez-Cuevas for helpful suggestions on the figure, and Dr. Dorothy Pless for reviewing and helping us to improve the manuscript. Some experiments described in this article were financed by the National Council of Science and Technology of México (Grant CONACYT 128259) and by Dirección General de Asuntos del Personal Académico, Universidad Nacional Autónoma de México (Grant PAPIIT IN201415). This work was carried out in partial fulfillment of the requirements to obtain the Doctoral Degree (Doctorado en Ciencias Biomédicas, UNAM) by S. González-Salinas, who was a recipient of a Graduate Scholarship from CONACYT (Becario 229335).

REFERENCES

Abel, T. & Lattal, K.M. (2001) Molecular mechanisms of memory acquisition, consolidation and retrieval. *Curr. Opin. Neurobiol.,* 11, 180–187.

Abel, T., Nguyen, P.V., Barad, M., Deuel, T.A., Kandel, E.R. & Bourtchouladze, R. (1997) Genetic demonstration of a role for PKA in the late phase of LTP and in hippocampus-based long-term memory. *Cell,* 88, 615–626.

Alberini, C.M. (2008) The role of protein synthesis during the labile phases of memory: Revisiting the skepticism. *Neurobiol. Learn. Mem.,* 89, 234–246.

Alberini, C.M. (2009) Transcription factors in long-term memory and synaptic plasticity. *Physiol. Rev.,* 89, 121–145.

Arlt, W. & Stewart, P.M. (2005) Adrenal corticosteroid biosynthesis, metabolism, and action. *Endocrinol. Metab. Clin. North Am.,* 34, 293–313.

Atkins, C.M., Selcher, J.C., Petraitis, J.J., Trzaskos, J.M. & Sweatt, J.D. (1998) The MAPK cascade is required for mammalian associative learning. *Nat. Neurosci., 1*, 602–609.

Barros, D.M., Izquierdo, L.A., Mello e Souza, T., Ardenghi, P.G., Pereira, P., Medina, J.H. & Izquierdo, I. (2000) Molecular signalling pathways in the cerebral cortex are required for retrieval of one-trial avoidance learning in rats. *Behav. Brain Res.,* 114, 183–192.

Barros, D.M., Ramirez, M.R., dos Reis, E.A. & Izquierdo, I. (2004) Participation of hippocampal nicotinic receptors in acquisition, consolidation and retrieval of memory for one trial inhibitory avoidance in rats. *Neuroscience,* 126, 651–656.

Barsegyan, A., Mackenzie, S.M., Kurose, B.D., McGaugh, J.L. & Roozendaal, B. (2010) Glucocorticoids in the prefrontal cortex enhance memory consolidation and impair working memory by a common neural mechanism. *Proc. Natl. Acad. Sci.,* 107, 16655–16660.

Bast, T., da Silva, B.M. & Morris, R.G.M. (2005) Distinct contributions of hippocampal NMDA and AMPA receptors to encoding and retrieval of one-trial place memory. *J. Neurosci.,* 25, 5845–5856.

Bayer, S.A., Altman, J., Russo, R.J. & Zhang, X. (1993) Timetables of neurogenesis in the human brain based on experimentally determined patterns in the rat. *Neurotoxicology*, 14, 83–144.

Bejar, R., Yasuda, R., Krugers, H., Hood, K. & Mayford, M. (2002) Transgenic calmodulin-dependent protein kinase II activation: dose-dependent effects on synaptic plasticity, learning, and memory. *J. Neurosci. Off. J. Soc. Neurosci.,* 22, 5719–5726.

Berlau, D.J. & McGaugh, J.L. (2006) Enhancement of extinction memory consolidation: The role of the noradrenergic and GABAergic systems within the basolateral amygdala. *Neurobiol. Learn. Mem.,* 86, 123–132.

Besnard, A., Laroche, S. & Caboche, J. (2013) Comparative dynamics of MAPK/ERK signalling components and immediate early genes in the hippocampus and amygdala following contextual fear conditioning and retrieval. *Brain Struct. Funct.,* 1–16.

Beylin, A.V. & Shors, T.J. (1998) Stress enhances excitatory trace eyeblink conditioning and opposes acquisition of inhibitory conditioning. *Behav. Neurosci.,* 112, 1327–1338.

Beylin, A.V. & Shors, T.J. (2003) Glucocorticoids are necessary for enhancing the acquisition of associative memories after acute stressful experience. *Horm. Behav.,* 43, 124–131.

Blum, S., Moore, A.N., Adams, F. & Dash, P.K. (1999) A mitogen-activated protein kinase cascade in the CA1/CA2 subfield of the dorsal hippocampus is essential for long-term spatial memory. *J. Neurosci. Off. J. Soc. Neurosci.,* 19, 3535–3544.

Boccia, M.M., Blake, M.G., Baratti, C.M. & McGaugh, J.L. (2009) Involvement of the basolateral amygdala in muscarinic cholinergic modulation of extinction memory consolidation. *Neurobiol. Learn. Mem.,* 91, 93–97.

Buccafusco, J.J. ed. (2009) Methods of behavior analysis in neuroscience 2nd ed. *CRC Press, Boca Raton* (FL).

Cammarota, M., Barros, D.M., Vianna, M.R., Bevilaqua, L.R., Coitinho, A., Szapiro, G., Izquierdo, L.A., Medina, J.H. & Izquierdo, I. (2004) The transition from memory retrieval to extinction. *An. Acad. Bras. Ciênc.*, 76, 573–582.

Canal, C.E., Chang, Q. & Gold, P.E. (2007) Amnesia produced by altered release of neurotransmitters after intraamygdala injections of a protein synthesis inhibitor. *Proc. Natl. Acad. Sci.,* 104, 12500–12505.

Chauveau, F., Tronche, C., Piérard, C., Liscia, P., Drouet, I., Coutan, M. & Béracochéa, D. (2010) Rapid stress-induced corticosterone rise in the hippocampus reverses serial memory retrieval pattern. *Hippocampus,* 20, 196–207.

Chhatwal, J.P., Myers, K.M., Ressler, K.J. & Davis, M. (2005) Regulation of gephyrin and gabaa receptor binding within the amygdala after fear acquisition and extinction. *J. Neurosci.,* 25, 502–506.

Chhatwal, J.P., Stanek-Rattiner, L., Davis, M. & Ressler, K.J. (2006) Amygdala BDNF signaling is required for consolidation but not encoding of extinction. *Nat. Neurosci.,* 9, 870–872.

Cobos-Zapiaín, G.G., Salado-Castillo, R., Sánchez-Alavez, M., Quirarte, G.L., Roldán-Roldán, G., Díaz del Guante, M.A. & Prado-Alcalá, R.A. (1996) High level of footshock during inhibitory avoidance training prevents amnesia induced by intranigral injection of GABA antagonists. *Neurobiol. Learn. Mem.,* 65, 202–206.

Cole, B.J. & Robbins, T.W. (1987) Dissociable effects of lesions to the dorsal or ventral noradrenergic bundle on the acquisition, performance, and extinction of aversive conditioning. *Behav. Neurosci.*, 101, 476–488.

Cordero, M.I., Venero, C., Kruyt, N.D. & Sandi, C. (2003) Prior exposure to a single stress session facilitates subsequent contextual fear conditioning in rats: Evidence for a role of corticosterone. *Horm. Behav.,* 44, 338–345.

De Quervain, D.J.F., Roozendaal, B. & McGaugh, J.L. (1998) Stress and glucocorticoids impair retrieval of long-term spatial memory. *Nature,* 394, 787–790.

Díaz-Trujillo, A., Contreras, J., Medina, A.C., Silveyra-Leon, G.A., Antaramian, A., Quirarte, G.L. & Prado-Alcalá, R.A. (2009) Enhanced inhibitory avoidance learning prevents the long-term memory-impairing effects of cycloheximide, a protein synthesis inhibitor. *Neurobiol. Learn. Mem.,* 91, 310–314.

Dudai, Y. (2004) The neurobiology of consolidations, or, how stable is the engram? *Annu. Rev. Psychol.*, 55, 51–86.

Durán-Arévalo, M., Cruz-Morales, S.E. & Prado-Alcalá, R.A. (1990) Is acetylcholine involved in memory consolidation of over-reinforced learning? *Brain Res. Bull.,* 24, 725–727.

Edo Izquierdo, S., Aldavert Vera, L., Coll Andreu, M., Garau Florit, A. & Segura Torres, P. (1994) A parametrical study of two-way active avoidance acquisition and long-term retention: new approaches for data analyses. *Psicothema,* 6, 49–69.

Edwards, D.R. & Mahadevan, L.C. (1992) Protein synthesis inhibitors differentially superinduce c-fos and c-jun by three distinct mechanisms: lack of evidence for labile repressors. *EMBO J.,* 11, 2415–2424.

Eisenberg, M., Kobilo, T., Berman, D.E. & Dudai, Y. (2003) Stability of retrieved memory: inverse correlation with trace dominance. *Science,* 301, 1102–1104.

El-Ghundi, M., O'Dowd, B.F. & George, S.R. (2011) insights into the role of dopamine receptor systems in learning and memory. *Rev. Neurosci.,* 18, 37–66.

Everitt, B.J., Robbins, T.W., Gaskin, M. & Fray, P.J. (1983) The effects of lesions to ascending noradrenergic neurons on discrimination learning and performance in the rat. *Neuroscience,* 10, 397–410.

Falls, W.A., Miserendino, M.J. & Davis, M. (1992) Extinction of fear-potentiated startle: blockade by infusion of an NMDA antagonist into the amygdala. *J. Neurosci.,* 12, 854–863.

Ferry, B., Roozendaal, B. & McGaugh, J.L. (1999) Involvement of α1-adrenoceptors in the basolateral amygdala in modulation of memory storage. *Eur. J. Pharmacol.*, 372, 9–16.

Flores, L.C. & Disterhoft, J.F. (2013) Caudate nucleus in retrieval of trace eyeblink conditioning after consolidation. *J. Neurosci.,* 33, 2828–2836.

Galindo, L.E., Garín-Aguilar, M.E., Medina, A.C., Serafín, N., Quirarte, G.L. & Prado-Alcalá, R.A. (2008) Acquisition and retention of enhanced active avoidance are unaffected by interference with serotonergic activity. *Behav. Brain Res.,* 195, 153–158.

Giordano, M. & Prado-Alcalá, R.A. (1986) Retrograde amnesia induced by post-trial injection of atropine into the caudate-putamen. Protective effect of the negative reinforcer. *Pharmacol. Biochem. Behav.*, 24, 905–909.

Gkogkas, C., Sonenberg, N. & Costa-Mattioli, M. (2010) Translational control mechanisms in long-lasting synaptic plasticity and memory. *J. Biol. Chem.,* 285, 31913–31917.

Gold, P.E. (2003) Acetylcholine modulation of neural systems involved in learning and memory. *Neurobiol. Learn. Mem.,* 80, 194–210.

Gold, P.E. (2008) Protein synthesis inhibition and memory: Formation vs amnesia. *Neurobiol. Learn. Mem.,* 89, 201–211.

González-Salinas, S., Medina, A.C., Marín-Vignando, V.E., Ruiz-López, C.X., Quirarte, G.L. & Prado-Alcalá, R.A. (2015) Protein synthesis is not required for acquisition, consolidation, and extinction of high foot-shock active avoidance training. *Behav. Brain Res.,* 287, 8–14.

Goto, Y., Otani, S. & Grace, A.A. (2007) The Yin and Yang of dopamine release: a new perspective. *Neuropharmacology*, 53, 583–587.

Gusev, P.A., Cui, C., Alkon, D.L. & Gubin, A.N. (2005) Topography of Arc/Arg3.1 mRNA expression in the dorsal and ventral hippocampus induced by recent and remote spatial memory recall: Dissociation of CA3 and CA1 activation. *J. Neurosci.,* 25, 9384–9397.

Guzowski, J.F., Setlow, B., Wagner, E.K. & McGaugh, J.L. (2001) Experience-dependent gene expression in the rat hippocampus after spatial learning: A comparison of the immediate-early genes arc, c-fos, and zif268. *J. Neurosci.,* 21, 5089–5098.

Hall, J., Thomas, K.L. & Everitt, B.J. (2001a) Cellular imaging of zif268 expression in the hippocampus and amygdala during contextual and cued fear memory retrieval: selective activation of hippocampal CA1 neurons during the recall of contextual memories. *J. Neurosci.,* 21, 2186–2193.

Hall, J., Thomas, K.L. & Everitt, B.J. (2001b) Fear memory retrieval induces CREB phosphorylation and Fos expression within the amygdala. *Eur. J. Neurosci.,* 13, 1453–1458.

Han, J.-H., Kushner, S.A., Yiu, A.P., Cole, C.J., Matynia, A., Brown, R.A., Neve, R.L., Guzowski, J.F., Silva, A.J. & Josselyn, S.A. (2007) Neuronal competition and selection during memory formation. *Science,* 316, 457–460.

Hatfield, T. & McGaugh, J.L. (1999) Norepinephrine infused into the basolateral amygdala posttraining enhances retention in a spatial water maze task. *Neurobiol. Learn. Mem.,* 71, 232–239.

Herry, C. & Mons, N. (2004) Resistance to extinction is associated with impaired immediate early gene induction in medial prefrontal cortex and amygdala. *Eur. J. Neurosci.*, 20, 781–790.

Herry, C., Trifilieff, P., Micheau, J., Lüthi, A. & Mons, N. (2006) Extinction of auditory fear conditioning requires MAPK/ERK activation in the basolateral amygdala. *Eur. J. Neurosci.,* 24, 261–269.

Huang, C.-H., Chiang, Y.-W., Liang, K.-C., Thompson, R.F. & Liu, I.Y. (2010) Extracellular signal-regulated kinase 1/2 (ERK1/2) activated in the hippocampal CA1 neurons is critical for retrieval of auditory trace fear memory. *Brain Res.,* 1326, 143–151.

Igaz, L.M., Bekinschtein, P., Vianna, M.M.R., Izquierdo, I. & Medina, J.H. (2004) Gene expression during memory formation. *Neurotox. Res.*, 6, 189–204.

Igaz, L.M., Vianna, M.R.M., Medina, J.H. & Izquierdo, I. (2002) Two time periods of hippocampal mRNA synthesis are required for memory consolidation of fear-motivated learning. *J. Neurosci.*, 22, 6781–6789.

Jöels, M. & Baram, T.Z. (2009) The neuro-symphony of stress. *Nat. Rev. Neurosci.*, 10, 459–466.

Kandel, E.R. (2001) The molecular biology of memory storage: a dialogue between genes and synapses. *Science,* 294, 1030–1038.

Kandel, E.R., Schwartz, J. & Jessell, T. (2000) Learning and memory In, Principles of Neural Science, Fourth Edition *McGraw-Hill Professional.*

Kang, H., Sun, L.D., Atkins, C.M., Soderling, T.R., Wilson, M.A. & Tonegawa, S. (2001) An important role of neural activity-dependent CaMKIV signaling in the consolidation of long-term memory. *Cell,* 106, 771–783.

Karssen, A.M., Meijer, O.C., van der Sandt, I.C., Lucassen, P.J., de Lange, E.C., de Boer, A.G. & de Kloet, E.R. (2001) Multidrug resistance P-glycoprotein hampers the access of cortisol but not of corticosterone to mouse and human brain. *Endocrinology,* 142, 2686–2694.

Kim, J., Lee, S., Park, H., Song, B., Hong, I., Geum, D., Shin, K. & Choi, S. (2007) Blockade of amygdala metabotropic glutamate receptor subtype 1 impairs fear extinction. *Biochem. Biophys. Res. Commun.,* 355, 188–193.

Kishioka, A., Uemura, T., Fukushima, F. & Mishina, M. (2013) Consolidation of auditory fear memories formed by weak unconditioned stimuli requires NMDA receptor activation and de novo protein synthesis in the striatum. *Mol. Brain,* 6, 17.

Kobayashi, K. & Yasoshima, Y. (2001) The central noradrenaline system and memory consolidation. *Neurosci. Rev. J. Bringing Neurobiol. Neurol. Psychiatry,* 7, 371–376.

Liang, K.C., Hu, S.J. & Chang, S.C. (1996) Formation and retrieval of inhibitory avoidance memory: differential roles of glutamate receptors in the amygdala and medial prefrontal cortex. *Chin. J. Physiol.,* 39, 155–166.

Lin, C.-H., Yeh, S.-H., Lu, H.-Y. & Gean, P.-W. (2003) The similarities and diversities of signal pathways leading to consolidation of conditioning and consolidation of extinction of fear memory. *J. Neurosci.*, 23, 8310–8317.

Linthorst, A.C.E. & Reul, J.M. (2008) Stress and the brain: solving the puzzle using microdialysis. *Pharmacol. Biochem. Behav.,* 90, 163–173.

Lozano, Y.R., Serafín, N., Prado-Alcalá, R.A., Roozendaal, B. & Quirarte, G.L. (2013) Glucocorticoids in the dorsomedial striatum modulate the consolidation of spatial but not procedural memory. *Neurobiol. Learn. Mem.,* 101, 55–64.

Makkar, S.R., Zhang, S.Q. & Cranney, J. (2010) Behavioral and neural analysis of GABA in the acquisition, consolidation, reconsolidation, and extinction of fear memory. *Neuropsychopharmacology*, 35, 1625–1652.

Mamiya, N., Fukushima, H., Suzuki, A., Matsuyama, Z., Homma, S., Frankland, P.W. & Kida, S. (2009) Brain region-specific gene expression activation required for reconsolidation and extinction of contextual fear memory. *J. Neurosci.,* 29, 402–413.

Martinez, J.L., Jr, Jensen, R.A. & McGaugh, J.L. (1981) Attenuation of experimentally-induced amnesia. *Prog. Neurobiol.,* 16, 155–186.

Mayford, M., Bach, M.E., Huang, Y.Y., Wang, L., Hawkins, R.D. & Kandel, E.R. (1996) Control of memory formation through regulated expression of a CaMKII transgene. *Science,* 274, 1678–1683.

McGaugh, J.L. (1973) Learning and memory: an introduction. Albion Pub. Co.

McGaugh, J.L. (2000) Memory–a century of consolidation. *Science,* 287, 248–251.

McIntyre, C.K., Ragozzino, M.E. & Gold, P.E. (1998) Intra-amygdala infusions of scopolamine impair performance on a conditioned place preference task but not a spatial radial maze task. *Behav. Brain Res.,* 95, 219–226.

Medina, A.C., Charles, J.R., Espinoza-González, V., Sánchez-Resendis, O., Prado-Alcalá, R.A., Roozendaal, B. & Quirarte, G.L. (2007) Glucocorticoid administration into the dorsal striatum facilitates memory consolidation of inhibitory avoidance training but not of the context or footshock components. *Learn. Mem.,* 14, 673–677.

Meneses, A. & Liy-Salmeron, G. (2012) Serotonin and emotion, learning and memory. *Rev. Neurosci.,* 23, 543–553.

Milad, M.R. & Quirk, G.J. (2012) Fear extinction as a model for translational neuroscience: Ten years of progress. *Annu. Rev. Psychol.,* 63, 129–151.

Miranda, M.I., Quirarte, G.L., Rodriguez-Garcia, G., McGaugh, J.L. & Roozendaal, B. (2008) Glucocorticoids enhance taste aversion memory via actions in the insular cortex and basolateral amygdala. *Learn. Mem. Cold Spring Harb.* N, 15, 468–476.

Myskiw, J.C., Fiorenza, N.G., Izquierdo, L.A. & Izquierdo, I. (2010) Molecular mechanisms in hippocampus and basolateral amygdala but not in parietal or cingulate cortex are involved in extinction of one-trial avoidance learning. *Neurobiol. Learn. Mem.,* 94, 285–291.

Nader, K. & Einarsson, E.O. (2010) Memory reconsolidation: an update. *Ann. N. Y. Acad. Sci.,* 1191, 27–41.

Noguès, X., Jaffard, R. & Micheau, J. (1996) Investigations on the role of hippocampal protein kinase C on memory processes: pharmacological approach. *Behav. Brain Res., 75*, 139–146.

O'Sullivan, N.C., McGettigan, P.A., Sheridan, G.K., Pickering, M., Conboy, L., O'Connor, J.J., Moynagh, P.N., Higgins, D.G., Regan, C.M. & Murphy, K.J. (2007) Temporal change in gene expression in the rat dentate gyrus following passive avoidance learning. *J. Neurochem.*, 101, 1085–1098.

Pavlov, I.P. (1927) Conditioned reflexes Courier Dover Publications.

Paylor, R., Rudy, J.W. & Wehner, J.M. (1991) Acute phorbol ester treatment improves spatial learning performance in rats. *Behav. Brain Res.*, 45, 189–193.

Pereira, P., Medina, J.H. & Izquierdo, I. (2000) Participation of hippocampal metabotropic glutamate receptors, protein kinase A and mitogen-activated protein kinases in memory retrieval. *Neuroscience,* 99, 1–5.

Pedreira, M.E. & Maldonado, H. (2003) Protein synthesis subserves reconsolidation or extinction depending on reminder duration. *Neuron*, 38, 863–869.

Peng, S., Zhang, Y., Zhang, J., Wang, H. & Ren, B. (2010) ERK in learning and memory: A review of recent research. *Int. J. Mol. Sci.,* 11, 222–232.

Phelps, E.A. & LeDoux, J.E. (2005) Contributions of the amygdala to emotion processing: from animal models to human behavior. *Neuron,* 48, 175–187.

Prado-Alcalá, R.A., Fernández-Samblancat, M. & Solodkin-Herrera, M. (1985) Injections of atropine into the caudate nucleus impair the acquisition and the maintenance of passive avoidance. *Pharmacol. Biochem. Behav.,* 22, 243–247.

Prado-Alcalá, R.A., Haiek, M., Rivas, S., Roldán-Roldán, G. & Quirarte, G.L. (1994) Reversal of extinction by scopolamine. *Physiol. Behav.,* 56, 27–30.

Prado-Alcalá, R.A., Medina, A.C., Serafin, N. & Quirarte, G.L. (2012) Intense emotional experiences and enhanced training prevent memory loss induced by post-training amnesic treatments administered to the striatum, amygdala, hippocampus or substantia nigra. *Rev. Neurosci.,* 23, 501–508.

Quirarte, G.L., Galvez, R., Roozendaal, B. & McGaugh, J.L. (1998) Norepinephrine release in the amygdala in response to footshock and opioid peptidergic drugs. *Brain Res.,* 808, 134–140.

Quirarte, G.L., Ledesma de la Teja, I.S, Casillas, M., Serafín, N., Prado-Alcalá, R.A. & Roozendaal, B. (2009) Corticosterone infused into the dorsal striatum selectively enhances memory consolidation of cued water-maze training. *Learn. Mem.,* 16, 586–589.

Quirk, G.J. & Mueller, D. (2007) Neural mechanisms of extinction learning and retrieval. *Neuropsychopharmacology,* 33, 56–72.

Rapanelli, M., Frick, L.R. & Zanutto, B.S. (2009) Differential gene expression in the rat hippocampus during learning of an operant conditioning task. *Neuroscience,* 163, 1031–1038.

Rapanelli, M., Lew, S.E., Frick, L.R. & Zanutto, B.S. (2010) Plasticity in the rat prefrontal cortex: linking gene expression and an operant learning with a computational theory. *PLoS ONE,* 5, e8656.

Rau, V. & Fanselow, M.S. (2009) Exposure to a stressor produces a long lasting enhancement of fear learning in rats. *Stress Amst. Neth.,* 12, 125–133.

Rauch, S.L., Shin, L.M. & Phelps, E.A. (2006) Neurocircuitry models of posttraumatic stress disorder and extinction: human neuroimaging research--past, present, and future. *Biol. Psychiatry*, 60, 376–382.

Reul, J.M. & de Kloet, E.R. (1985) Two receptor systems for corticosterone in rat brain: microdistribution and differential occupation. *Endocrinology,* 117, 2505–2511.

Riedel, G., Platt, B. & Micheau, J. (2003) Glutamate receptor function in learning and memory. *Behav. Brain Res.,* 140, 1–47.

Riedemann, T., Patchev, A.V., Cho, K. & Almeida, O.F. (2010) Corticosteroids: way upstream. *Mol. Brain*, 3, 1–20.

Rodrigues, S.M., LeDoux, J.E. & Sapolsky, R.M. (2009) The influence of stress hormones on fear circuitry. *Annu. Rev. Neurosci.*, 32, 289–313.

Rodriguez-Ortiz, C.J., De la Cruz, V., Gutiérrez, R. & Bermudez-Rattoni, F. (2005) Protein synthesis underlies post-retrieval memory consolidation to a restricted degree only when updated information is obtained. *Learn. Mem.,* 12, 533–537.

Rogers, J.L. & Kesner, R.P. (2003) Cholinergic modulation of the hippocampus during encoding and retrieval. *Neurobiol. Learn. Mem*., 80, 332–342.

Roldán-Roldán, G., Cobos-Zapiain, G., Quirarte, G.L. & Prado-Alcalá, R.A. (2001) Dose- and time-dependent scopolamine-induced recovery of an inhibitory avoidance response after its extinction in rats. *Behav. Brain Res.,* 121, 173–179.

Roozendaal, B. (2002) Stress and Memory: Opposing effects of glucocorticoids on memory consolidation and memory retrieval. *Neurobiol. Learn. Mem.,* 78, 578–595.

Roozendaal, B., Hahn, E.L., Nathan, S.V., de Quervain, D.J.-F. & McGaugh, J.L. (2004) Glucocorticoid effects on memory retrieval require concurrent noradrenergic activity in the hippocampus and basolateral amygdala. *J. Neurosci.,* 24, 8161–8169.

Roozendaal, B., McEwen, B.S. & Chattarji, S. (2009) Stress, memory and the amygdala. *Nat. Rev. Neurosci*., 10, 423–433.

Roozendaal, B. & McGaugh, J.L. (1997) Glucocorticoid receptor agonist and antagonist administration into the basolateral but not central amygdala modulates memory storage. *Neurobiol. Learn. Mem.,* 67, 176–179.

Routtenberg, A. & Rekart, J.L. (2005) Post-translational protein modification as the substrate for long-lasting memory. *Trends Neurosci.,* 28, 12–19.

Sakaguchi, M. & Hayashi, Y. (2012) Catching the engram: strategies to examine the memory trace. *Mol. Brain,* 5, 32.

Sanders, M.J., Wiltgen, B.J. & Fanselow, M.S. (2003) The place of the hippocampus in fear conditioning. *Eur. J. Pharmacol.,* 463, 217–223.

Sandi, C., Loscertales, M. & Guaza, C. (1997) Experience-dependent facilitating effect of corticosterone on spatial memory formation in the water maze. *Eur. J. Neurosci.,* 9, 637–642.

Santini, E., Sepulveda-Orengo, M. & Porter, J.T. (2012) Muscarinic receptors modulate the intrinsic excitability of infralimbic neurons and consolidation of fear extinction. *Neuropsychopharmacol. Off. Publ. Am. Coll. Neuropsychopharmacol.,* 37, 2047–2056.

Schafe, G.E., Atkins, C.M., Swank, M.W., Bauer, E.P., Sweatt, J.D. & LeDoux, J.E. (2000) Activation of ERK/MAP kinase in the amygdala is required for memory consolidation of pavlovian fear conditioning. *J. Neurosci.,* 20, 8177–8187.

Schafe, G.E. & LeDoux, J.E. (2000) Memory consolidation of auditory pavlovian fear conditioning requires protein synthesis and protein kinase A in the amygdala. *J. Neurosci. Off. J. Soc. Neurosci.,* 20, RC96.

Sharma, A.V., Nargang, F.E. & Dickson, C.T. (2012) Neurosilence: Profound suppression of neural activity following intracerebral administration of the protein synthesis inhibitor anisomycin. *J. Neurosci.,* 32, 2377–2387.

Sierra-Mercado, D., Padilla-Coreano, N. & Quirk, G.J. (2011) Dissociable roles of prelimbic and infralimbic cortices, ventral hippocampus, and basolateral amygdala in the expression and extinction of conditioned fear. neuropsychopharmacology, 36, 529–538.

Solana-Figueroa, R., Salado-Castillo, R., Quirarte, G.L., Galindo, L.E. & Prado-Alcalá, R.A. (2002) Enhanced inhibitory avoidance training protects against the amnesic effect of p–chloroamphetamine. *Life Sci.,* 71, 391–399.

Sotres-Bayon, F., Bush, D.E.A. & LeDoux, J.E. (2007) Acquisition of fear extinction requires activation of nr2b-containing nmda receptors in the lateral amygdala. *Neuropsychopharmacology,* 32, 1929–1940.

Squire, L.R. (1986) Mechanisms of memory. *Science,* 232, 1612–1619.

Steckler, T., Kalin, N.H. & Reul, J.M.H.M. (2005) Handbook of stress and the brain: *The neurobiology of stress Elsevier.*

Suzuki, A., Josselyn, S.A., Frankland, P.W., Masushige, S., Silva, A.J. & Kida, S. (2004) Memory reconsolidation and extinction have distinct temporal and biochemical signatures. *J. Neurosci.,* 24, 4787–4795.

Sweatt, J.D. (2004) Mitogen-activated protein kinases in synaptic plasticity and memory. *Curr. Opin. Neurobiol.,* 14, 311–317.

Szapiro, G., Galante, J.M., Barros, D.M., de Stein, M.L., Vianna, M.R., Izquierdo, L.A., Izquierdo, I. & Medina, J.H. (2002) Molecular mechanisms of memory retrieval. *Neurochem. Res.,* 27, 1491–1498.

Szapiro, G., Izquierdo, L.A., Alonso, M., Barros, D., Paratcha, G., Ardenghi, P., Szapiro, G., Vianna, M.R.M., McGaugh, J.L., Medina, J.H. & Izquierdo, I. (2003) The role of NMDA glutamate receptors, PKA, MAPK, and CAMKII in the hippocampus in extinction of conditioned fear. *Hippocampus,* 13, 53–58.

Tronson, N.C., Corcoran, K.A., Jovasevic, V. & Radulovic, J. (2012) Fear conditioning and extinction: emotional states encoded by distinct signaling pathways. *Trends Neurosci.,* 35, 145–155.

Tronson, N.C., Schrick, C., Fischer, A., Sananbenesi, F., Pagès, G., Pouysségur, J. & Radulovic, J. (2007) Regulatory mechanisms of fear extinction and depression-like behavior. *Neuropsychopharmacology,* 33, 1570–1583.

Tronson, N.C., Schrick, C., Guzman, Y.F., Huh, K.H., Srivastava, D.P., Penzes, P., Guedea, A.L., Gao, C. & Radulovic, J. (2009) Segregated populations of hippocampal principal ca1 neurons mediating conditioning and extinction of contextual fear. *J. Neurosci. Off. J. Soc. Neurosci.,* 29, 3387–3394.

Tulving, E. & Thomson, D.M. (1973) Encoding specificity and retrieval processes in episodic memory. *Psychol. Rev.,* 80, 352–373.

Ulrich-Lai, Y.M. & Herman, J.P. (2009) Neural regulation of endocrine and autonomic stress responses. *Nat. Rev. Neurosci.,* 10, 397–409.

Vianna, M.R., Barros, D.M., Silva, T., Choi, H., Madche, C., Rodrigues, C., Medina, J.H. & Izquierdo, I. (2000) Pharmacological demonstration of the differential involvement of protein kinase C isoforms in short- and long-term memory formation and retrieval of one-trial avoidance in rats. *Psychopharmacology* (Berl.), 150, 77–84.

Vianna, M.R., Igaz, L.M., Coitinho, A.S., Medina, J.H. & Izquierdo, I. (2003) Memory extinction requires gene expression in rat hippocampus. *Neurobiol. Learn. Mem.,* 79, 199–203.

Wallenstein, G.V. & Vago, D.R. (2001) Intrahippocampal scopolamine impairs both acquisition and consolidation of contextual fear conditioning. *Neurobiol. Learn. Mem.,* 75, 245–252.

Wang, H., Hu, Y. & Tsien, J.Z. (2006) Molecular and systems mechanisms of memory consolidation and storage. *Prog. Neurobiol.,* 79, 123–135.

Yang, Y.L., Chao, P.K. & Lu, K.T. (2005) Systemic and intra-amygdala administration of glucocorticoid agonist and antagonist modulate extinction of conditioned fear. *Neuropsychopharmacology,* 31, 912–924.

Zeng, H., Shen, E.H., Hohmann, J.G., Oh, S.W., Bernard, A., Royall, J.J., Glattfelder, K.J., Sunkin, S.M., Morris, J.A., Guillozet-Bongaarts, A.L., Smith, K.A., Ebbert, A.J., Swanson, B., Kuan, L., Page, D.T., Overly, C.C., Lein, E.S., Hawrylycz, M.J., Hof, P.R., Hyde, T.M., Kleinman, J.E. & Jones, A.R. (2012) Large-scale cellular-resolution gene profiling in human neocortex reveals species-specific molecular signatures. *Cell,* 149, 483–496.

Zoladz, P.R., Woodson, J.C., Haynes, V.F. & Diamond, D.M. (2010) Activation of a remote (1-year old) emotional memory interferes with the retrieval of a newly formed hippocampus-dependent memory in rats. *Stress,* 13, 36–52.

In: Synaptic Fundamentals of Memory Performance
Editor: Ignacio González-Burgos
ISBN: 978-1-63483-279-3

Chapter 6

MEMORY IN MUSIC AND EMOTIONS

Christian Mikutta[1,*], Werner K. Strik[2], Robert Knight[1] and Andreas Altorfer[2]
[1]University of California Berkeley,
Helen Wills Institute of Neuroscience, Berkeley, CA, US
[2]University Hospital of Psychiatry,
Translational Research Center, Bern, Switzerland

ABSTRACT

Music is a basic and ancient feature of human socialization. Music is a powerful inducer of emotions, and humans appear to listen to music specifically because of this. It was shown that emotion is a powerful modulator of memory encoding. The following chapter provides an overview over music specific encoding mechanisms in the short- and long-term memory. Hereby music specific features of working memory model as well as the interaction of the acceding auditory pathways, music processing and memory encoding are discussed. Furthermore, we show the overlap and the differences between language and music memory. The impact of music-induced emotions on memory encoding is explored. Finally music's ability to reveal autobiographic memories is summarized.

Keywords: memory, music, language, emotions

1. INTRODUCTION

Music is a basic and ancient feature of human socialization (Koelsch, 2014). Music is a powerful inducer of emotions (Meyer, 1956; Blood et al., 1999; Koelsch, 2014), and humans appear to listen to music specifically because of this (Menon et al., 2005). It was shown that emotion is a powerful modulator of memory encoding (Hamann, 2001). Therefore the

* Send correspondence to: Christian Mikutta MD, University of California Berkeley, Helen Wills Institute of Neuroscience, 132 Barker Hall, Berkeley, CA 9472 US; Email: christian.mikutta@spk.unibe.ch.

interaction of memory encoding and music induced emotions provide an interesting field of research. The following chapter provides an overview over music specific encoding mechanisms in the short- and long-term memory. Furthermore, the interaction and overlap between verbal and musical memory is discussed. The impact of music-induced emotions on memory encoding is explored. Finally music's ability to reveal autobiographic memories is summarized.

2. Encoding Music in the Short-Term Memory

Working memory / short-term memory comprise a brain system, which enables temporary storage and simultaneous manipulation of information (Baddeley, 1992). The terms Short-term memory (STM) and working memory (WM) have not been used consistently in the literature. One possibility is to use the term STM to refer to the simple temporary storage of information, and WM to refer to the maintenance and manipulation of information (Schulze et al., 2012). For music -as for all audio stimuli- a translation of the wave-like sound impulses into neuronal impulses is needed before a possible storage into the STM can take place (Koelsch et al., 2005). Predictive timing processes are related to auditory-motor, fronto-parietal, and medial limbic systems and underlie metrical representation and its transitions (Fujioka et al., 2014). During the extraction of the musical features, the acoustic information enters the sensory memory. After that, the acoustic information is formed into auditory patterns ("Gestalten", e.g., representations comprising several perceptual elements) in the auditory sensory memory (Figure 1). Arrangement of acoustic events follows "Gestalt" principles such as similarity, proximity and continuity. In everyday life, such operations are not only important for music processing, but also, for instance, for separating a speaker's voice during a conversation from other sound sources in the environment. Previous EEG studies have provided evidence that mismatch negativities (MMN) seem to be the electrophysiological correlates of these processes in the EEG, occurring about 100- 200ms after introduction of the stimulus (Koelsch et al., 2005). The main contributors to the MMN are located in the auditory cortex and to a lesser extent in the frontal cortex. The involvement of the frontal cortex seems to indicate the sequencing of the WM. Therefore, it seems likely that the sensory auditory memory is connected with the auditory working memory as well as the long-term memory (LTM).

The interaction of auditory stimuli with memory is aptly described in the working memory model by Baddeley & Hitch (2000), which is organized around an attentional control system (the "central executive") that operates in connection with two subsystems: the visuospatial sketchpad and the phonological loop. The visuospatial sketchpad encodes and stores visual and spatial information; the phonological loop represents a verbal STM memory. The episodic buffer represents the interaction between the STM and the LTM (Baddeley, 2003).

Berz suggests in his model, that the encoding of music into the STM is specifically influenced by schemata, which are held in the LTM (Berz, 1995). The best available evidence for a separate component for musical WM, according to Berz (1995), is shown by the 'unattended music effect': If there would be only one acoustic store covering music as well as language, unattended instrumental music would cause the same disruptions on verbal performance as would unattended speech or unattended vocal music; this was shown not to be the case.

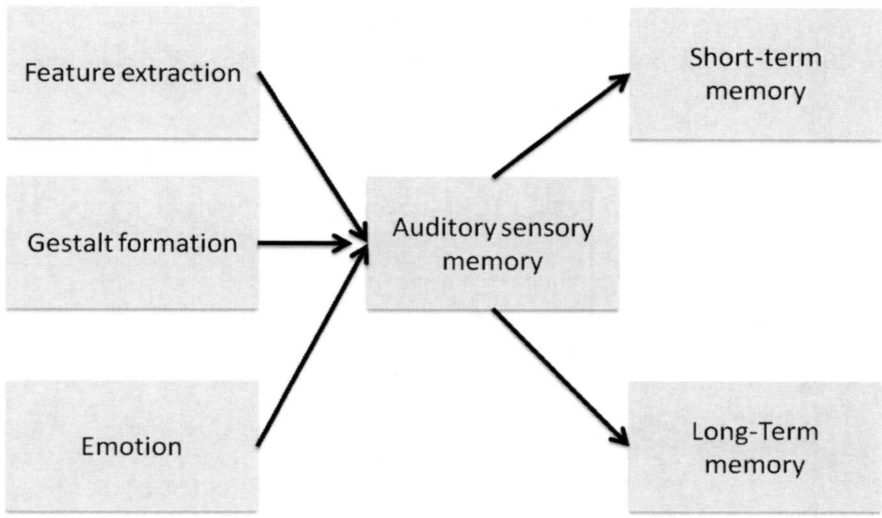

Figure 1. Input sources and the connections of the auditory sensory memory (Adapted from Koelschet al., 2005).

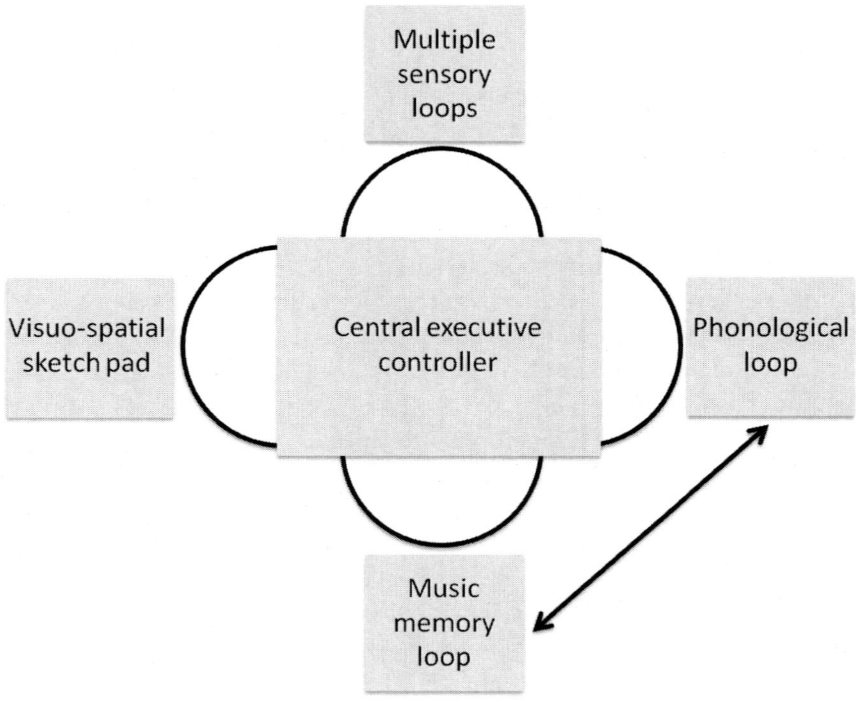

Figure 2. The working memory model from Baddeley, with the suggested additive 'music memory loop.'

Therefore, Berz (1995) suggests an additive slave system specific to music for the WM model (Figure 2). He proposes a similar model like the phonological loop including a musical store and a control process, which is based on musical inner speech.

Although there is a considerable overlap in anatomic structures involved in WM processing (Broca's area, premotor cortex, and inferior parietal lobe), it appears that music is stored differently in the WM, than verbal information (Roberts, 1986; Schulze et al., 2011).

3. Interaction of Short- and Long-Term Memory in Music

As mentioned above the interaction of sensory memory, WM and LTM are crucial for certain tasks. An everyday application of this interaction would be the recognition of familiar music. However, music recognition is a complex procedure. At least recognition of a familiar piece comprises a mapping procedure between certain features of the input stimulus and stored long-term representations that encompass constant properties of the stimulus. In terms of the "Gestalt" Theory, the separate features of the music are bound into events. These events are organized into groupings based on the similarity and proximity concepts. Those grouped events activate the specific parts of the LTM, which store similar events.

Hebert and colleagues (1997) explored in a comprehensive study which musical features are apt for this interaction. 32 participants listened to stimuli with either varying pitch or rhythm to differentiate the informative content for memorization for those two basic musical features. The lesser effectiveness of rhythmic structure as compared to melody appears to be related to its lesser encoding clarity relative to melodic structures. But in conclusion the most effective cue for music identification involved the proper combination of pitches and rhythm, of which the latter would be the most informative (Hebert et al., 1997). The process of music recognition seems to be mainly located in the right temporal lobe as demonstrated by lesion studies by Zatorre (1985). In a very interesting case study (Peretz, 1996), the observation of patient C.N. showed several years after having sustained bilateral temporal lesions, that this patient was unable to memorize new musical tunes. Furthermore, there was a lack of priming effect for musical material in this patient, which suggested diminished access and encoding specific to music. For the author, this clinical case argues for the existence of a LTM subsystem specific to musical material. The LTM is divided into implicit (unconscious) and explicit (conscious) memory (Baird et al., 2009). The explicit memory is then subdivided into an episodic and semantic part. Focusing on music, episodic musical memory can be defined as the ability to retrieve the spatiotemporal, personal and emotional contexts of the music. On the other hand, semantic musical memory can be defined as memory for factual musical knowledge or memory for associative or emotional concepts that is not linked to the retrieval of a specific personal experience or autobiographical event.

Implicit memory involves 'knowing how' and is mediated by non-conscious processes, including priming, procedural memory or motor skill learning, which is critical for e.g., playing a musical instrument (Wheeler et al., 1997).

Halpern and colleagues (2008) concluded that there seems to be a difference in memorization between verbal and musical material. Therefore, music, which cannot be named by the participants, is a better method for testing 'level of processing.' To measure implicit memory, Halpern and colleagues (2008) used a rating of the pleasantness of old and new melodies, whereas to measure explicit memory the researchers used the difference between the recognition confidence ratings of old and new melodies. Half of the 40 previously heard musical excerpts differed in timbre or tempo in comparison with the first exposure. Change in timbre and tempo both impaired explicit memory, and change in tempo also made implicit tune recognition worse. Halpern and colleagues (2008) concluded that indeed music is as well stored in two different types of memory: one implicit and the other explicit.

In a lesion study with patients suffering from unilateral medial temporal lobe dysfunction, Peretz and colleagues (2009) required the 37 patients to listen to 20 familiar and 20 unfamiliar musical excerpts. In the task, they judged the familiarity of the musical excerpt. Afterwards they were presented with the same stimuli, half of which were the same as the stimuli that were presented before. The subjects were asked to rate their liking (valence). In the second task, they had to rate their recognition. The results showed that memory effects were maximal on affect ratings for unfamiliar melodies, whereas recognition memory was better for familiar melodies. Implicit retrieval of melodies can still be preserved despite disrupted explicit retrieval abilities in patients with left temporal lesions, whereas both implicit and explicit tasks were impaired in patients with right temporal lesions patients. In conclusion Peretzet al., (2009) showed on the one hand that the right temporal lobe has an important role of creating melody representations, which support memory recognition (implicit process). On the other hand left-sided temporal lobe structures are more involved in the explicit retrieval of melodies (Samson et al., 2005).

In a high-resolution positron emission tomography study, Platelet al., (2003) outlined different brain networks involved in processing semantic and episodic memory. The participants had to judge if the musical extract was felt as "familiar." The experiment included two delayed recognition tasks, one containing only familiar and the other only non-familiar music excerpts. For episodic musical memory they found increases in cerebral blood flow bilaterally in the middle and superior frontal gyrus region and the precuneus, whereas for semantic musical memory there was a blood flow increase bilaterally in the medial and the orbitofrontal cortex, the left angular gyrus, and the left anterior part of the middle temporal cortex. From findings of Platelet al., (2003) and Peretzet al., (2009) one can conclude that these two different musical memory systems have a different neural representation. In a fMRI study, Groussardet al., (2010) explored the impact of musical expertise on the LTM. 20 musicians and 20 non-musicians were required to perform a familiarity task on 60 melody excerpts, i.e., semantic memory for music. Results showed that musical expertise induced supplementary activations in the hippocampus, medial frontal gyrus, and superior temporal areas on both sides, suggesting a constant interaction between episodic and semantic memory during this task in musicians. This activation pattern seems to overlap with those of the neural networks involved in episodic and semantic memory. In conclusion, the results indicate that trained musicians encode more contextual and perceptual details while listening to a familiar piece of music. Therefore, musical training may enable specific memory abilities.

4. Music and Language Memory Interactions

The interaction between music and language processing has been discussed intensively in literature. Research has found evidence for partly overlapping encoding procedures within memory processes. Peynirciogluet al., (1998) showed in a study that 60 healthy participants were better at recalling the titles of the 144 musical excerpts, when they are presented in an instrumental version as compared to remembering a melody by simply reading or hearing its title. However, if participants were given the titles as cues they recalled melodies better, just as if they were given the melodies as cues (Peynircioglu et al., 1998).

In conclusion Peynirciogluet al., (1998) showed that there is at least an interaction between semantic memory and musical memory. In 2002, Koelsch and colleagues showed that short musical pieces with particular characteristics could prime the semantic language memory system, thereby yielding faster and more efficient recognition of specific words. In a comprehensive design, Koelsch et al., (2002) primed the 44 target words (German nouns e.g., wideness, narrowness, needle, cellar, stairs, river, king, illusion) either with related sentences (e.g., wideness -the gaze wandered into the distance), unrelated sentences (the manacles allow only little movement), or with related music (e.g., Strauss Op. 54 Salome) or unrelated music (Valpola, E-minor piece accordion). They were able to show that target words that were semantically unrelated to prime sentences elicited a larger N400 in the EEG than did target words that were preceded by semantically related sentences. In addition, target words that were preceded by semantically unrelated musical primes showed a similar N400 effect, as compared to target words. The results show that music cannot only influence the processing of words, but it can also prime representations of meaningful concepts, independent of the emotional content of these concepts. In conclusion, the results of this group indicate that both music and language can prime the meaning of a word, and that music can determine physiological indices of semantic processing (Koelsch et al., 2004).

Groussard and colleagues (Groussard et al., 2010) showed in a PET study that the verbal semantic and musical semantic memory share common areas. 11 participants were required to perform a musical semantic memory task, where the subjects heard the first part of familiar melodies and had to decide whether the second part they heard matched to the first and a verbal semantic memory task with the same design, but with well-known expressions or proverbs as stimuli. Verbal and musical semantic processes activated a common network comprised of the left temporal cortex. The musical task showed a more anterior activation while the verbal task showed a predominantly posterior one. Another argument in favor of a separate LTM subsystem between language and music comes from event-related brain potential (ERP) studies (e.g., Besson, 2001), which show different ERP effects for semantic processes when subjects focus their attention only to the lyrics or to the music of opera excerpts. In conclusion, there is evidence for a considerable overlap within verbal and musical memory processes. However, within this system, sub-divisions for both categories seem to exist.

5. Emotions and Memory in Music

Music is a universal feature of human societies, partly owing to its power to evoke strong emotions and influence moods. Therefore, music is a powerful inducer of emotions (Meyer, 1956; Blood et al., 1999; Koelsch, 2014). Besides music, also emotional verbal and pictorial stimuli are remembered better than non-emotional ones (Heuer et al., 1990; Burke et al., 1992; Cahill et al., 1995; LaBar, 1998; Kensinger et al., 2003). This is probably due to the interaction of emotional and memory processes in limbic structures (Hamann, 2001) and might be explained by the semantic associative network model of memory by Bower (1981). The semantic associative network model assumes that emotions are represented in a network of nodes together with words, pictures, or music. Stimulation of emotion nodes creates spreading activation that lowers the threshold of excitation of all associatively linked nodes and thus helps to retrieve an emotional item from memory. In his famous study, Bower (1981) showed that subjects exhibited mood-state-dependent memory in recall of word lists, personal experiences recorded in a daily diary, and childhood experiences. Participants recalled a greater percentage of those experiences that were affectively congruent with the mood they were in during recall.

A study by Eschrich and colleagues (Eschrich et al., 2008) showed exactly this connection in particular for music. 24 participants listened to 40 musical pieces with different grades of valence and arousal. One week later, participants listened to the 40 old and 40 new musical excerpts randomly mixed and were asked to make an 'old/new' decision as well as to indicate arousal and valence for each of the pieces. Musical pieces that were rated as positive in terms of valence were recognized significantly better.

On the other hand, a better memory encoding and therefore, a higher familiarity, seem to alter the emotions induced by the music. Thus, it can result in an increase of positive affect toward the presented music.

In addition to the emotion inducing effect of music itself, music has been shown to be associated with other personal memories, so called autobiographical memories. Everybody knows the feeling memories from the past coming up associated with certain music. For example, one might not remember the exact title of a song but that it was played, when one met his wife the first time. This effect seems to be quite obvious considering the tremendous importance of music in all cultures and the frequency in which music is played in our everyday lives (Koelsch, 2014). We hear music at parties, clubs, concerts, restaurants, movies, and in television commercials, it is to be expected that pieces of music integrate with specific episodes in our lives (Janata et al., 2007). Janata and colleagues (2007) provided evidence that music is able to revive memories of events, people, and places that were formed while listening to a specific piece in the past. In their study, the group used 1515 short excerpts from 100 pop and R&B songs from the Billboard charts. Each participant listened to 30 randomly chosen excerpts. After music representation participants filled out specifically designed questionnaires concerning memories and emotions. Results showed that those brief musical excerpts serve as potent retrieval cues for autobiographical memories that include general memories for lifetime periods and detailed memories for specific events. Further they observed highly significant correlations between image vividness and autobiographical salience in 75% of the participants. The experienced emotions tended to be positive in valence, corroborating the results of emotional responses to music in everyday life that showed as well a positive valence in most of the cases (Juslin et al., 2003). This finding seems to be consistent with general findings that a better recall is achieved for positive valence and high arousal stimuli/events (Conway, 1993; Conway et al., 1999). Thus, positive emotions and high arousal levels that are associated with specific events act as a memory enhancer for these particular events. In the context of associative memory models, this memory-enhancing effect of emotions and arousal can be explained as a strengthening of the associations between the memories due to strong emotions (Janata et al., 2007).

In a follow-up study, Janata (2009) used fMRI to explore the psychophysiological representation of music induced autobiographical memories. In a similar approach he used excerpts at random from the Billboard Top 100 Pop and R&B charts for the years when the subjects were between 7 and 19 years of age. In the 13 healthy participants (mean age 20), the dorsal regions of the medial prefrontal cortex (MPFC) were shown to respond to the degree of autobiographical salience experienced during the 30 sec. musical excerpts. The present results demonstrate that this area shows a generalized increase to the degree of familiarity and autobiographical salience but also that this region follows the structural aspects of the music. The MPFC is part of a mechanism, which associates structural aspects of a retrieval cue with episodic memories.

Ford and colleagues (2011) subdivided the concept of autobiographical memories described above into 3 levels i.e., lifetime period, general event, and event-specific as proposed by Conwayet al., (2000). 'Lifetime' period encompasses abstract knowledge about oneself during a given period of time, 'general event' is comprised of memory for events that have been repeated or extended beyond one day, and 'event specific' includes memory for an event isolated in place and time. For exploring neurophysiological differences, 16 healthy participants listened to 30 sec. clips from popular songs between 1998 and 2007, and were studied in the fMRI scanner. After each musical excerpt, participants had to judge in which of the 3 categories their retrieved memories fitted best. Results revealed regions like ventromedial prefrontal cortex (PFC), medial temporal lobe (MTL), and posterior cingulate, which were recruited during a general search for autobiographical memories. Other regions were specific for the subcategories of autobiographical memories. Dorsolateral and dorsomedial PFC showed engagement in event based memories, while the dorsomedial PFC and bilateral MTL were activated during temporally specific events. The strongest activation was achieved by event-based autobiographical memories. Thus, both neuroimaging studies showed a particular activation of the ventromedial PFC. Moreover, those regions identified by Janata (2009) being modulated by salience (ventromedial, dorsomedial ventrolateral PFC) were in the Fordet al., (2011) study more active, the more specific the subjective memories were. In conclusion, it seems that the salience of autobiographical memories and the richness of specific memories are interdependent.

A concept standing nearby autobiographical memories is 'nostalgia.' Nostalgia is defined as an affective process that can accompany autobiographical memories (Wildschut et al., 2006). It has been described as a complex emotion that gives rise primarily (albeit not exclusively) to positive affect, and serves to counteract sadness and loneliness (Wildschut et al., 2006). The group around Janata (Barrett et al., 2010) explored the influence of personality traits on the feeling of 'nostalgia' evoked by music. The conceptual model of music-induced nostalgia included 'context-level constructs', i.e., aspects of a person's relationship to a given song as well as attributes of a person's experience while listening to a given song. Context-level constructs help determine why the same person experiences varying levels of nostalgia when listening to different songs. The second part are 'person-level constructs', i.e., individual differences between listeners, such as the degree to which a person is inclined to experience nostalgia and the level to which individuals differ on personality traits (such as extraversion or neuroticism). Person-level variables help to understand why some persons feel more nostalgic than others when listening to music. This basic concept is depicted in Figure 3.

In their experiment, a group consisting of 226 participants listened to randomly selected excerpts of popular music and rated how nostalgic each song made them feel. They used the specific questionnaires for assessing mood, nostalgia proneness, the 'big five' personality trades. Results within the context level constructs showed, that autobiographical salience of a particular song was the strongest predictor of the intensity of music evoked nostalgia. In addition, participants' familiarity with a song also significantly predicted the strength of nostalgia experienced while listening to that song. These effects were moderated by individual differences (nostalgia proneness, mood state, and factors of the Big Five trades). Concerning the personal level constructs they showed that that nostalgia proneness was the most robust person-level predictor of music-evoked nostalgia. The authors found as well a pattern of interactions between the nostalgia proneness and context-level constructs, suggesting that nostalgia proneness generally heightens the potency of context-level variables. Notably, the authors showed that nostalgia was not exclusively associated with positive valence emotions. Therefore, arguing that music induced nostalgia is more than successful remembering and the mixed valence may explain the sweet-bitter taste of nostalgia.

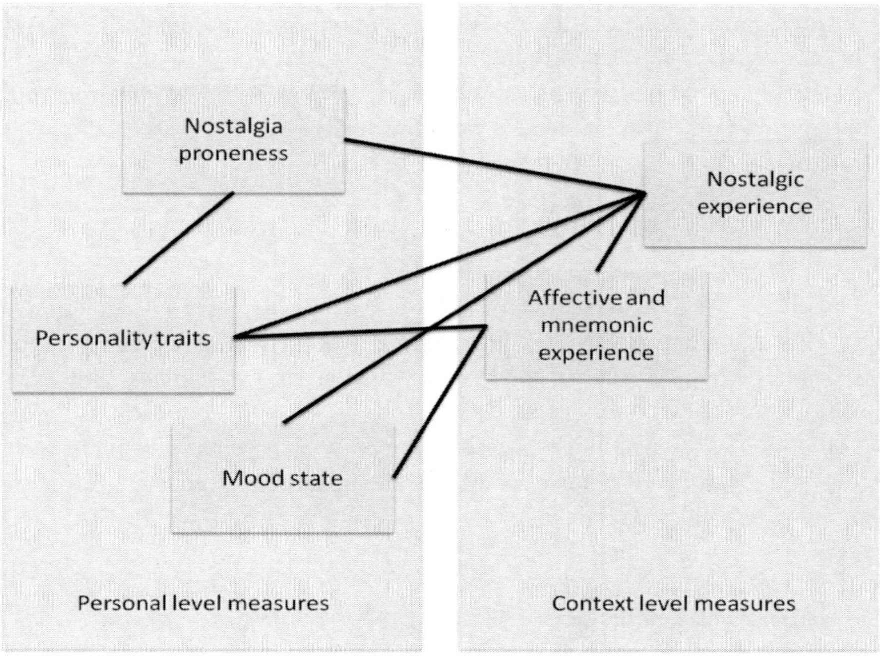

Figure 3. Summary of the interaction of the context level and personal level constructs in the heuristic model (Adapted from Barrettet al., 2010).

Krummhanslet al., (2013) went further and tried to explore which period of music showed the highest correlation between autobiographical memories and musical memories for each generation. Furthermore, the group explored that music transmitted over one-generation shapes as well autobiographical memories. As a basic concept they embraced the reminiscence bump, i.e., the notion that autobiographical memories are more frequently recalled for events in late adolescence and early adulthood. Studies have found that the music encountered during the late adolescence and early adulthood has the deepest impact on individuals throughout their lives (Schulkind et al., 1999). In their experiment, 62 college-age participants listened to two top Billboard hits per year from 1955 to 2009. Participants rated their recognition of the piece the preference for, quality judgments of, and emotional reactions to that music. First all measures showed an increase for music released during the first two decades of their lives. This finding fits to the literature of music and autobiographical memories (see above). Strikingly the authors found as well that the same response measures showed two distinct bumps for the music from 1960 to 1969 and from 1980 to 1984, music that was popular before the participants were born. So those participants revealed an affinity to the music of their parents' generation. The bump for music popular from 1980 to 1984 might be explained in terms of intergenerational influences. The participants' parents averaged 20 to 25 years of age in the early eighties. Therefore, it is assumed that in this period they established their own preferences. Assuming that this music was played during the child rearing years of those parents, it might make an imprint in the children (the actual participants). Concerning the other bump (1960-1969) the authors speculate about a transmission through 2 generations. Furthermore, they argue that the musical quality of this period might be higher.

In conclusion, music is a potent retriever of autobiographical memories as well as a reliable inducer of nostalgia. The vast interaction of music with general autobiographical memories and several subtypes of autobiographical memories reflect the importance and overwhelming presence of music in modern western society.

Conclusion

Music has different encoding ways in the STM as well as in the LTM as compared to other stimuli. This separate pathways account for tremendous importance of music in history of mankind. Music seems to share mechanisms with the speech domain. However, fMRI studies showed distinguished subsystems. Music -as a powerful modulator of emotions- is able to alter emotion-based encoding processes. Finally, music seems to be an important part of autobiographical memories. Therefore, music is an apt stimulus to engage further research within the emotional memory domain.

Grants:

1) Swiss National Foundation Grant P2SKP3_148497
2) NINDS, NIBIB, US Army Research Office, The Nielsen Corporation, SNF

REFERENCES

Baddeley, A. (1992) Working memory. *Science,* 255, 556-559.

Baddeley, A. (2003) Working memory: looking back and looking forward. *Nat. Rev. Neurosci.,* 4, 829-839.

Baird, A. & Samson, S. (2009) Memory for music in Alzheimer's disease: unforgettable? *Neuropsychol. Rev.,* 19, 85-101.

Barrett, F.S., Grimm, K.J., Robins, R.W., Wildschut, T., Sedikides, C. & Janata, P. (2010) Music-evoked nostalgia: affect, memory, and personality. *Emotion,* 10, 390-403.

Berz, W.L. (1995) Working Memory in Music: A Theoretical Model. *Music Perception,* 12, 353-364.

Besson, M. & Schoen, D. (2001) Comparison between language and music. In The Biological Foundations of Music, R.J. Zatorre, I. Peretz, I. (Eds.). *Ann. N.Y. Acad. Sci.* pp. 232–258.

Bharucha, J. & Krumhansl, C.L. (1983) The representation of harmonic structure in music: hierarchies of stability as a function of context. *Cognition,* 13, 63-102.

Blood, A.J., Zatorre, R.J., Bermudez, P., & Evans, A.C. (1999) Emotional responses to pleasant and unpleasant music correlate with activity in paralimbic brain regions. *Nat. Neurosci.,* 2, 382-387.

Bower, G.H. (1981) Mood and memory. Am. Psychol., 36, 129-148.

Burke, A., Heuer, F. & Reisberg, D. (1992) Remembering emotional events. *Mem. Cognit.,* 20, 277-290.

Cahill, L., Babinsky, R., Markowitsch, H.J. & McGaugh, J.L. (1995) The amygdala and emotional memory. *Nature,* 377, 295-296.

Conway, M.A. (1993) Emotion and memory. Science, 261, 369-370.

Conway, M.A. & Pleydell-Pearce, C.W. (2000) The construction of autobiographical memories in the self-memory system. *Psychol. Rev.,* 107, 261-288.

Conway, M.A., Turk, D.J., Miller, S.L., Logan, J., Nebes, R.D., Meltzer, C.C. & Becker, J.T. (1999) A positron emission tomography (PET) study of autobiographical memory retrieval. *Memory*, 7, 679-702.

Eschrich, S., Munte, T.F. & Altenmuller, E.O. (2008) Unforgettable film music: the role of emotion in episodic long-term memory for music. *BMC Neurosci.,* 9, 48.

Ford, J.H., Addis, D.R. & Giovanello, K.S. (2011) Differential neural activity during search of specific and general autobiographical memories elicited by musical cues. *Neuropsychologia,* 49, 2514-2526.

Fujioka, T., Fidali, B.C. & Ross, B. (2014) Neural correlates of intentional switching from ternary to binary meter in a musical hemiola pattern. *Front. Psychol.,* 5, 1257.

Groussard, M., Viader, F., Hubert, V., Landeau, B., Abbas, A., Desgranges, B., Eustache, F. & Platel, H. (2010) Musical and verbal semantic memory: two distinct neural networks? *Neuroimage,* 49, 2764-2773.

Halpern, A.R. & Mullensiefen, D. (2008) Effects of timbre and tempo change on memory for music. *Q J Exp. Psychol.* (Colchester), 61, 1371-1384.

Hamann, S. (2001) Cognitive and neural mechanisms of emotional memory. *Trends Cogn. Sci.,* 5, 394-400.

Hebert, S. & Peretz, I. (1997) Recognition of music in long-term memory: are melodic and temporal patterns equal partners? *Mem. Cognit.,* 25, 518-533.

Heuer, F. & Reisberg, D. (1990) Vivid memories of emotional events: the accuracy of remembered minutiae. *Mem. Cognit.,* 18, 496-506.

Janata, P. (2009) The neural architecture of music-evoked autobiographical memories. *Cereb. Cortex,* 19, 2579-2594.

Janata, P., Tomic, S.T. & Rakowski, S.K. (2007) Characterization of music-evoked autobiographical memories. *Memory,* 15, 845-860.

Juslin, P.N. & Laukka, P. (2003) Emotional expression in speech and music: evidence of cross-modal similarities. *Ann. N Y Acad. Sci.,* 1000, 279-282.

Kensinger, E.A. & Corkin, S. (2003) Memory enhancement for emotional words: are emotional words more vividly remembered than neutral words? *Mem. Cognit.,* 31, 1169-1180.

Koelsch, S. (2014) Brain correlates of music-evoked emotions. *Nat. Rev. Neurosci.*, 15, 170-80.

Koelsch, S., Kasper, E., Sammler, D., Schulze, K., Gunter, T. & Friederici, A.D. (2010) Music, language and meaning: brain signatures of semantic processing. *Nat. Neurosci.,* 7, 302-307.

Koelsch, S. & Siebel, W.A. (2005) Towards a neural basis of music perception. *Trends Cogn. Sci.*, 9, 578-584.

Krumhansl, C.L. & Zupnick, J.A. (2013) Cascading reminiscence bumps in popular music. *Psychol. Sci.,* 24, 2057-2068.

LaBar, K.P. (1998) Arousal-mediated memory consolidation: Role of the medial temporal lobe in humans. *Psychol. Sci.,* 9, 490-493.

Menon, V. & Levitin, D.J. (2005) The rewards of music listening: response and physiological connectivity of the mesolimbic system. *Neuroimage,* 28, 175-184.

Meyer, L. (1956) Emotion and meaning in music. Chicago: *University of Chicago Press.*

Pantev, C., Roberts, L.E., Schulz, M., Engelien, A. & Ross, B. (2001) Timbre-specific enhancement of auditory cortical representations in musicians. *Neuroreport,* 12, 169-174.

Peretz, I. (1996) Can we lose memory for music? A case of music agnosia in a non-musician. *J. Cogn. Neurosci.*, 8, 481-496.

Peynircioglu, Z.F., Tekcan, A.I., Wagner, J.L., Baxter, T.L. & Shaffer, S.D. (1998) Name or hum that tune: feeling of knowing for music. *Mem. Cognit.,* 26, 1131-1137.

Platel, H., Baron, J.C., Desgranges, B., Bernard, F. & Eustache, F. (2003) Semantic and episodic memory of music are subserved by distinct neural networks. *Neuroimage,* 20, 244-256.

Roberts, L. (1986) Modality and suffix effects in memory for melodic and harmonic musical materials. *Cogn. Psychol.*, 18, 123-157.

Samson, S. & Peretz, I. (2005) Effects of prior exposure on music liking and recognition in patients with temporal lobe lesions. *Ann. N Y Acad. Sci.,* 1060, 419-428.

Schulkind, M.D., Hennis, L.K. & Rubin, D.C. (1999) Music, emotion, and autobiographical memory: they're playing your song. *Mem. Cognit.,* 27, 948-955.

Schulze, K. & Koelsch, S. (2012) Working memory for speech and music. *Ann. N Y Acad. Sci.,* 1252, 229-236.

Schulze, K., Mueller, K. & Koelsch, S. (2011) Neural correlates of strategy use during auditory working memory in musicians and non-musicians. *Eur. J. Neurosci.,* 33, 189-196.

Wheeler, M.A., Stuss, D.T. & Tulving, E. (1997) Toward a theory of episodic memory: the frontal lobes and autonoetic consciousness. *Psychol. Bull.,* 121, 331-354.

Wildschut, T., Sedikides, C., Arndt, J. & Routledge, C., Nostalgia: content, triggers, functions. *J. Pers. Soc. Psychol.,* 91, 975-993.

Zatorre, R.J. (1985) Discrimination and recognition of tonal melodies after unilateral cerebral excisions. *Neuropsychologia,* 23, 31-41.

In: Synaptic Fundamentals of Memory Performance
Editor: Ignacio González-Burgos
ISBN: 978-1-63483-279-3

Chapter 7

Estrogen Actions on Glial Reactivity and Inflammation-Mediated Memory Impairment: Sex Differences and Interaction with Other Neurotrophic Factors

María José Bellini*
Institute for Biochemical Research (INIBIOLP) –
National University of La Plata, La Plata, Argentina

Abstract

There is growing evidence that documents profound effects of estrogens on learning, memory, and mood as well as neurodevelopment and neurodegenerative diseases. However, the ability of estradiol to influence synaptic plasticity, neurotransmission, neurodegeneration and cognition, could be different depending on sex dimorphisms. It emerges that estrogens have different, even opposite, effects as well as similar effects in male and female brains. The protective effects of estradiol on neural cells are mediated in part by modulation of neurotrophic factors such as insulin like growth factor (IGF-l), tyrosine kinase A (Trk A), nerve growth factors (NGF), and the like. Also, it modulates the action of neurotrophins, which in turn regulate the synaptogenesis, synaptic plasticity and synaptic functions. By these actions estrogen prevents or slows down the neurodegenerative process. Another described effect of estradiol is the capacity to modulate inflammatory response mediated by glial cells. Neuroinflammation is a feature not only of many neurological disorders but also of aging, and it is accompanied by activation of glial cells and the release of proinflammatory cytokines and chemokines. Such activation is a normal response oriented to protect neural tissue. However, excessive and chronic activation of glia may lead to neurotoxicity and may be harmful for neural tissue. Estrogenic compounds may be candidates to counteract brain inflammation under neurodegenerative conditions by targeting the production and release of pro-inflammatory molecules by glial cells. In this chapter we will review different mechanisms that may be implicated in the diverse actions of estradiol, the differences

* Send correspondence to: Maria Jose Bellini, INIBIOLP, Faculty of Medicine, UNLP, CC 455, 1900 La Plata, Argentina, tel: (54-221) 425-6735, fax: (54-221) 425-0924/ 425-8988, e-mail: mariajosebellini@yahoo.com.

according to gender and we empathize in the anti-inflammatory action on glial cell. We will also explore the interaction of estradiol with others neurotrophic factors, such as IGF-I in the regulation of neurodegeneration and memory impairment. Finally, the possibility of using selective estrogen receptor modulators (SERMs) to exert estradiol-like neuroprotective actions in the brain as an alternative to estrogen will be discussed.

Keywords: estrogen, inflammation, cognition, sex differences, glia

1. Introduction

Estrogen is a potent steroid of both gonadal and neuronal origin that exerts profound and enduring effects on cognitive function during development, adulthood and aging. Estrogen has traditionally been referred to as the ''female'' hormone whose principal source is the ovary and consists principally of three forms: 17β-estradiol, estrone, and estriol. However, the male also produces estrogen. In fact, while estrogen levels in the male are quantitatively lower than those in the female, many developmental actions of testosterone in the brain of both sexes depend upon initial intraneuronal conversion by the cytochrome P450 enzyme aromatase to the estrogenic metabolite 17β-estradiol. This steroid subsequently exerts its action on neurons or glia cells by classical or non-classical receptors. Among its various effects estrogen is capable of enhancing synaptic plasticity, neurite growth, hippocampal neurogenesis, and long-term potentiation. It also protects against neuron apoptosis and neural injury in a variety of experimental settings, including toxicity-induced by excitatory neurotransmitters, β-amyloid, oxidative stress, and ischemia (Petrovska et al., 2012). Estrogen can be generated not only from circulating testosterone by local aromatase but synthesized de novo by neurons and glia (Garcia-Segura, 2008).

Many estrogen actions are potentially relevant to cognitive changes occurring after menopause, but for most, the clinical implications are yet unclear (Luine, 2008; Frick, 2009). In theory, estrogen holds great clinical potential for central nervous system (CNS) disorders because of its proven neuroprotective and neuroactivating properties (McEwen & Alves, 1999; Wise et al., 2001; Brann et al., 2007; Garcia-Segura et al., 2008). However, as discussed in detail in the remainder of this chapter, there is mounting evidence that estrogen may have opposite effects in male and female brains which could be due principally to differences in brain organization (for review see Gillies & McArthur, 2010).

2. Estrogen and Memory

2.1. General Aspects

Memory comprises acquisition, consolidation and retrieval of information (for review see McGaugh, 2000). Many substances can influence these different phases.

It is well demonstrated that sex hormones, mainly estrogen, impact cognitive function. Estrogen works synergistically with many biologic systems to promote physical, cognitive, and affective function. Basic science reveals that administration of estrogen (estrogen alone and estrogen plus Progesterone) results in increased levels of antioxidants, reduces free radicals, and substantially lowers oxidative damage to mitochondrial DNA (Irwin et al., 2008). Critical to neuronal health, estrogen also regulates glucose and oxidative metabolism, mitochondrial function, and promotes adenosine triphosphate (ATP) (Brinton, 2008a) Indeed, declines in these processes are characteristic of neurodegenerative diseases such as Alzheimer disease (AD) (Brinton, 2008b). Estrogen treatment promotes the growth of long thin spines in the hippocampus and prefrontal cortex (Wang et al., 2010; Srivastava, 2012; Luine & Frankfurt, 2013), which reduction is correlated with impaired memory function (Luine et al., 2011). Higher levels of presynaptic estrogen receptor α (ERα) are associated with stronger memory performance in ovariectomized animals treated with exogenous estrogen (Wang et al., 2010). Neurotrophins, such as nerve growth factor (NGF) and brain-derived neurotrophic factor (BDNF), represent another mechanism of neural plasticity in the brain. These substances facilitate the growth of dendritic spines in the hippocampus (Luine et al., 2011). In vitro investigations support a favorable effect of estrogens on the activity of neurotropins (Green et al., 2000; Solum & Handa, 2002). By rising hippocampal BDNF levels, estrogen transiently increases dendritic spines, thereby potentiating opportunity for increased connectivity and plasticity (Srivastava, 2012).

Estrogen also interacts with a number of neurotransmitters affecting cognition and mood. Animal research reveals that long-term use of estrogen prevented declines in cholinergic nerve cell fiber length and density at menopause (Tinkler et al., 2004). In humans, the negative effect of cholinergic challenge on cognitive performance and neural activation patterns was counteracted by prior exposure to estradiol (Dumas et al., 2006; 2012). Of note, naturally occurring higher levels of estriol were associated with poorer cognition, specifically working memory performance (Dumas et al., 2012).

2.2. Sex Differences

Many estrogen effects differ qualitatively or quantitatively between the sexes, suggesting that they may be subject to sexual differentiation during pre- or early postnatal development. In addition, circulating hormone levels may contribute differentially in adult males and females.

It is well documented that men and women have different types of cognitive function, and the sex differences in cognition are associated with brain estrogen and testosterone actions in the regions important for cognition, memory and mood such as the cortex, hippocampus and amygdala (Wilson & Davies,1973; Cahill, 2006; Cosgrove et al., 2007).

Gender differences in cognitive function have been well demonstrated in adulthood as well as ageing. For example, men demonstrated larger amygdala and thalamus volumes compared to women (Neufang et al., 2009; Bramen et al., 2011; Koolschijn & Crone, 2013), whereas the size of the hippocampus is larger in females compared to males (Neufang et al., 2009; Giedd et al., 1996). It is also worth noticing that there are a relatively higher number of androgen receptors in the amygdala (Clark et al., 1988) and a relatively higher number of estrogen receptors in the hippocampus (Morse et al., 1986). The sex differences in regional brain structure might be responsible for the sex differences in specific cognitive and behavioral tasks (De Vries, 2004; Cahill, 2006; Cosgrove et al., 2007).

Sex differences in brain function also include gender differences in the incidence of psychopathologies such as depressive illness, which is more common in women; substance abuse and antisocial behavior, which are more common in men, as well as pain sensitivity. The diversity of these effects implies that regions of the brain are involved outside of the hypothalamus, which has been the traditional site for the study of ovarian steroid receptors and their role in the control of reproductive function. The actions of estrogen could be mediated by intracellular receptors, which modulate genomic actions, or by membrane receptors or indirectly by their actions on glial cells (the mechanisms of action will be discuss in another section of this chapter).

Due to the hippocampus is one of the major areas related to memory process, this section emphasizes in the sex differences and estradiol actions concerning to this region even so it will also be discuss the differences in the prefrontal cortex (PFC), another brain area involved in memory.

In experimental mammalian species, such as rats, and in humans, males perform better than females, on average, in the acquisition of tasks involving spatial memory, which are highly dependent on the hippocampus (Luine, 2008; Mitsushima et al., 2009). The activation influences of adult gonadal steroids play an important role in maintaining sexually differentiated cognitive behaviors.

Many studies investigating only females report a positive effect of estrogens on hippocampal- dependent tasks in rats, mice, and rhesus monkeys (Foster et al., 2008; Luine, 2008; Spencer et al., 2008). Relatively few studies have made direct comparisons of males and females, but in some tests of hippocampal spatial discrimination (the Morris water maze), hormone treatment of gonadectomized mice revealed that estradiol selectively impaired performance in females but had no effect in males (Fugger et al., 1998). Several reports suggest that functional sex differences are related to organizational influences in early development (Roof, 1993; McEwen & Alves, 1999; Romeo et al., 2004).

For example, exposure to high levels of estradiol during development improves (masculinizes) spatial behavior in adult female rats to levels seen in normal males. It seems therefore that sex differences in aspects of hippocampal function are determined by testosterone acting after conversion to estrogen by aromatase in a manner similar to that established for the hypothalamus, indicating that non-reproductive brain regions are subject to hormonal processes of sex differentiation similar to those in brain regions intimately associated with reproduction.

It should be noted, however, that in other tests of hippocampal function (a delayed matching-to-position task), estradiol treatment of rats gonadectomized as adults enhanced task acquisition in both sexes and, although testosterone treatment of males was without effect on this component of the task, testosterone did affect delay-dependent working memory (Gibbs, 2005).

Furthermore, both human and animal studies showed that administration of androgens to females may induce male-typical cognition and behavior, and the male-type cognition disappearing when the treatment was withdrawn (Cahill, 2006). For example, one recent cross-sectional human study showed that women with polycystic ovary syndrome characterized by elevated endogenous testosterone performed significantly better at three-dimensional mental rotation, a male favored cognitive behavior, than a female control group (Barry et al., 2013).

Another study also demonstrated that a single administration of testosterone improves 3D mental rotation abilities in young women (Aleman et al., 2004).

On balance, it seems that estrogens and androgens influence different aspects of cognitive tasks or domains in males and females, with indications that these effects are sex-specific (Warren & Juraska, 1997; Gibbs, 2005).

Indeed, it is generally thought that males and females use different strategies, underpinned by different organization of the underlying neural substrate, to solve similar spatial tasks; females tend to rely more on local cues and landmarks, whereas males rely more on the spatial relationships between two fixed points (Raber, 2008). The available evidence also suggests that hormonal influences can differ with the type of task, the aspect of the task under investigation (acquisition, consolidation, retrieval), and the degree to which the task relies on input from brain regions other than the hippocampus, such as the prefrontal cortex, which is associated more with working memory tasks requiring visual object information (Torres-Aleman et al., 1990; Takase et al., 2009).

Concerning the prefrontal cortex, it plays an important role in working or short-term memory in various mammalian species, including rats, nonhuman primates, and humans. Tests of prefrontal functions reveal many sex differences: females generally outperform males in the acquisition of tasks that rely more heavily on this region, such as visual object recognition (Kritzer et al., 2007; Luine, 2007; Mitsushima et al., 2009). Although the organizational and activational influences of sex hormones have not be studied as extensively in this region as the hippocampus, emerging evidence suggests the impact of both estrogens and androgens in both sexes (Gibbs, 2005). For example, estradiol promotes performance in memory tasks in women (Berman et al., 1997; Keenan et al., 2001), female rhesus monkeys (Wang et al., 2010), and rats (Wallace et al., 2006), and circulating levels of both estradiol and testosterone correlate with certain spatial and mnemonic tasks in female rats (Kritzer et al., 2007). In adult male rats, gonadectomy impairs performance in various tasks of working memory and other types of cognitive tasks that are known to rely on the PFC, but the hormone responsiveness depends on the task and probably the neurotransmitter pathways involved.

Hence, testosterone, but not estradiol, reversed the effects of castration on performance in tests of spatial working memory, and this correlated with the density of dopaminergic terminals in the medial PFC. Like the hippocampus, the PFC retains the capacity for synaptic remodeling, which is also critical for learning and memory that is lost in AD (Scheff & Price, 2003).

Estradiol also maintains dendritic spines in specific cortical regions of female nonhuman primates (Tang et al., 2004) and rats (Wallace et al., 2006), in parallel with positive effects on working memory; preliminary studies indicate that androgens may also positively affect spine synapses in the female PFC (Hajszan et al., 2008).

Although work in this brain region is still at an early stage, both morphological and behavioral studies suggests that the PFC uses sex hormones in a manner different from that seen in the hippocampus and hypothalamus, suggesting that hormonal therapeutic strategies to modulate the function of each of these brain regions could be achieved by a different cocktail of hormone supplementation that might be unique to males or females.

Therefore, at behavioral level it is very difficult to reach simple interpretations on the influences of estradiol or testosterone on cognition in males and females. In contrast, striking sexually dimorphic responses to estradiol have been reported for neuroanatomical, morphological, neurochemical, and electrophysiological correlates of learning and memory.

3. MECHANISMS OF ACTION

3.1. Nuclear and Extra-Nuclear Mechanisms for Genomic and Rapid, Non-Genomic Mechanisms of Estrogen Signaling in the Brain

The last decade or so has seen very rapid advances in our understanding of the mechanisms of action of estrogen in the brain, as evidenced by many excellent reviews (McEwen & Alves 1999; Toran-Allerand et al., 1999; Wise et al., 2001; Brann et al., 2007; Tetel, 2009; Arevalo et al., 2015). Here there are summarizing some basic background information on cellular signaling mechanisms and ER expression patterns:

1. Classic Estrogen Receptors. Classic ERs are located in the nucleus and cytoplasm of the cell and belong to the nuclear receptor superfamily, members of which act as nuclear ligand-gated transcription factors, binding to estrogen response elements (EREs) within specific genes to alter their rate of transcription (Mangelsdorf et al., 1995). The two known isoforms, ERa and ERb are coded by separate genes and are located throughout the brain, but have a differential distribution. ERα mRNA is widely distributed in many brain regions, including the hippocampus, hypothalamus, amygdala, and brainstem nuclei, and co-localizes with ERβ mRNA in many regions. ERβ has a more restricted distribution and is found in particular abundance in human, nonhuman primate, and rodent hippocampus and selected hypothalamic nuclei, especially the supraoptic and paraventricular nuclei (PVN) (Shughrue et al., 1997, 1998; Register et al., 1998; Gundlah et al., 2000; Osterlund et al., 2000a,b; Mitra et al., 2003; Ostlund et al., 2003; Merchenthaler et al., 2004; Suzuki and Handa, 2005; Gonzalez et al., 2007; Weiser et al., 2008). The two forms of ER are structurally and functionally distinct, each regulating unique sets of target genes in a tissue- and cell type-specific manner (Kian Tee et al., 2004). This may be the net effect of homo- or hetero-dimerization of ERα and ERβ. Steroid receptor-mediated transcription is also modulated by corregulators (activator and repressor proteins and protein complexes). There are vast numbers of these corregulator proteins, and various selective combinations associate with ERs and critically determine the region and cell-type specificity of the effects of ER ligands, as well as potential interactions of ER with other nuclear receptors, such as those for progesterone (PR), testosterone, androgen receptors (AR), and glucocorticoids (Tetel, 2009). As well as acting directly through EREs, ligand-activated classic ERs can also modulate gene transcription indirectly at alternative response elements by influencing the activity of other transcription factors. Specifically, estradiol can activate transcription via the activated protein-1 response element in the presence of ERα but fails to do so when linked with ERβ (Kushner et al., 2000). The expression, co-expression, and ratio of ERα / ERβ, as well as the presence of any given combination of co-regulatory proteins in any given cell, will therefore greatly influence the estrogen response.

2. Membrane Signaling. In addition to classic genomic actions, it is now recognized that estrogens can initiate rapid signaling via actions at the cell membrane in many brain regions. Because there is no clear consensus on the molecular identity of the membrane receptors, it is not possible to define their expression patterns in the brain. However, pharmacological and emerging ultrastructural evidence demonstrates that classic "nuclear" ERα and ERβ, and probably other novel receptors (such as GPR30), can also be localized at the cell membrane to effect rapid activation of intracellular brain signaling pathways and modulatory proteins

within seconds to minutes of exposure to steroid (McEwen & Alves, 1999; Gorosito et al., 2008; Vasudevan & Pfaff, 2008; Mermelstein, 2009) These include effects on calcium channels and intracellular stores to increase intracellular [Ca2], which may lead to activation of calcium-calmodulin-dependent kinases, and activation of other protein kinases in 1) the cAMP/cAMP-dependent protein kinase pathway, 2) the mitogen-activated protein kinase (MAPK or extracellular signal-regulated kinases, ERK) pathway (also named MEK), and 3) the phosphoinositide 3-kinase (PI3K)/Akt (also termed PKB) pathway. In parallel or in series, these pathways may interact and converge, finally to affect gene transcription and protein synthesis via the rapid downstream activation of transcription factors, such as the cAMP response element binding protein (CREB) or nuclear factor κB (Toran-Allerand et al., 1999, 2002; Boulware et al., 2005; Vasudevan & Pfaff, 2008; Mermelstein, 2009). Thus, although referred to as non-genomic mechanisms to distinguish them from the classic mode of action, it is now understood that actions initiated at the plasma membrane may also ultimately affect gene transcription. The mechanisms by which activated membrane ERs elicit cellular responses are not yet understood, but interactions with other cell-surface receptors and their associated molecules, such as G-proteins, insulin-like growth factor 1 (IGF-I), and metabotropic glutamate receptors (which are linked to G-proteins) have emerged as means by which membrane ERs can trigger intracellular second- messenger signaling systems and affect cellular responses (Garcia-Segura et al., 2001; Wyckoff et al., 2001; Mermelstein, 2009). Estrogen-activated signaling pathways can also increase mitochondrial efficiency and lead to a reduction in free radical generation in the brain and mitochondrial-dependent apoptosis (Nilsen et al., 2007; Brinton, 2008a). Furthermore, membrane- initiated and genomic actions of hormones may be coupled, so the distinctions are not as clear-cut as was first thought (Vasudevan & Pfaff, 2008). It is noteworthy that most of the cellular mechanisms described for estrogen actions, especially MEK/ERK and PI3K/Akt signaling and mitochondrial function, have important roles in cell survival, apoptosis, function, and neurodevelopment and may sub-serve the critical neuroregulatory, neurotrophic, and neuroprotective effects of estrogens in brain physiology and pathological conditions of the brain. There is, however, no simple rule to predict which mode of estrogenic action will prevail and whether estrogens will exert positive/enhancing or negative/ suppressing influences on any given signaling pathway because, notoriously, these vary between neural phenotype and brain region.

3.2. Interaction with Other Neurotrophic Factors

Estradiol exerts its actions via different mechanisms, one of which involves interacting with different neurotrophic factor receptors. Among them is IGF-I, that is a potent neuroprotective hormone (Torres Aleman, 2012). There is a substantial body of evidence of a close interdependence between the actions of IGF-I and estradiol in the brain (Mendez et al., 2005). Both factors have in common the duality of being hormones, as well as locally produced neuromodulators, and they exert similar pleiotropic actions in the developing and adult brain. There are several potential points of convergence between estradiol and IGF-I receptor (IGF-IR) signaling in the brain. Estrogen activates the mitogen-activated protein kinase (MAPK) pathway and has a synergistic effect with IGF-I on the activation of Akt, a kinase downstream phosphoinositol-3 kinase. In addition, IGF-IR is necessary for the estradiol induced expression of the anti-apoptotic molecule Bcl-2 in hypothalamic neurons. The interplay of ERs and IGF-IR in the brain may depend on interactions between neural cells expressing ERs with neural cells expressing IGF-IR, or on direct interactions of the signaling pathways of ERs and IGF-IR in the same cell, since most neurons expressing IGF-IR also express at least one of the ER subtypes (Cardona-Gómez et al., 2001; Cardona-Gómez et al., 2002; Garcia-Segura et al., 2010). It is also known that IGF-I regulates ER transcriptional activity and, as we mentioned above, estradiol regulates IGF-I receptor signaling in neural cells and some details on the molecular mechanisms involved in this cross-talk have been established. IGF-I is required to maintain a broad range of brain functions (Carro et al., 2003) regarding modulation of cognition, IGF-I is associated with increases in speed of information processing and working memory (Aleman et al., 1999; Bellar et al., 2011). Future directions may include the assessment of the interaction of ERs and IGF-I receptors with other signaling systems.

Another neurotrophic factor of relevance is BDNF. It was shown that estrogen can induce BDNF expression via an estrogen-sensitive response element on the BDNF gene. It was subsequently shown that BDNF mRNA levels increase in many brain areas of ovariectomized rats treated with estradiol (Singh et al., 1995; Sohrabji et al., 1995; Solum & Handa, 2002). BDNF is a member of the neurotrophin family, which includes nerve growth factor, neurotrophin-3, and neurotrophin-4/5. All neurotrophins have potent actions at tropomyosin receptor kinases (trk). BDNF binds with high specificity to trkB. It is well documented that BDNF potentiates synaptic transmission in hippocampal area CA1, area CA3, and the dentate gyrus, and is critical to the late phase of long-term potentiation (Patterson et al., 1996; Pang and Lu, 2004). In area CA3, BDNF potentiates a major glutamatergic input to pyramidal cells, the mossy fiber pathway (Scharfman, 1997). These studies suggested that BDNF might be a mediator of estrogen action.

4. Inflammation and Cognitive Impairment

4.1. Overviews

The neural cell response to injury is known as neuroinflammation. Two types of inflammatory responses are known to occur in the CNS, acute and chronic. Acute inflammation comprises a rapid activation of glial cells: microglia and astrocytes and the release of a set of growth factors and proinflammatory molecules in the surrounding and within the damaged tissue. These factors restore the stability and function of adjacent nervous cells in a paracrine way; it is basically a defensive response directed to repair the damaged site. Nevertheless as time progresses, chronic proinflammatory cytokines and chemokines attract macrophages/microglia and T cells to the focus of inflammation that promote further injury and propagate a feed-forward inflammatory response resulting in a progressive neurodegeneration and cognitive decline. Neurodegenerative disorders, such as Alzheimer's and Parkinson's diseases and stroke are often accompanied by chronic inflammatory events (Hensley, 2010; Baune, 2015).

Also, it has been described that pro-inflammatory markers increase with age, and correlate with deleterious cognitive outcomes in late life (Franceschi et al., 2000; Kravitz et al., 2009; Bettcher et al., 2012). In terms of underlying mechanisms, older adults with higher systemic levels of inflammatory markers have been shown to evidence smaller hippocampi and medial temporal lobes relative to those with low levels of inflammation (Bettcher et al., 2012). Although much of the injury caused by chronic inflammation is irreversible, the progressive nature of this reaction allows interferences at delayed time points when anti-inflammatory agents can inhibit glial cell activation and release of proinflammatory cytokines.

4.2. Estrogen and Inflammation

The neuroprotective and anti-inflammatory effects of estradiol in the brain are mediated, at least in part, by a reduction of reactive gliosis (Arevalo et al., 2010). Estradiol exerts anti-inflammatory effects on astrocytes and microglia by mechanisms involving estrogen receptors (Arevalo et al., 2010). For instance, estrogens decrease the expression of nitric oxide and the inflammatory markers TNFa, IL-1b, IL-6, matrix metalloproteinase- 9, and interferon-inducible protein-10 in cultured astrocytes incubated with bacterial LPS (Kipp et al., 2007; Lewis et al., 2008; Cerciat et al., 2010) by mechanisms that involve the inhibition of NFκB-induced transcription of proinflammatory chemokines and cytokines (Dodel et al., 1999; Cerciat et al., 2010). Furthermore, estrogens decrease the number of reactive astrocytes in vivo, after excitotoxic-induced neurodegeneration (Ciriza et al., 2004), in experimental Parkinson's disease (Tripanichkul et al., 2006), in experimental diabetic central neuropathy (Saravia et al., 2006), after lesion of the cholinergic basal forebrain (Martinez & de Lacalle, 2007), and after stab wound brain lesions (García-Estrada et al., 1999; Barreto et al., 2007; Barreto et al., 2009).

4.3. Glial Cells Mediate Hormonal Signaling

It is becoming increasingly apparent that glial cells of the central and peripheral nervous system are key participants because they are capable of both sending and receiving hormonal signals. Hormones are also a critical component of neuronal/glial cross talk, leading to neuromodulatory and neurotrophic actions under physiological and pathological conditions (Garcia-Ovejero et al., 2005).

Both Schwann cells, in the peripheral nervous system, and oligodendroglia, astroglia, NG2 cells and microglia, in CNS, are targets of the hormone. Glial cells are involved in a large variety of functions, including the regulation of neuronal metabolism, neuronal activity and synaptic transmission and plasticity. In addition, Schwann cells and oligodendrocytes produce myelin, which is essential for the quick propagation of impulses in axons (Volterra et al., 2002).

Glial cells express classical ERs (Garcia-Ovejero et al., 2005) and this expression is enhanced under different pathological conditions (Blurton-Jones & Tuszynski, 2001; Savaskan et al., 2001; García-Ovejero et al., 2002; Takahashi et al., 2004); this may facilitate actions of estradiol to reduce neuronal damage (Carbonaro et al., 2009). Estradiol also exerts rapid signaling events in glia via membrane-associated ERs (Grove-Strawser et al., 2010), the regulation of the activation of kinase signaling pathways (Ivanova et al., 2001; Zhang et al.,

2002; Dhandapani et al., 2005; Hirahara et al., 2009), and the modification of intracellular calcium levels (Chaban et al., 2004; Arnold, 2005). Furthermore, ER independent antioxidant actions of estradiol may reduce oxidative stress mechanisms involved in glial activation (Wang et al., 2006). The reaction of glial cells to neurodegenerative damage is a complex phenomenon that includes a mixture of positive and negative responses for neuronal survival and regeneration.

After peripheral nerve injury Schwann cells proliferate, form a permissive environment for axonal growth and re-myelinate the growing axons (Fawcett & Keynes, 1990; Chen et al., 2007). In the injured CNS oligodendrocyte precursor cells are activated to generate re-myelinating oligodendrocytes, which restore myelin in demyelinated damaged axons (Franklin et al., 2008). Astrocytes become reactive, increasing their volume and the expression of intermediate filaments such as glial fibrillary acidic protein (GFAP), vimentin and nestin. Reactive astrocytes maintain the integrity of the blood–brain barrier and the survival of peri-lesion tissue by the release of molecules, including estradiol (Garcia-Segura et al., 2003; Saldanha et al., 2009), that exert neuroprotective actions on neurons. However, reactive astrocytes interfere with axonal regeneration and contribute to local brain inflammation (Laird et al., 2008). Reactive microglia exerts important positive functions by remodeling the damaged tissue, but release proinflammatory cytokines and may exacerbate neuronal damage (Hanisch & Kettenmann, 2007).

Anti-inflammatory effects of estradiol on astrocytes may also contribute to the neuroprotective effects of the hormone. Under pathological conditions, astrocytes release a number of proinflammatory cytokines and chemokines that attract macrophages/microglia and T cells to CNS inflammatory sites.

The downregulation of the production of cytokines and chemokines by reactive astrocytes may be involved in the neuroprotective mechanisms of estradiol, at least under chronic neurodegenerative conditions. The anti-inflammatory effects of estradiol may involve ERs expressed in astrocytes. A study using selective ERα and ERβ specific ligands suggests that both receptor subtypes are involved in the anti-inflammatory action of estradiol on astrocytes in vitro (Lewis et al., 2008).

Estradiol also reduces CNS inflammation acting on microglia. Activation of microglia is a normal response from neural tissue to cope with infections and neurodegeneration and it is oriented to protect neural tissue. However, exaggerated and chronic activation of microglia may lead to neurotoxicity and may be detrimental for neural tissue (Streit, 2002; Block et al., 2007; Lehnardt, 2010; Baune, 2015). Therefore, the regulation of the response of microglial cells to inflammation may represent a therapeutic approach to control neurodegeneration. Studies in microglia cultures have shown that estradiol inhibits the induction of inducible nitric oxide synthase and several other inflammatory mediators in response to LPS and to proinflammatory cytokines (Bruce-Keller et al., 2000; Drew & Chavis, 2000; Dimayuga et al., 2005; Vegeto et al., 2008). Studies in vivo have also demonstrated that estradiol reduces microglia reactivity and the expression of cytokines and chemokines induced by an acute intracerebroventricular injection of LPS in female mice (Vegeto et al., 2003; Vegeto et al., 2006; Vegeto et al., 2008) and by the systemic administration of LPS (Tapia-Gonzalez et al., 2008). The hormone also reduces microglia activation after a stab wound injury.

Recent studies have investigated the actions of estradiol on oligodendrocytes and myelin integrity after different forms of white matter injury. The results have shown that estradiol is able to reduce, at least partially, oligodendrocyte cell loss and demyelination and to facilitate remyelination (Crawford et al., 2010). The protective actions of estradiol on oligodendrocytes and myelin may be mediated by the hormonal control of peripheral immune cells (Du et al., 2011) and by direct actions on oligodendrocytes (Hirahara et al., 2009).

Therefore the actions of estradiol on glial cells are important to maintain physiological homeostasis, control the inflammation and ameliorate the cognitive impairment observed with aging or under pathological conditions.

5. Potential for Estradiol or Brain-Selective Estrogen Receptor Modulators-Therapies

As it has already discussed, there are numerous neuroprotective actions of estrogens that have direct relevance to neurodegenerative diseases and inflammation-associated decline in cognition. Despite these actions, the promise of estrogen-based therapies for reducing the risk for neurodegeneration remains to be fulfilled. The application of estradiol as a neuroprotectant in humans presents numerous limitations, mainly due to the endocrine actions of the molecule on peripheral tissues, including estrogen dependent tumors. Therefore, as ongoing research continues to address these crucial and immediate concerns, an emerging area of investigation is the development of natural and synthetic hormone mimetics that will preferentially activate estrogen neuroprotective mechanisms while minimizing adverse effects in other tissues.

The possibility of using selective estrogen receptor modulators (SERMs) to exert estradiol-like neuroprotective actions in the brain has emerged as an alternative to estradiol (DonCarlos et al., 2009). According to chemical family, SERMs are classified as first-generation SERMs, such as tamoxifen and its derivatives, second-generation SERMs, such as raloxifene, and third-generation SERMs. Fourth-generation SERMs are benzopyran compounds (Dowers et al., 2006). SERMs bind to estrogen receptors (ERs) and induce specific changes in their three-dimensional conformation (Brzozowski et al., 1997; Paige et al., 1999) allowing a tissue-selective recruitment of transcriptional cofactors (Klinge, 2000; McKenna & O'Malley, 2002; Belandia & Parker, 2003). Therefore, SERMs may act as ER agonists in the brain and as antagonists in others tissues, such as breast tumors.

The neuroprotective actions of tamoxifen and raloxifene, have been assessed in different experimental models of neural dysfunction. These include animal models of traumatic injury of the central nervous system and peripheral nerves, stroke, multiple sclerosis, Parkinson's disease, Alzheimer's disease, cognitive decline, and mood disorders.

In general, there is still poor knowledge of the precise molecular targets of SERMs in the nervous system. Although some key molecules have been identified, such as MAPK, PI3K/Akt, CREB, and NF-kB, the molecular mechanisms involved in the neuroprotective actions of SERMs should be investigated with more detail in the different cellular populations of the nervous system. Ideally, SERMs with cellular specificity for neurons, astrocytes, oligodendrocytes, and microglia may promote cell-specific responses to decrease neuronal death, increase re-myelination, enhance the production of neuroprotective growth factors by astrocytes, and reduce the chronic proinflammatory response of astrocytes and microglia.

There are considerable precedents to fuel efforts to develop SERMs with selectivity for the brain, and not peripheral targets, which could eliminate unwanted peripheral actions of estrogens, including their feminizing actions, thereby making them accessible for men as well as women.

Conclusion

The studies reviewed here clearly support that estrogens exert their neuroprotective effects in part by regulating the brain inflammation under physiological conditions, like aging; or neurodegenerative diseases, like Alzheimer or Parkinson. These actions are mediated, in part, by glia cells.

The ability of estradiol to influence cognitive impairment associated with aging or neurodegenerative diseases, depends on the sex or the brain area under study.

However, there are many aspects that still need to be addressed, including determination of the best estrogenic formulations and whether cyclic versus continuous hormone therapy delivery is most suitable for promoting brain function and cognition. In addition, it is important to understand the role that other factors, such as IGF-I and the different cellular and subcellular targets of estradiol, play in the neuroprotective mechanisms of the hormone. Another important consideration is that although estradiol is neuroprotective, its peripheral actions limit its use for the treatment or prevention of neurodegenerative diseases and affective disorders. Therefore, new alternatives to estradiol therapy based on the neuroprotective mechanisms of the hormone are being explored. SERM's, may represent an alternative to estradiol and may also be used in males.

Further developments may include the use of aromatase modulators to selectively increase brain estradiol synthesis as an alternative to the administration of estrogenic compounds. Given the importance of the interactions of estradiol and IGF-I neuroprotective mechanisms, the outcome of the modulation of IGF-I levels in parallel with administration of estrogenic therapies should also be explored in experimental neurodegenerative models.

References

Aleman, A., Bronk, E., Kessels, R.P.C., Koppeschaar, H.P.F. & van Honk, J. (2004) A single administration of testosterone improves visuospatial ability in young women. *Psychoneuroendocrinology,* 29, 612–617.

Aleman, A., Verhaar, H.J.J., de Haan, E.H.F., de Vries, W.R., Samson, M.M., Drent, M.L., van der Veen, E.A. & Koppeschaar, H.P.F. (1999) Insulin-like growth factor-I and cognitive function in healthy older men. *J. Clin. Endocrinol. Metab.,* 84, 471–475.

Arevalo, M.A., Azcoitia, I. & Garcia-Segura, L.M. (2015) The neuroprotective actions of oestradiol and oestrogen receptors. *Nat. Rev. Neurosci.*, 16, 17–29.

Arevalo, M.A., Santos-Galindo, M.., Bellini, M.J., Azcoitia, I. & Garcia-Segura, L.M. (2010) Actions of estrogens on glial cells: implications for neuroprotection. *Biochim. Biophys. Acta*, 1800, 1106–12.

Arnold, S. (2005) Estrogen suppresses the impact of glucose deprivation on astrocytic calcium levels and signaling independently of the nuclear estrogen receptor. *Neurobiol. Dis.*, 20, 82–92.

Barreto, G., Santos-Galindo, M., Diz-Chaves, Y., Pernía, O., Carrero, P., Azcoitia, I. & Garcia-Segura, L.M. (2009) Selective estrogen receptor modulators decrease reactive astrogliosis in the injured brain: effects of aging and prolonged depletion of ovarian hormones. *Endocrinology,* 150, 5010–5015.

Barreto, G., Veiga, S., Azcoitia, I., Garcia-Segura, L.M. & Garcia-Ovejero, D. (2007) Testosterone decreases reactive astroglia and reactive microglia after brain injury in male rats: role of its metabolites, oestradiol and dihydrotestosterone. *Eur. J. Neurosci.,* 25, 3039–3046.

Barry, J.A., Parekh, H.S.K. & Hardiman, P.J. (2013) Visual-spatial cognition in women with polycystic ovarian syndrome: the role of androgens. *Hum. Reprod.,* 28, 2832–2837.

Baune, B.T. (2015) Inflammation and neurodegenerative disorders: is there still hope for therapeutic intervention? *Curr. Op. Psych.*, 28, 148-154.

Belandia, B. & Parker, M.G. (2003) Nuclear receptors : a rendezvous for chromatin remodeling factors. *Cell,* 114, 277–280.

Bellar, D., Glickman, E.L., Juvancic-Heltzel, J. & Gunstad, J. (2011) Serum insulin like growth factor-1 is associated with working memory, executive function and selective attention in a sample of healthy, fit older adults. *Neuroscience,* 178, 133–137.

Berman, K.F., Schmidt, P.J., Rubinow, D.R., Danaceau, M.A., Van Horn, J.D., Esposito, G., Ostrem, J.L. & Weinberger, D.R. (1997) Modulation of cognition-specific cortical activity by gonadal steroids: a positron-emission tomography study in women. *Proc. Nat. Acad. Sci. USA*, 94, 8836–8841.

Bettcher, B.M., Wilheim, R., Rigby, T., Green, R., Miller, J.W., Racine, C.A., Yaffe, K., Miller, B.L. & Kramer, J.H. (2012) C-reactive protein is related to memory and medial temporal brain volume in older adults. *Brain Behav. Imm.,* 26, 103–108.

Block, M.L., Zecca, L. & Hong, J.S. (2007) Microglia-mediated neurotoxicity: uncovering the molecular mechanisms. *Nat. Rev. Neurosci.*, 8, 57–69.

Blurton-Jones, M. & Tuszynski, M.H. (2001) Reactive astrocytes express estrogen receptors in the injured primate brain. *J. Comp. Neurol.*, 433, 115–123.

Boulware, M.I., Weick, J.P., Becklund, B.R., Kuo, S.P., Groth, R.D. & Mermelstein, P.G. (2005) Estradiol activates group I and II metabotropic glutamate receptor signaling, leading to opposing influences on cAMP response element-binding protein. *J. Neurosci.*, 25, 5066–5078.

Bramen, J.E., Hranilovich, J.A., Dahl, R.E., Forbes, E.E., Chen, J., Toga, A.W., Dinov, I.D., Worthman, C.M. & Sowell, E.R. (2011) Puberty influences medial temporal lobe and cortical gray matter maturation differently in boys than girls matched for sexual maturity. *Cereb. Cortex,* 21, 636–646.

Brann, D.W., Dhandapani, K., Wakade, Ch., Mahesh, V.B. & Khan, M.M. (2007) Neurotrophic and neuroprotective actions of estrogen: basic mechanisms and clinical implications. *Steroids,* 72, 381–405.

Brinton, R.D. (2008a) Estrogen regulation of glucose metabolism and mitochondrial function: therapeutic implications for prevention of Alzheimer's disease. *Adv. Drug Del. Rev.*, 60, 1504–1511.

Brinton, R.D. (2008b) The healthy cell bias of estrogen action: mitochondrial bioenergetics and neurological implications. *TINS*, 31, 529–537.

Bruce-Keller, A.J., Keeling, J.L., Keller, J.N., Huang, F.F. Camondola, S. & Mattson, M.P. (2000) Antiinflammatory effects of estrogen on microglial activation. *Endocrinology,* 141, 3646–3656.

Brzozowski, A.M., Pike, A.C.W., Dauter, Z., Hubbard, R.E., Bonn, T., Engstrom, O., Ohman, L., Greene, G.L., Gustafsson, J.A. & Carlquist, M. (1997) Molecular basis of agonism and antagonism in the oestrogen receptor. *Nature,* 389, 753–758.

Cahill, L. (2006) Why sex matters for neuroscience. *Nat. Rev. Neurosci*., 7, 477–484.

Carbonaro, V., Caraci, F., Giuffrida, M.L., Merlo, S., Canonico, P.L., Drago, F., Copani, A. & Sortino, M.A. (2009) Enhanced expression of ERalpha in astrocytes modifies the response of cortical neurons to beta-amyloid toxicity. *Neurobiol. Dis*., 33, 415–421.

Cardona-Gómez, G.L., Mendez, P., DonCarlos, L.L., Azcoitia, I. & Garcia-Segura, L.M. (2001) Interactions of estrogens and insulin-like growth factor-I in the brain: implications for neuroprotection. *Brain Res. Rev*., 37, 320–334.

Cardona-Gómez, G.P., Mendez, P., DonCarlos, L.L., Azcoitia, I. & Garcia-Segura, L.M. (2002) Interactions of estrogen and insulin-like growth factor-I in the brain: molecular mechanisms and functional implications. *J. Steroid Biochem. Mol. Biol*., 83, 211–217.

Carro, E., Trejo, J.L., Núñez, A. & Torres-Aleman, I. (2003) Brain repair and neuroprotection by serum insulin-like growth factor I. *Mol. Neurobiol*., 27, 153–162.

Cerciat, M., Unkila, M., Garcia-Segura, L.M. & Arevalo, M.A. (2010) Selective estrogen receptor modulators decrease the production of Interleukin-6 and Interferon-γ-inducible protein-10 by astrocytes exposed to inflammatory challenge in vitro. *Glia*, 58, 93–102.

Chaban, V.V., Lakhter, A.J. & Micevych, P. (2004) A membrane estrogen receptor mediates intracellular calcium release in astrocytes. *Endocrinology*, 145, 3788–3795.

Chen, Z.L., Yu, W.M. & Strickland, S. (2007) Peripheral regeneration. *Ann. Rev. Neurosci.* 30, 209–233.

Ciriza, I., Carrero, P., Azcoitia, I., Lundeen, S.G. & Garcia-Segura, L.M. (2004) Selective estrogen receptor modulators protect hippocampal neurons from kainic acid excitotoxicity: differences with the effect of estradiol. *J. Neurobiol.,* 61, 209–221.

Clark, A.N.N.S., Maclusky, N.J. & Goldman-Rakic, P.S. (1988) Androgen binding and metabolism in the cerebral cortex of the developing Rhesus monkey. *Endocrinology*, 123, 932–940.

Cosgrove, K.P., Mazure, C.M. & Staley, J.K. (2007) Evolving knowledge of sex differences in brain structure, function, and chemistry. *Biol. Psych*., 62, 847–855.

Crawford, D.K., Mangiardi, M., Song, B., Patel, R., Du, S., Sofroniew, M.V., Voskuhl, R.R. & Tiwari-Woodruff, S.K. (2010) Oestrogen receptor B ligand: a novel treatment to enhance endogenous functional remyelination. *Brain*, 133, 2999–3016.

De Vries, G.J. (2004). Minireview: sex differences in adult and developing brains: compensation, compensation, compensation. *Endocrinology*, 145, 1063–1068.

Dhandapani, K.M., Wade, F.M., Mahesh, V.B. & Brann, D.W. (2005) Astrocyte-derived transforming growth factor-B mediates the neuroprotective effects of 17β-Estradiol: involvement of nonclassical genomic signaling pathways. *Endocrinology*, 146, 2749–2759.

Dimayuga, F.O., Reed, J.L., Carnero, G.A., Wang, Ch., Dimayuga, E.R., Dimayuga, V.M., Perger, A., Wilson, M.E., Keller, J.N. & Bruce-Keller, A.J. (2005) Estrogen and brain inflammation: effects on microglial expression of MHC, costimulatory molecules and cytokines. *J. Neuroimmunol.,* 161, 123–36.

Dodel, R., Du, Y., Bales, K.R., Gao, F. & Paul, S. (1999) Sodium salicylate and 17β-Estradiol attenuate nuclear transcription factor NF-κB translocation in cultured rat astroglial cultures following exposure to amyloid Aβ1-40 and lipoplysaccharides. *J. Neurochem.*, 73, 1453–1460.

DonCarlos, L.L., Azcoitia, I. & Garcia-Segura, L.M. (2009) Neuroprotective actions of selective estrogen receptor modulators. *Psychoneuroendocrinology,* 34, S113–S122.

Dowers, T.S., Qin, Z.H., Thatcher, G.R.J. & Bolton, J.L. (2006) Bioactivation of selective estrogen receptor modulators (SERMs). *Chem. Res. Toxicol.* 19, 1125–1137.

Drew, P.D. & Chavis, J.A. (2000) Female sex steroids: effects upon microglial cell activation. *J. Neuroimmunol.*, 111, 77–85.

Du, S., Sandoval, F., Trinh, P., Umeda, E. & Voskuhl, R. (2011) Estrogen receptor-B ligand treatment modulates dendritic cells in the target organ during autoimmune demyelinating disease. *Eur. J. Immunol.*, 41, 140–150.

Dumas, J.A., Kutz, A.M., Naylor, M.R., Johnson, J.V. & Newhouse, P.A. (2012) Estradiol treatment altered anticholinergic-related brain activation during working memory in postmenopausal women. *Neuroimage,* 60, 1394–1403.

Dumas, J.A., Hancur-Bucci, C., Naylor, M., Sites, C. & Newhouse, P. (2006) Estrogen treatment effects on anticholinergic-induced cognitive dysfunction in normal postmenopausal women. *Neuropsychopharmacology,* 31, 2065–2078.

Fawcett, J.W. & Keynes, R.J. (1990) Peripheral nerve regeneration. *Ann. Rev.* Neurosci., 13, 43–60.

Foster, T.C., Rani, A., Kumar, A., Cui, L. & Semple-Rowland, S.L. (2008) Viral vector – mediated delivery of estrogen receptor-A to the hippocampus improves spatial learning in estrogen receptor-A knockout mice. *Mol. Ther.,* 16, 1587–1593.

Franceschi, C., Bonafè M., Valensin, S., OlivierI, F., de Luca, M., Ottaviani, E. & de Benedictis, G. (2000) Inflamm-aging: an evolutionary perspective on immunosenescence. *Ann. NY Acad. Sci.*, 908, 244–254.

Franklin, R.J.M. & ffrench-Constant, Ch. (2008) Remyelination in the CNS: from biology to therapy. *Nat. Rev. Neurosci.*, 9, 839–855.

Frick, K.M. (2009) Estrogens and age-related memory decline in rodents: what have we learned and where do we go from here? *Horm. Behav.*, 55, 2–23.

Fugger, H.N., Cunningham, S.G., Rissman, E.F. & Foster, T.C. (1998) Sex differences in the activational effect of ERalpha on spatial learning. *Horm. Behav.*, 34, 163–170.

García-Estrada, J., Luquín, S., Fernández, A.M. & Garcia-Segura, L.M. (1999) Dehydroepiandrosterone, pregnenolone and sex steroids down-regulate reactive astroglia in the male rat brain after a penetrating brain injury. *Int. J. Dev. Neurosci.*, 17, 145–151.

Garcia-Ovejero, D., Azcoitia, I., DonCarlos, L.L., Melcangi, R.C. & Garcia-Segura, L.M. (2005) Glia-neuron crosstalk in the neuroprotective mechanisms of sex steroid hormones. *Brain Res. Rev.*, 48, 273–286.

García-Ovejero, D., Veiga, S., García-Segura, L.M. & DonCarlos, L.L. (2002) Glial expression of estrogen and androgen receptors after rat brain injury. *J. Comp. Neurol.,* 450, 256–271.

Garcia-Segura, L.M. (2008) Aromatase in the brain: not just for reproduction anymore. *J. Neuroendocrinol.*, 20, 705–712.

Garcia-Segura, L.M., Arévalo, M.A. & Azcoitia, I. (2010) Interactions of estradiol and insulin-like growth factor-I signalling in the nervous system: new advances, in:

Neuroendocrinology: the normal neuroendocrine system. L. Martini (Ed.). *Prog. Brain Res. Series. Elsevier, Holland*. 181, 251–272.

Garcia-Segura, L.M., Veiga, S., Sierra, A., Melcangi, R.C. & Azcoitia, I. (2003) Aromatase: a neuroprotective enzyme. *Prog. Neurobiol.*, 71, 31–41.

Garcia-Segura, L.M., Azcoitia, I. & DonCarlos, L.L. (2001) Neuroprotection by estradiol. *Prog. Neurobiol.*, 63, 29–60.

Garcia-Segura, L.M., Lorenz, B. & DonCarlos, L.L. (2008) The role of glia in the hypothalamus: implications for gonadal steroid feedback and reproductive neuroendocrine output. *Reproduction,* 135, 419–429.

Gibbs, R.B. (2005) Testosterone and estradiol produce different effects on cognitive performance in male rats. *Horm. Behav.*, 48, 268–277.

Giedd, J.N., Snell, J.W., Lange, N., Jagath, C., Casey, B.J., Kozuch, P.L. Catherine, A., Vauss, Y.C. & Hamburger, S.D. (1996) Quantitative magnetic resonance imaging of human brain development: ages, 4-18. *Cereb. Cortex,* 6, 551–560.

Gillies, G.E. & McArthur, S. (2010) Estrogen actions in the brain and the basis for differential action in men and women: a case for sex-specific medicines. *Pharmacol. Rev.*, 62, 155–198.

Gorosito, S.V., Lorenzo, A.G. & Cambiasso, M.J. (2008) Estrogen receptor alpha is expressed on the cell-surface of embryonic hypothalamic neurons. *Neuroscience,* 154, 1173–1177.

Green, P.S. & Simpkins, J.W. (2000) Neuroprotective effects of estrogens: potential mechanisms of action. *Int. J. Dev. Neurosci.*, 18, 347–358.

Grove-Strawser, D., Boulware, M.I. & Mermelstein, P.G. (2010) Membrane estrogen receptors activate the metabotropic glutamate receptors mGluR5 and mGluR3 to bidirectionally regulate CREB phosphorylation in female rat striatal neurons. *Neuroscience,* 170, 1045–1055.

Hajszan, T., MacLusky, N.J. Leranth, C. (2008) Role of androgens and the androgen receptor in remodeling of spine synapses in limbic brain areas. *Horm. Behav.,* 53, 638–646.

Hanisch, U.K. & Kettenmann, H. (2007) Microglia: active sensor and versatile effector cells in the normal and pathologic brain. *Nat. Neurosci.*, 10, 1387–1394.

Hensley, K. (2010) Neuroinflammation in Alzheimer's disease: mechanisms, pathologic consequences, and potential for therapeutic manipulation. *J. Alz. Dis.* 21, 1–14.

Irwin, R.W., Yao, J., Hamilton, R.T., Cadenas, E., Brinton, R.D. & Nilsen, J. (2008) Progesterone and estrogen regulate oxidative metabolism in brain mitochondria. *Endocrinology,* 149, 3167–3175.

Ivanova, T., Karolczak, M. & Beyer, C. (2001) Estrogen stimulates the mitogen-activated protein kinase pathway in midbrain astroglia. *Brain* Res., 889, 264–269.

Keenan, P.A., Ezzat, W.H., Ginsburg, K. & Moore, G.J. (2001) Prefrontal cortex as the site of estrogen's effect on cognition. *Psychoneuroendocrinology,* 26, 577–590.

Kipp, M., Karakaya, S., Johann, S., Kampmann, E., Mey, J. & Beyer, C. (2007) Oestrogen and progesterone reduce lipopolysaccharide-induced expression of tumour necrosis factor-A and interleukin-18 in midbrain astrocytes. *J. Neuroendocrinol.*, 19, 819–822.

Klinge, C.M. (2000) Estrogen receptor interaction with co-activators and co-repressors. *Steroids,* 65, 227–251.

Koolschijn, P., Cédric, M.P. & Crone, E.A. (2013) Sex differences and structural brain maturation from childhood to early adulthood. *Dev. Cogn. Neurosci.,* 5, 106–118.

Kravitz, B.A., Corrada, M.M. & Kawas, C.H. (2009) Elevated c-reactive protein levels are associated with prevalent dementia in the oldest-old. *Alz. Dem.*, 5, 318–323.

Kritzer, M.F., Brewer, A., Montalmant, F., Davenport, M. & Robinson, J.K. (2007) Effects of gonadectomy on performance in operant tasks measuring prefrontal cortical function in adult male rats. *Horm. Behav.*, 51, 183–194.

Kushner, P.J., Agard, D.A., Greene, G.L., Scanlan, T.S., Shiau, A.K., Uht, R.M. & Webb, P. (2000) Estrogen receptor pathways to AP-1. *J. Steroid Biochem. Mol. Biol.* 74, 311–317.

Laird, M.D., Vender, J.R. & Dhandapani, K.M. (2008) Opposing roles for reactive astrocytes following traumatic brain injury. *Neurosignals,* 16, 154–164.

Lehnardt, S. (2010) Innate immunity and neuroinflammation in the CNS: the role of microglia in toll-like receptor-mediated neuronal injury. *Glia,* 58, 253–263.

Lewis, D.K., Johnson, A.B., Stohlgren, S., Harms, A. & Sohrabji, F. (2008) Effects of estrogen receptor agonists on regulation of the inflammatory response in astrocytes from young adult and middle-aged female rats. *J. Neuroimmunol.* 195, 47–59.

Luine, V.N. & Frankfurt, M. (2013) Interactions between estradiol, BDNF and dendritic spines in promoting memory. *Neuroscience,* 239, 34–45.

Luine, V.N. (2008) Sex steroids and cognitive function. *J. Neuroendocrinol.* 20, 866–872.

Luine, V.N. (2007) The prefrontal cortex, gonadal hormones and memory. *Horm. Behav.* 51, 181–182.

Luine, V.N., Wallace, M.E. & Frankfurt, M. (2011) Age-related deficits in spatial memory and hippocampal spines in virgin, female Fischer 344 rats. Curr. Gerontol. *Ger. Res., January*: 316386.

Mangelsdorf, D.J., Thummel, C., Beato, M., Herrlich, P., Schütz, G., Umesono, K., Blumberg, B., Kastner, P., Mark, M., Chambon, P., Evans, R.M. (1995) The nuclear receptor superfamily: the second decade. *Cell,* 83, 835–839.

Martinez, L. & de Lacalle, S. (2007) Astrocytic reaction to a lesion, under hormonal deprivation. *Neurosci. Lett.*, 415, 190–193.

McEwen, B.S. & Alves, S.E. (1999) Estrogen actions in the central nervous system. *Endoc. Rev.*, 20, 279–307.

McGaugh, J.L. (2000) Neuroscience - Memory - a century of consolidation. *Science,* 287, 248–251.

McKenna, N.J. & O'Malley, B.W. (2002) Combinatorial control of gene expression by nuclear receptors and coregulators. *Cell,* 108, 465–474.

Mendez, P., Cardona-Gomez, G.P. & Garcia-Segura, L.M. (2005) Interactions of insulin-like growth factor-I and estrogen in the brain, in: The growth hormone/insulin-like growth factor axis during development. I. Varela-Nieto & J.A. Chowen (Eds.). *Adv. Exp. Med. Biol.* 567:285–303. Springer, USA.

Mermelstein, P.G. (2009) Membrane-localised oestrogen receptor A and B influence neuronal activity through activation of metabotropic glutamate receptors. *J. Neuroendocrinol.*, 21, 257–262.

Mitsushima, D., Takase, K., Takahashi, T. & Kimura, F. (2009) Activational and organisational effects of gonadal steroids on sex-specific acetylcholine release in the dorsal hippocampus. *J. Neuroendocrinology*, 21, 400–405.

Morse, J.K., Scheff, S.W. DeKosky, S.T. (1986) Gonadal steroids influence axon sprouting in the hippocampal dentate gyrus: a sexually dimorphic response. *Exp. Neurol.*, 94, 649–658.

Neufang, S., Specht, K., Hausmann, M. & Konrad, K. (2009) Sex differences and the impact of steroid hormones on the developing human brain. *Cereb. Cortex*, 19, 464-473.

Nilsen, J., Irwin, R.W., Gallaher, T.K. & Brinton, R.D. (2007) Estradiol in vivo regulation of brain mitochondrial proteome. *J. Neurosci.,* 27, 14069–14077.

Paige, L.A., Christensen, D.J., Grøn, H., Norris, J.D., Gottlin, E.B., Padilla, K.M., Chang, C.Y. Ballas, L.M., Hamilton, P.T., McDonnell, D.P. & Fowlkes, D.M. (1999) Estrogen receptor (ER) modulators each induce distinct conformational changes in ER A and ER B. *Proc. Nat. Acad. Sci.,* 96, 3999–4004.

Pang, P.T. & Lu, B. (2004) Regulation of late-phase LTP and long-term memory in normal and aging hippocampus: role of secreted proteins tPA and BDNF. *Ageing Res. Rev.* 3, 407–30.

Patterson, S.L., Abel, T., Deuel, T.A.S., Martin, K.C., Rose, J.C. & Kandel, E.R. (1996) Recombinant BDNF rescues deficits in basal synaptic transmission and hippocampal LTP in BDNF knockout mice. *Neuron,* 16, 1137–1145.

Petrovska, S., Dejanova, B. & Jurisic, V. (2012) Estrogens: mechanisms of neuroprotective effects. *J. Physiol. Biochem*., 68, 455–460.

Raber, J. (2008) AR, apoE, and cognitive function. *Horm. Behav*., 53, 706–715.

Romeo, R.D., Waters, E.M. & Mcewen, B.S. (2004) Steroid-induced hippocampal synaptic plasticity: sex differences and similarities. *Neuron Glia Biol*., 1, 219–229.

Roof, R.L. (1993) The dentate gyrus is sexually dimorphic in prepubescent rats: testosterone plays a significant role. *Brain Res*., 610, 148–151.

Saldanha, C.J., Duncan, K.A. & Walters, B.J. (2009) Neuroprotective actions of brain aromatase. *Front. Neuroendocrinol*., 30, 106–118.

Saravia, F.E., Beauquis, J., Revsin, Y., Homo-Delarche, F., de Kloet, E.R. &. De Nicola, A.F. (2006) Hippocampal neuropathology of diabetes mellitus is relieved by estrogen treatment. *Cell. Mol. Neurobiol*., 26, 941–955.

Savaskan, E., Olivieri, G., Meier, F., Ravid, R. & Müller-Spahn, F. (2001) Hippocampal estrogen B-receptor immunoreactivity is increased in Alzheimer's disease. *Brain Res*., 908, 113–119.

Scharfman, H.E. (1997) Hyperexcitability in combined entorhinal/hippocampal slices of adult rat after exposure to brain-derived neurotrophic factor. *J. Neurophysiol*., 78, 1082–1095.

Scheff, S.W. & Price, D.A. (2003) Synaptic pathology in Alzheimer's disease: a review of ultrastructural studies. *Neurobiol. Aging*, 24, 1029–1046.

Singh, M., Meyer, E.M. & Simpkins, J.W. (1995) The effect of ovariectomy and estradiol replacement on brain-derived neurotrophic factor messenger ribonucleic acid expression in cortical and hippocampal brain regions of female Sprague-Dawley rats. *Endocrinology,* 136, 2320–2324.

Sohrabji, F., Miranda, R.C. & Toran-Allerand, C.D. (1995) Identification of a putative estrogen response element in the gene encoding brain-derived neurotrophic factor. *Proc. Nat. Acad. Sci. USA*, 92, 11110–11114.

Solum, D.T. & Handa, R.J. (2002) Estrogen regulates the development of brain-derived neurotrophic factor mRNA and protein in the rat hippocampus. *J. Neurosci*. 22, 2650–2659.

Spencer, J.L., Waters, E.M., Romeo, R.D., Wood, G.E., Milner, T.A. & McEwen, B.S. (2008) Uncovering the mechanisms of estrogen effects on hippocampal function. *Front. Neuroendocrinol*. 29, 219–237.

Srivastava, D.P. (2012) Two-step wiring plasticity--a mechanism for estrogen-induced rewiring of cortical circuits. *J. Steroid Biochem. Mol. Biol.* 131, 17–23.

Streit, W.J. 2002) Microglia as neuroprotective, immunocompetent cells of the CNS. *Glia,* 40, 133-139.

Takahashi, N., Tonchev, A,B., Koike, K., Murakami, K., Yamada, K., Yamashima, T. & Inoue, M. (2004) Expression of estrogen receptor-beta in the postischemic monkey hippocampus. *Neurosci. Lett.*, 369, 9–13.

Takase, K., Kimura, F., Yagami, T. & Mitsushima, D. (2009) Sex-specific 24-h acetylcholine release profile in the medial prefrontal cortex: simultaneous measurement of spontaneous locomotor activity in behaving rats. *Neuroscience,* 159, 7–15.

Tang, Y., Janssen, W.G.M., Hao, J., Roberts, J.A., McKay, H., Lasley, B., Allen, P.B., Greengard, P., Rapp, P.R., Kordower, J.H., Hof, P.R. & Morrison, J.H. (2004) Estrogen replacement increases spinophilin-immunoreactive spine number in the prefrontal cortex of female Rhesus monkeys. *Cereb. Cortex*, 14, 215–223.

Tapia-Gonzalez, S., Carrero, P., Pernia, O., Garcia-Segura, L.M. & Diz-Chaves, Y. (2008) Selective oestrogen receptor (ER) modulators reduce microglia reactivity in vivo after peripheral inflammation: potential role of microglial ERs. *J. Endocrinol.* 198, 219–230.

Tetel, M.J. (2009) Nuclear receptor coactivators: essential players for steroid hormone action in the brain and in behaviour. *J. Neuroendocrinol.* 21, 229–237.

Tinkler, G.P., Tobin, J.R. & Voytko, M.L. (2004) Effects of two years of estrogen loss or replacement on nucleus basalis cholinergic neurons and cholinergic fibers to the dorsolateral prefrontal and inferior parietal cortex of monkeys. *J. Comp. Neuro.,* 521, 507–521.

Toran-Allerand, C.D., Singh, M. & Sétáló, G. (1999) Novel mechanisms of estrogen action in the brain: new players in an old story. *Front. Neuroendocrinol.* 20, 97–121.

Toran-Allerand, C.D., Guan, X., MacLusky, N.J., Horvath, T.L., Diano, S., Singh, M., Connolly, E.S., Nethrapalli, I.S. & Tinnikov, A.A. (2002) ER-X: a novel, plasma membrane-associated, putative estrogen receptor that is regulated during development and after ischemic brain injury. *J. Neurosci.,* 22, 8391–8401.

Torres-Aleman, I. (2012) Insulin-like growth factor-1 and central neurodegenerative diseases. *Endocrinol. Metab. Clin. North Am.* 41, 395–408.

Torres-Aleman, I., Naftolin, F. & Robbins, R.J. (1990) Trophic effects of basic fibroblast growth factor on fetal rat hypothalamic cells. Interactions with insulin-like growth factor I. *Dev. Brain Res.*, 52, 253–257.

Tripanichkul, W., Sripanichkulchai, K. & Finkelstein, D.I. (2006) Estrogen down-regulates glial activation in male mice following 1-methyl-4-phenyl-1, 2, 3, 6-tetrahydropyridine intoxication. *Brain Res.,* 1084, 28–37.

Vasudevan, N. & Pfaff, D.W. (2008) Non-genomic actions of estrogens and their interaction with genomic actions in the brain. *Front. Neuroendocrinol.,* 29, 238–57.

Vegeto, E., Belcredito, S., Etteri, S., Ghisletti, S., Brusadelli, A., Meda, C., Krust, A., Dupont, S., Ciana, P., Chambon, P. & Maggi, A. (2003) Estrogen receptor-A mediates the brain antiinflammatory activity of estradiol. *Proc. Nat. Acad. Sci.* 100, 9614–9619.

Vegeto, E., Belcredito, S., Ghisletti, S., Meda, C., Etteri, S. & Maggi, A. (2006) The endogenous estrogen status regulates microglia reactivity in animal models of neuroinflammation. *Endocrinology*, 147, 2263–2272.

Vegeto, E., Benedusi, V. & Maggi, A. (2008) Estrogen anti-inflammatory activity in brain: a therapeutic opportunity for menopause and neurodegenerative diseases. *Front. Neuroendocrinol.* 29, 507–519.

Volterra, A., Magistrett, P.J. Haydon, P.J. (2002) The tripartite synapse-glia in synaptic transmission. Oxford University Press. USA.

Hirahara, Y., Matsuda, K., Gao, W., Arvanitis, D.N., Kawata, M. & Boggs, J.M. The localization and non-genomic function of the membrane-associated estrogen receptor in oligodendrocytes. *Glia,* 57, 153-165.

Wallace, M., Luine, V., Arellanos, A. & Frankfurt, M. (2006) Ovariectomized rats show decreased recognition memory and spine density in the hippocampus and prefrontal cortex. *Brain Res.,* 1126, 176–182.

Wang, A.C.J., Hara, Y., Janssen, W.G.M., Rapp, P.R. & Morrison, J.H. (2010) Synaptic estrogen receptor-A levels in prefrontal cortex in female Rhesus monkeys and their correlation with cognitive performance. *J. Neurosci.*, 30, 12770–12776.

Wang, J.Y., Wen, L.L., Huang, Y.N., Chen, Y.T. & Ku, M.C. (2006) Dual effects of antioxidants in neurodegeneration: direct neuroprotection against oxidative stress and indirect protection via suppression of glia-mediated inflammation. *Curr. Pharm. Des.*, 12, 3521–3533.

Warren, S.G. & Juraska, J.M. (1997) Spatial and nonspatial learning across the rat estrous cycle. *Behav. Neurosci.*, 111, 259–266.

Wilson, C.A. & Davies, D.C. (1973) The control of sexual differentiation of the reproductive system and brain. *Reproduction,* 133, 331–359.

Wise, P.M., Dubal, D.B., Wilson, M.E., Rau, S.W. & Liu, Y. (2001) Estrogens: trophic and protective factors in the adult brain. *Front. Neuroendocrinol.* 22, 33–66.

Wyckoff, M.H., Chambliss, K.L., Mineo, C., Yuhanna, I.S., Mendelsohn, M.E., Mumby, S.M. & Shaul, P.W. (2001) Plasma membrane estrogen receptors are coupled to endothelial nitric-oxide synthase through Galpha(i). *J. Biol. Chem.,* 276, 27071–27076.

Zhang, L., Li, B.S., Zhao, W., Chang, Y.H., Ma, W., Dragan, M., Barker, J.L., Hu, Q. & Rubinow, D.R. (2002) Sex-related differences in MAPKs activation in rat astrocytes: effects of estrogen on cell death. *Mol. Brain Res.,* 103, 1–11.

In: Synaptic Fundamentals of Memory Performance
Editor: Ignacio González-Burgos ISBN: 978-1-63483-279-3

Chapter 8

NEUROTOXICITY OF Aβ EXPLAINED BY ITS ASSOCIATION TO PLASMA MEMBRANES

Christian Peters[1], Eduardo Fernandez-Perez[1], Jorge Fuentealba[2] and Luis G. Aguayo[1,*]

[1]Laboratory of Neurophysiology, Department of Physiology, Universidad de Concepción, Chile

[2]Screening of Neuroactive Compounds Laboratory, Department of Physiology, Faculty of Biological Sciences, University of Concepcion, Chile

ABSTRACT

Cortical and hippocampal synapse densities are reduced in Alzheimer's disease (AD), and this strongly appears to correlate with memory dysfunction. It is now believed that the changes in neuronal networking that occur at the onset of AD and that lead to the neuronal loss displayed in later stages of the disease is what causes the severe cognitive and behavioral impairments. Mounting evidence indicates that amyloid-β (Aβ) oligomers are the main species responsible for synaptic disconnections and neuronal death.

Aβ toxicity depends on its primary sequence, motifs, structure and state of aggregation, membrane association and damage. For example, Aβ associates to the plasma membrane of neurons, interacting with lipids like GM1 and cholesterol, and proteins like APP, cellular Prion and NMDA receptors. One of the main consequences of Aβ oligomer interaction with neurons is an increase in intracellular Ca^{2+} concentration that could, when prolonged, cause a marked alteration in ionic homeostasis. There is ample evidence that Ca^{2+} influx is enhanced when Aβ oligomers induce the disruption of the plasma membrane. In fact, Aβ perforates the membrane similar to pore-forming toxins, inducing a dyshomeostasis in intracellular calcium that leads to a delayed synaptic failure.

Here, we discuss the role of Aβ residues and its interaction with different membrane components, such as lipids and proteins, in the toxicity induced by Aβ. The inhibition of

* Send correspondence to: Luis G. Aguayo, PhD, Department of Physiology, Universidad de Concepción, P.O. Box 160-C, Concepción, Chile. Telephone: 56-41-2203380, Fax: 56-41-2245975, Email: laguayo@udec.cl

these processes might serve as a novel approach to slow down the disease, which currently does not have efficacious therapy.

Keywords: Alzheimer's disease, neurotoxicity, membrane, amyloid

1. INTRODUCTION

1.1. Alzheimer´s Disease

Alzheimer´s disease (AD) is one of the most common brain disorders (Reitz et al., 2011) characterized by alterations at the cellular and molecular levels that lead to cerebral dysfunctions that worsen over the years as the disease advances (Selkoe, 2002). AD is a progressive, neurodegenerative pathology that affects the central nervous system (CNS) in the elderly causing significant cognitive and behavioral disorders. Currently, the molecular and cellular mechanisms that lead to AD are largely unknown hindering the development of effective symptomatic or modifying therapies for this disease. Interestingly, a major histopathological feature of this disease is the presence of macroscopic structures in the brain parenchyma called senile plaques, which consist mainly of oligomers of β-amyloid peptide (Aβ) (Kawahara et al., 2000). Presently, with the objective of alleviating and deterring the symptoms of AD, most studies have been aimed at trying to restore the altered synaptic transmission and intracellular signaling pathways encountered during the disease (Selkoe, 2002; Demuro et al., 2010). However, this approach to identify anti AD compounds has not been productive since once the symptoms are apparent in the clinical stage, there appears to already be a significant degree of cerebral damage making recovery of synaptic deterioration ineffective (Selkoe, 2002). Therefore, we focus on identifying the early stages of Aβ-induced neurodegeneration that we believe occurs at the neuronal membrane level which should be one of the initial steps in its toxicity-signaling pathway.

Aβ PRODUCES SYNAPTIC FAILURE IN THE CENTRAL NERVOUS SYSTEM

It can be postulated that in its most incipient clinical form, the early symptoms of AD, confusion and loss of episodic and working memory, are due to network disconnections produced by oligomeric forms of Aβ (Selkoe, 2002). Therefore, in the context of a primarily synaptic disease, it is possible that this early form of brain dysfunction is similar to that induced by synaptically active drugs, such as benzodiazepines and ethanol (Ticku, 1990; Cagetti et al., 2003). In agreement with this idea, it has been previously reported that aggregated, oligomeric Aβ can affect complex events in brain synaptic transmission; such as long term potentiation (LTP), which is believed to be essential for neuronal plasticity and learning phenomena (Oddo et al., 2003; Shankar et al., 2007). In agreement, Aβ dimers were found to inhibit LTP, suggesting a large complexity on the nature of the neuroactive forms (Shankar et al., 2008). Thus, it is now accepted that diverse forms of Aβ are responsible for producing synaptic failure, but the cellular mechanisms underlying this malfunction are largely unknown.

So far, the data supporting inhibitory effects of Aβ on neurotransmission correlate well with structural alterations at both pre and postsynaptic sites. For example, Aβ oligomers, but not monomers, produce alterations in dendrite spine morphology in hippocampal neurons (Shankar et al., 2007). Additionally, the structural change was associated to a decrease in the frequency of miniature excitatory postsynaptic currents (mEPSCs), and smaller effects on their amplitude. Also, Aβ promoted NMDA receptor endocytosis without affecting the trafficking of $GABA_A$ receptors in cortical neurons. Presynaptically, several proteins such as SNAP-25, synaptophysin, and synaptotagmin have also been reported to be reduced in AD brains and after treatment with Aβ (Kelly et al., 2005; Reddy et al., 2005). Additionally, Aβ oligomers altered dynamin-1, a neuron-specific mechanochemical GTPase that pinches off synaptic vesicles allowing them to re-enter the synaptic vesicle pool (Kelly et al., 2005; Kelly, 2006). More recently, it was reported that the initial step in synaptic failure produced by Aβ is a consequence of membrane perforation and pore formation (Arispe et al., 2007; Arispe, 2004), and vesicular depletion caused by intracellular calcium increase (Parodi et al., 2009; Sepulveda et al., 2010; Sepúlveda et al., 2014).

3. Importance of Aβ Structure and Its Toxicity in AD

The current approaches that are being used to evaluate the effects of Aβ in the central nervous system (CNS) have centered on the use of transgenic animals and neuronal preparations exposed to distinct types of Aβ amyloid peptides. In relation to the latter, experimental evidence support the idea that the major portion of neurotoxic forms of Aβ aggregates is found in the fraction between 4 and 90 kDa (Demuro et al., 2005). This population of amyloid forms has been termed soluble Aβ aggregates and within this group there is a further separation known as Aβ oligomers (Aβo) that have an average molecular weight of 85-90 kDa and are characterized by a spherical conformation (diameter 2-5 nm) in solution (Demuro et al., 2005; Jang et al., 2008). In addition, another type of soluble Aβ aggregate called ADDLs (Aβ-Derived Diffusible Ligands) has been described under more restricted laboratory conditions and that are made up of trimeric, tetrameric and pentameric conformations of the Aβ peptide (Lambert et al., 1998; Chromy et al., 2003). Both Aβo and ADDLs have been found in the cerebral spinal fluid of AD patients (Kuo et al., 1996; Georganopoulou et al., 2005) and are believed to play complementary roles altering complex synaptic phenomenons, such as long term potentiation (LTP) (Demuro et al., 2005). Of course, this separation is somewhat arbitrary since under physiological conditions the inter-conversion of the species is probabilistic in nature due to its unstable conformational property (Glabe, 2008). Nevertheless, recent confocal microscopy studies localized ADDLs, derived from the brains of AD patients, together with PSD-95 and synaptophysin (Gong et al., 2003; Lacor et al., 2004; Deshpande et al., 2006; Lacor et al., 2007). Additionally, this form of amyloid peptide co-immunoprecipitated with subcellular fractions from rat brains (Verdier et al., 2005). More specifically, it was found that synapsin I and II, and β-tubulin, among others, co-immunoprecipitated with fibrillar fragments of the Aβ42 peptide indicating that Aβ42 is capable of interacting with proteins present in presynaptic zones.

Several species of Aβ have now been described depending on the site of proteolysis made by the γ-secretase (Zhao et al., 2005). The most abundant Aβ peptides are the Aβ40 and Aβ42, the latter being the more aggregative and toxic (Selkoe, 2008). Furthermore, it has been suggested that alterations in the brain of patients with AD would relate primarily to the effects of Aβ soluble oligomers (Shankar et al., 2007). It is likely that the toxic effects of Aβ oligomers are associated to membrane receptors by altering their functions (Snyder et al., 2005), interfering with signaling pathways (De Ferrari & Inestrosa, 2000) and are also associated directly to the membrane to form pore-like structures (Arispe et al., 2007). In this regard, there is evidence that changes in membrane conductance are caused by Aβ oligomers of low molecular weight that bind to the membrane and form an ionic pore (Quist et al., 2005). However, other reports suggest the presence of Aβ aggregates of higher molecular mass that alter the stability of the membranes (Green et al., 2004).

The toxic action of Aβ effects also depend both on the state of aggregation and the species of Aβ used. Hartley and co-workers separated different fractions of Aβ40 aggregate by size exclusion chromatography. Through this methodology, the authors showed that fiber fractions, called protofibers, caused marked changes in electrical activity of neuronal cultures and neurotoxicity (Hartley et al., 1999).

4. Important Residues and Motifs for Membrane Actions of Aβ

4.1. Residues Important in Aggregation, Association and Perforation

In order to explain the phenomena occurring at the molecular and structural level of Aβ association to the membrane, it is necessary to understand the role of the residues involved in these processes (Figure 1). Studies have shown that residues F19 and F20 are crucial in the early stages of Aβ aggregation (Tjernberg et al., 1996). Moreover, G33 and G37 have been described as important in the process of Aβ association to artificial lipid membranes (Hung et al., 2008). Interestingly, these two glycines are also essential in the process of forming ion-permeable structures in lipid membranes (Kim et al., 2005), which could correspond to what we call pore-like structures in biological membranes.

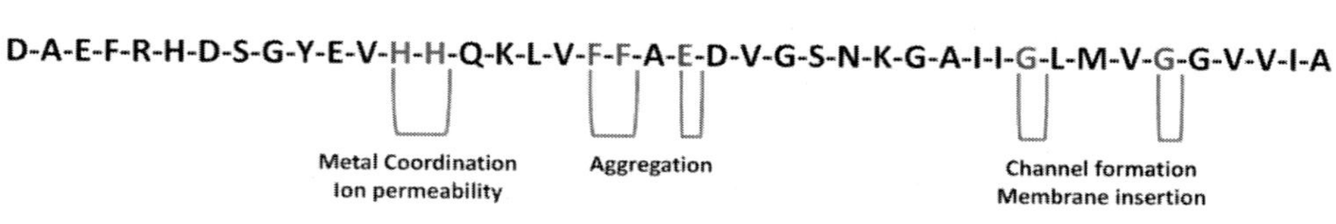

Figure 1. Primary sequence of Aβ. Important residues of Aβ are highlighted in red. H13 and H14 are present in the central region of the amyloid pore, allowing the flow of ions through the plasma membrane (Arispe et al., 2008) and the coordination of metals (Hung et al., 2009). F19 and F20 are critical in the aggregation process of Aβ (Tjernberg et al., 1996), while the C-terminal G33 and G37 are important in the membrane insertion and pore formation of Aβ (Kim et al., 2005, Hung et al., 2008).

Residues H13 and H14 are believed to form part of the central pore structure, permitting the passage of Ca2+ and coordinating other ions like Cu2+ and Zn2+ (Arispe et al., 2008).

Interestingly, several mini peptides (NA7, NA4) with a similar primary sequence to the region which allows the influx of calcium ions (H13 and H14) blocked Aβ perforation in cell membranes (Sepulveda et al., 2010). Recent data using a high sensitivity patch clamp technique that allows the recording of the opening and closure of a single molecule (Hamill et al., 1981), indicated that the actual pore formation in the cell membrane is not of a classical type, but it could be more like an actual membrane breakage (Sepúlveda et al., 2013).

4.2. Role of GxxxG Motifs in APP and Aβ

The GxxxG motif present in the APP and Aβ sequence is a common sequence configuration in several membrane proteins and is known as the glycine zipper. Glycine zipper motifs are strongly overrepresented and conserved in membrane protein sequences, and mutations in glycine zipper motifs are deleterious to their function in several cases (Aguzzi & Haass, 2003; Kim et al., 2005). The glycine zipper has a significant structural impact, engendering a strong driving force for right-handed packing against a neighboring helix (Aguzzi & Haass, 2003). Thus, the presence of a glycine zipper motif leads directly to testable structural hypotheses, particularly for a subclass of glycine zipper proteins that form channels. For instance, Kim and co workers suggested that the membrane pores formed by the amyloid-beta peptide in vitro are made by glycine zipper packing and reported that mutations in the glycine zipper motif block channel formation (Kim et al., 2005). These findings highlight an important structural motif in a wide variety of normal and pathological processes.

Sequence patterns having GxxxG motifs, which are known to be important in homodimeric transmembrane segments, have glycines facing in direct contact (Russ & Engelman, 2000). The actual data suggest that the glycines of the glycine zipper motif of Aβ (between G25 and G37) are critical for Aβ toxicity. In fact, G33 represents an important residue in the assembly of neurotoxic Aβ42 aggregates (Harmeier et al., 2009). Furthermore, mutations in the G33 and/or G37 synthetic peptides for leucine reduced their toxicity and association to lipid membranes (Hung et al., 2008).

Some properties of these GxxxG motifs include the processing of APP and the consequent formation of several species of Aβ (Richter et al., 2010). The specific cut of APP by γ-secretase in the C-terminal fragment is influenced by a GxxxG dimerization motif located in the transmembrane sequence of APP (Munter et al., 2007).

Molecular docking analyses suggest that certain modulators of γ-secretase bind to GxxxG motifs in APP transmembrane segments, reducing the levels of Aβ42 (Richter et al., 2010).

Furthermore, it has been found that mutations at residues G29 and G33 of the GxxxG motif decreases the dimerization of the transmembrane segment, specifically reducing the formation of Aβ42 and increasing Aβ38 and shorter peptide species (Munter et al., 2007).

Since Aβ42 is recognized as the most toxic specie and the primary cause of neurodegeneration in AD (Selkoe, 2008), drugs designed to act on the GxxxG dimerization motif could be promising targets for treating AD. In agreement with this idea, a recent study using a pentapeptide showed a complete blockade of Aβ oligomer toxicity in hippocampal neurons (Peters et al., 2013).

5. Mechanisms of Membrane Permeabilization Mediated by Aβ

Aβ, similar to other amyloid proteins, binds to membranes accelerating the fibrillation process. This process depends on the lipid composition and the ratio of proteins and lipids (Butterfield & Lashuel, 2010).

Recent evidence indicates that the toxicity of amyloid proteins directly correlates with its ability to interfere with the function of the membrane (Butterfield & Lashuel, 2010).

The initial discovery by Rojas and collaborators that Aβ has ion channel activity in lipid bilayers, proposed mechanisms in which Aβ-mediated toxicity is based on the formation of ion channels that cause membrane depolarization, calcium influx, and disruption of ionic homeostasis (Lashuel & Lansbury, 2006).

It is important to consider that the mechanisms of Aβ action may vary according to the type of species used, the membrane composition and experimental conditions (Kawahara et al., 2011). Therefore, it is important to keep these considerations in mind in order to achieve a good understanding for the molecular basis of AD.

6. Membrane Interactions of Aβ and Synaptotoxicity

Although there exists some debate on whether Aβ can up or down regulate selective components of synaptic transmission, several studies point out that Aβ alters pre and postsynaptic components affecting long-term potentiation, NMDA/AMPA neurotransmissions and calcium homeostasis (Stephan et al., 2001; Glabe & Kayed, 2006; Parodi et al., 2009). Supporting the complexity of these effects, it appears that no single mechanism can explain all these actions, thus hindering the development of effective anti Aβ therapies. A plausible hypothesis to explain this pleiotropic effect of Aβ is that the membrane perforation induced by oligomeric forms of the peptide causes calcium ion entry into the neuron, producing a large release of synaptic vesicles after acute applications (Parodi et al., 2009). Subsequently, after sustained release, synaptic vesicles are depleted causing synaptic failure (Parodi et al., 2009). In support of this idea, there is evidence indicating that the changes in membrane conductance are caused by small molecular weight oligomers of Aβ that bind to the membrane forming pore-like structures (Quist et al., 2005). Atomic force microscopy (AFM) revealed the presence of large Aβ aggregates (400-500 nm) on the surface of artificial lipid membranes that produced a release of fluorescent compounds from liposomes suggesting that the membrane disruption was caused by Aβ (Green et al., 2004). Furthermore, AFM studies also demonstrated changes in membrane conductance related to large structures having a "donut" appearance with an exterior diameter of approximately 16 nm and an inside pore between 1-2 nm (Jang et al., 2007; Quist et al., 2005). Interestingly, these molecular entities are very similar to those produced by pore forming peptides such as amylin (Quist et al., 2005) or gramicidin A (Diociaiuti et al., 2002). Recent data from our laboratory allowed us to conclude that the effects of Aβ on a neuronal "native" membrane are more complex than in artificial membranes. For example, we detected a transition state from cationic-selective to non-selective pores, as detected by loss in the Cl^- gradient during prolonged interaction of the peptide with the membrane (Sepulveda et al., 2010). The data obtained with single cell imaging analysis showed that Aβ disruption allowed the entry of ethidium bromide (EtBr) and 6-NBDG, a glucose fluorescent analog, into the cell, thus providing additional support for this lack of ionic selectivity during the latter stage of membrane perforation. For gramicidin pores, on the other hand, a modest entry of both molecules into the cell suggests pore sizes smaller than those of Aβ. Our interpretation is that when Aβ binds to the cell membrane it may initiate its own nucleation, producing a large perforation allowing for the entry of large molecules. Thus, the "pore hypothesis" is widely supported by previous evidence (Arispe 2004; Kayed et al., 2004; Green et al., 2004; Quist et al., 2005; Sepulveda et al., 2010). It is also possible that Aβ pores are also inserted in some intracellular organelle membranes affecting their own functions. Nevertheless, it is still unclear what cellular determinants are involved in the synaptotoxic actions and what membrane components are important for association and pore formation at the plasma membrane. On the other hand, several studies have shown that Aβ associates to different membrane proteins to affect neuronal functions, which we detail below.

6.1. Membrane Proteins Affect the Toxicity of Aβ

It is becoming well accepted that Aβ interacts with membrane proteins to mediate several neurotoxic effects in brain neurons. For example, previous studies have shown that Aβ can interact and alter the signaling of membrane proteins like N-methyl-D-aspartate receptors (NMDAR) (Snyder et al., 2005), lipoprotein receptor-related protein 6 (LRP6) (De Ferrari et al., 2007), receptor for advanced glycation endproducts (RAGE) (Yan et al., 1996), metabotropic glutamate receptors (mGluR5), α-7 nicotinic acetylcholine receptors (α-7 AchR) (Wang et al., 2000), amyloid precursor proteins (APP) (Lorenzo et al., 2000), and Prion proteins (PrP) (Lauren et al., 2009). However, cellular and molecular mechanisms associated with the interaction of Aβ to these proteins are not fully understood.

6.1.1. NMDAR-Aβ Association

Previous studies suggested that Aβ preferentially binds to excitatory synapses at the postynaptic membrane, consistent with the deleterious effect of Aβ on NMDAR-dependent long-term potentiation (LTP) (Walsh et al., 2002; Wang et al., 2002; Townsend et al., 2006) and on learning and memory impairment in rodents (Billings et al., 2007; Holscher et al., 2007). It is not completely resolved if Aβ can directly or indirectly interact with specific NMDAR subunits. However, it was suggested that Aβ might interact with NMDA receptors (Lacor et al., 2007), inducing NMDA receptor internalization (Snyder et al., 2005) and deregulation of NMDA signaling pathways (Roselli et al., 2005; Shankar et al., 2007). Thus, it appears that Aβ can interact with NMDA receptors and affect their function, but it is unknown whether this interaction can cause other toxic effects (Parodi et al., 2009).

6.1.2. Prion-Aβ Association

PrP is a glycoprotein highly expressed in the brain and widely known for its involvement in prion diseases (Zou et al., 2011) that have an infectious, sporadic or genetic etiology characterized by the accumulation of pathologic PrPsc in the brain (Prusiner, 1998). It has recently been described that PrP could be acting as a membrane receptor for Aβ and that this interaction could be important for the effect of Aβ in synaptic plasticity (Lauren et al., 2009; Balducci et al., 2010; Chen et al., 2010; Um et al., 2013). The strong interaction reported could explain the high affinity (nanomolar) that Aβ has for PrP (Balducci et al., 2010). Furthermore, this receptor may also mediate the toxic effects of Aβ. Indeed, an antibody against residues 95-105 of PrP blocked the toxicity of Aβ (Lauren et al., 2009). In addition, the absence of PrP (Knockout) or its blockade using anti-PrP antibodies decreased the pathological effects in transgenic animals that overexpress APP and display amyloid deposits in the brain (Gimbel et al., 2010; Chung et al., 2010). However, results regarding the role of PrP on Aβ are controversial. Despite these differences, there is good agreement on the interaction between Aβ and PrP. Recently, it was demonstrated that Aβ oligomers increase the localization of PrP on the cell surface (Caetano et al., 2011). Moreover, recent work showed that Aβ-PrP interaction is important for membrane perforation and calcium increase induced by Aβ (Peters et al., 2015), suggesting an important role of PrP in the neurotoxicity of Aβ.

6.1.3. APP-Aβ Association

Another protein that interacts with Aβ is the amyloid precursor protein (APP). APP is found in the neuronal plasma membrane and when processed by β- and α- secretases, the Aβ peptide is generated. Mutations in APP are related to an increase in hereditary forms of AD (Kedikian et al., 2010). These mutations alter the processing of APP and/or the generation of Aβ, predisposing the aggregation and accumulation of Aβ (Tanzi & Bertram, 2005). An increase in the expression of wild type APP is sufficient to cause "AD-like" alterations (Rovelet-Lecrux et al., 2006). The protein structure and cellular functions of APP are consistent with its potential role as a surface membrane receptor implicated in cell adhesion, although a natural ligand for APP has still not been established (Zheng & Koo, 2006). Interestingly, APP binds fibrillar Aβ (fAβ) and modulates its toxicity (Lorenzo et al., 2000), suggesting that perhaps fAβ could be a pathological ligand for APP (Sola Vigo et al., 2009). Furthermore, the deposits of fAβ promote the accumulation of APP on the cell surface (Heredia et al., 2004), similarly to what occurs when extracellular ligands bind to cell adhesion receptors. Dystrophic neurites rich in APP are surrounded by senile plaques suggesting a role in the degenerative process (Phinney et al., 1999). Overexpression of APP sensitizes hippocampal neurons to the toxic action of Aβ through activation of Go proteins (Sola Vigo et al., 2009).

6.2. Participation of Membrane Lipids on Aβ Neurotoxicity

It is currently accepted that the insertion of different peptides in the plasma membrane is strongly affected by the lipid composition (i.e. negatively charged lipids, clusters of gangliosides, cholesterol, lipid rafts, and lipid/protein ratio) (Kawahara et al., 2011). It has been found that Aβ aggregates bind with high specificity to synaptic sites in the rat hippocampus (Lacor et al., 2004; Deshpande et al., 2006; Lacor et al., 2007) in ordered membrane microdomains composed of both lipids and proteins (Zampagni et al., 2010). Furthermore, it was observed that the fluidity and surface charge of the membrane can also alter the binding of Aβ and influence aggregation processes and amyloid pore formation (Kawahara et al., 2011). For example, various amino acid residues in Aβ such as arginine 5, lysine 16 and lysine 28 have a positive charge at neutral pH and therefore possess affinity for negatively charged lipids like phosphatidylglycerol, phosphatidylserine or ganglioside GM1, but not for neutral lipids like phoshphatidylcholine (Seelig et al., 1995). There exists evidence suggesting that lipid rafts provide a good substrate for Aβ aggregation (Yanagisawa et al., 1995). For example, it is known that the production of Aβ can occur in these structures (Ehehalt et al., 2003) and a significant quantity of peptide has been detected in regions resistant to detergents (DRMs) and rich in proteins, sphingolipids and cholesterol (Lee et al., 1998; Morishima-Kawashima & Ihara, 1998). Thus, depletion of lipid raft components could have an effect on the production of Aβ, making way for a possible AD therapy. Therefore, cholesterol, a major component of lipid rafts and a risk factor in AD, is an ideal candidate for these types of studies (Canevari & Clark, 2007). For example, it was found that cholesterol has the capacity to affect the binding of Aβ to artificial lipid membranes (Ji et al., 2002) and its content is inversely related to toxicity (Cecchi et al., 2009).

Cholesterol in neuronal membranes induces important changes in physical properties such as changes in fluidity and density packing of lipids, affecting the binding of Aβ to the cell membrane (Mirzabekov et al., 1996). Interestingly, previous results showed that as cholesterol increases the rigidity of the membrane, it inhibits the formation of pores (Allende et al., 2005). Moreover, cholesterol blocks the increase in intracellular calcium produced by Aβ, preventing its cytotoxic effects (Kawahara & Kuroda, 2001). Therefore, membranes enriched in cholesterol demonstrate a higher resistance to the toxicity induced by Aβ oligomers, in contrast to membranes depleted of cholesterol (Cecchi et al., 2009).

This is consistent with previous studies indicating that cholesterol homeostasis could be important since toxic Aβ aggregates interact readily with membranes having a low amount of cholesterol (Kawahara et al., 2000; Yip et al., 2001).

Other studies in human neuroblastoma cells showed that increases in cholesterol reduced the ability of Aβ to bind to the membranes as demonstrated by co-localization of Aβ with GM1 ganglioside, a known marker for lipid rafts (Cecchi et al., 2009). In addition, increases in cholesterol levels exerted a protective effect against the toxicity induced by Aβ oligomers in these cells (Cecchi et al., 2008).

Sphingolipids also play a key role in the toxicity induced by Aβ (van Echten-Deckert & Walter, 2012) because they are essential components of lipid rafts in the brain and have an important function in synaptic transmission (Nagai, 1995).

Gangliosides are widely described in the CNS where they are expressed in the extracellular face of the cell membrane. They are predominantly located in the lipid raft regions probably because their highly packed acyl chains are more stable in the liquid-ordered phase of the membrane (Fishman et al., 1975). Gangliosides correspond to glycosphingolipids that contain a ceramide molecule in the hydrophobic region and sialic acid residues in the hydrophilic region, with the ceramide portion being embedded in the extracellular face of the membrane and the chain of negatively charged oligosaccharides exposed to the extracellular matrix (van Echten-Deckert & Herget, 2006).

Yanagisawa and co workers (1995) demonstrated that Aβ was strongly associated to ganglioside GM1 in AD patients (Yanagisawa et al., 1995). It has been shown in vitro that Aβ is capable of binding to ganglioside GM1 and this interaction acts like a seed accelerating the process of oligomerization (Yanagisawa et al., 1995; Yanagisawa et al., 1997).

In addition, it was demonstrated that the process of amyloid fibril formation is accelerated in the presence of liposomes having a very similar composition to sphingomyelin, cholesterol and ganglioside GM1 lipid rafts (Kakio et al., 2002). Moreover, examination of the ability of GM1 to associate with Aβ revealed that Aβ exhibits a significantly higher binding affinity for sialic acid residues (hydrophilic) than for ceramide residues, suggesting that the association to GM1 is principally due to electrostatic interactions (Choo-Smith et al., 1997). Additionally, interaction between sialic acid residues and Aβ induced a reordering in the conformation of the Aβ peptidic chain (McLaurin et al., 1998) which could potentiate the oligomerization process. On the other hand, brain, but not liver, DRMs rich in gangliosides promoted Aβ oligomerization. The study revealed that this process also occurred when the membranes were depleted of cholesterol and protein indicating that neither cholesterol nor proteins are essential for aggregation (Kim et al., 2006). Similarly, interaction of Aβ oligomers with GM1 decreases membrane fluidity and at the same time stimulates APP processing resulting in a positive feedback that leads to production of more Aβ (Peters et al., 2009). Saavedra and collaborators (2007) found that Aβ oligomers could be internalized once co-localized with the B subunit of cholera toxin (CTB), a marker for lipid rafts that specifically binds to GM1, suggesting that Aβ internalization occurs in these lipid microdomains possibly through GM1 binding (Saavedra et al., 2007). Therefore, the interaction between GM1 and Aβ in the membrane could be fundamental in the regulation of aggregation processes and the binding of Aβ to the membrane, as well as in the neurotoxic consequences, including pore formation.

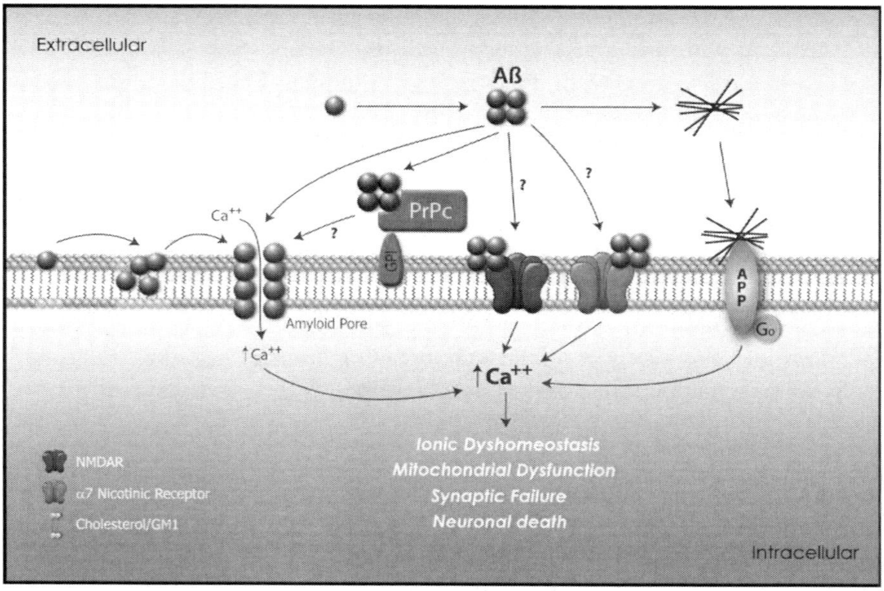

Figure 2. Neurotoxicity of Aβ explained by its association to plasma membranes. Aβ aggregate forming oligomers and fibers. The monomeric and small oligomers can associate to different lipids of the plasma membrane, specially to cholesterol and gangliosides GM1, forming amyloid pores that allow the flow of calcium ions (and others) into the cells. In parallel, the oligomeric species of Aβ can modulate, directly or indirectly, membrane proteins such as PrPc, NMDAR and nAChRs, inducing finally an increase in intracellular calcium. On the other hand, Aβ fibers can interact with APP, producing an increase of calcium though a process that involves the activation of Go protein. All of these actions of Aβ in the plasma membrane of the neurons have strong consequences on ionic homeostasis, mitochondrial function, synaptic activity and neuronal survival.

CONCLUSION

We reviewed data supporting the hypothesis that Aβ oligomers are able to associate and cause changes in the permeability of neuronal membranes, thus initiating a process of ionic and metabolic dyshomeostasis that leads to synaptic failure.

The association of Aβ to the membrane and its toxicity appears to be dependent on the presence of lipids and membrane proteins, making it possible to propose future therapeutic approaches to treat AD. A schematic proposal of these processes are resumed in Figure 2.

REFERENCES

Aguzzi, A. & Haass, C. (2003) Games played by rogue proteins in prion disorders and Alzheimer's disease. *Science*, 302, 814-818.

Allende, D., Simon, S.A. & McIntosh, T.J. (2005) Melittin-induced bilayer leakage depends on lipid material properties: evidence for toroidal pores. *Biophys. J.*, 88, 1828-1837.

Arispe, N. (2004) Architecture of the Alzheimer's A beta P ion channel pore. *J. Membr. Biol.*, 197, 33-48.

Arispe, N., Diaz, J.C. & Flora, M. (2008) Efficiency of histidine-associating compounds for blocking the alzheimer's Abeta channel activity and cytotoxicity. *Biophys. J.,* 95, 4879-4889.

Arispe, N., Diaz, J.C. & Simakova, O. (2007) Abeta ion channels. Prospects for treating Alzheimer's disease with Abeta channel blockers. *Biochim. Biophys. Acta*, 1768, 1952-1965.

Balducci, C., Beeg, M., Stravalaci, M., Bastone, A., Sclip, A., Biasini, E., Tapella, L., Colombo, L., Manzoni, C., Borsello, T., Chiesa, R., Gobbi, M., Salmona, M. & Forloni, G. (2010) Synthetic amyloid- oligomers impair long-term memory independently of cellular prion protein. *Proc. Natl. Acad. Sci.*, 107, 2295-2300.

Billings, L.M., Green, K.N., McGaugh, J.L. & LaFerla, F.M. (2007) Learning decreases A beta*56 and tau pathology and ameliorates behavioral decline in 3xTg-AD mice. *J. Neurosci.*, 27, 751-761.

Butterfield, S.M. & Lashuel, H.A. (2010) Amyloidogenic protein-membrane interactions: mechanistic insight from model systems. *Angew. Chem. Int. Ed. Engl.,* 49, 5628-5654.

Caetano, F.A., Beraldo, F.H., Hajj, G.N., Hajj, G.N., Guimaraes, A.L., Jürgensen, S., Wasilewska-Sampaio, A.P., Hirata, P.H., Souza, I., Machado, C.F., Wong, D.Y., De Felice, F.G., Ferreira, S.T., Prado, V.F., Rylett, R.J., Martins, V.R. & Prado, M.A. (2011) Amyloid-beta oligomers increase the localization of prion protein at the cell surface. *J. Neurochem.,* 117, 538-553.

Cagetti, E., Liang, J., Spigelman, I. & Olsen, R.W. (2003) Withdrawal from chronic intermittent ethanol treatment changes subunit composition, reduces synaptic function, and decreases behavioral responses to positive allosteric modulators of GABAA receptors. Mol. Pharmacol., 63, 53-64.

Canevari, L. & Clark, J.B. (2007) Alzheimer's disease and cholesterol: the fat connection. *Neurochem. Res.*, 32, 739-750.

Cecchi, C., Nichino, D., Zampagni, M. Bernacchioni, C., Evangelisti, E., Pensalfini, A., Liguri, G., Gliozzi, A., Stefani, M. & Relini, A. (2009) A protective role for lipid raft cholesterol against amyloid-induced membrane damage in human neuroblastoma cells. *Biochem. Biophys. Acta*, 1788, 2204-2216.

Cecchi, C., Rosati, F., Pensalfini, A. Formigli, L., Nosi, D., Liguri, G., Dichiara, F., Morello, M., Danza, G., Pieraccini, G., Peri, A., Serio, M. & Stefani, M. (2008) Seladin-1/DHCR24 protects neuroblastoma cells against Abeta toxicity by increasing membrane cholesterol content. *J. Cell. Mol. Med.*, 12, 1990-2002.

Chen, S., Yadav, S.P. & Surewicz, W.K. (2010) Interaction between human prion protein and amyloid-beta (Abeta) oligomers: role OF N-terminal residues. *J. Biol. Chem.*, 285, 26377-26383.

Choo-Smith, L.P., Garzon-Rodriguez, W., Glabe, C.G. & Surewicz, W.K. (1997) Acceleration of amyloid fibril formation by specific binding of Abeta-(1-40) peptide to ganglioside-containing membrane vesicles. *J. Biol. Chem.*, 272, 22987-22990.

Chromy, B.A., Nowak, R.J., Lambert, M.P. Viola, K.L., Chang, L., Velasco, P.T., Jones, B.W., Fernandez, S.J., Lacor, P.N., Horowitz, P., Finch, C.E., Krafft, G.A. & Klein, W.L. (2003) Self-assembly of Abeta(1-42) into globular neurotoxins. *Biochemistry*, 42, 12749-12760.

Chung, E., Ji, Y., Sun, Y., Kascsak, R.J., Kascsak, R.B., Mehta, P.D., Strittmatter, S.M. & Wisniewski, T. (2010) Anti-PrPC monoclonal antibody infusion as a novel treatment for cognitive deficits in an Alzheimer's disease model mouse. *BMC Neuroscience*, 11, 130.

De Ferrari, G.V. & Inestrosa, N.C. (2000) Wnt signaling function in Alzheimer's disease. *Brain Res. Rev.*, 33, 1-12.

De Ferrari, G.V., Papassotiropoulos, A., Biechele, T., Wavrant De-Vrieze, F., Avila, M.E., Major, M.B., Myers, A., Sáez, K., Henríquez, J.P., Zhao, A., Wollmer, M.A., Nitsch, R.M., Hock, C., Morris, C.M., Hardy, J. & Moon, R.T. (2007) Common genetic variation within the low-density lipoprotein receptor-related protein 6 and late-onset Alzheimer's disease. *Proc. Natl. Acad. Sci. USA*, 104, 9434-9439.

Demuro, A., Mina, E., Kayed, R., Milton, S.C., Parker, I. & Glabe, C.G. (2005) Calcium dysregulation and membrane disruption as a ubiquitous neurotoxic mechanism of soluble amyloid oligomers. *J. Biol. Chem.*, 280, 17294-17300.

Demuro, A., Parker, I. & Stutzmann, G.E. (2010) Calcium signaling and amyloid toxicity in Alzheimer disease. *J. Biol. Chem.*, 285, 12463-12468.

Deshpande, A., Mina, E., Glabe, C. & Busciglio, J. (2006) Different conformations of amyloid beta induce neurotoxicity by distinct mechanisms in human cortical neurons. *J. Neurosci.*, 26, 6011-6018.

Diociaiuti, M., Bordi, F., Motta, A., Carosi, A., Molinari, A., Arancia, G. & Coluzza, C. (2002) Aggregation of gramicidin A in phospholipid Langmuir-Blodgett monolayers. *Biophys. J.*, 82, 3198-3206.

Ehehalt, R., Keller, P., Haass, C., Thiele, C. & Simons, K. (2003) Amyloidogenic processing of the Alzheimer beta-amyloid precursor protein depends on lipid rafts. *J. Cell Biol.*, 160, 113-123.

Fishman, P.H., Max, S.R., Tallman, J.F., Brady, R.O., Maclaren, N.K. & Cornblath, M. (1975) Deficient Ganglioside Biosynthesis: a novel human sphingolipidosis. *Science*, 187, 68-70.

Georganopoulou, D.G., Chang, L., Nam, J.M., Thaxton, C.S., Mufson, E.J., Klein, W.L. & Mirkin, C.A. (2005) Nanoparticle-based detection in cerebral spinal fluid of a soluble pathogenic biomarker for Alzheimer's disease. *Proc. Natl. Acad. Sci. USA*, 102, 2273-2276.

Gimbel, D.A., Nygaard, H.B., Coffey, E.E., Gunther, E.C., Lauren, J., Gimbel, Z.A. & Strittmatter, S.M. (2010) Memory impairment in transgenic Alzheimer mice requires cellular prion protein. *J. Neurosci.*, 30, 6367-6374.

Glabe, C.G. (2008) Structural classification of toxic amyloid oligomers. *J. Biol. Chem.*, 283, 29639-29643.

Glabe, C.G. & Kayed, R. (2006) Common structure and toxic function of amyloid oligomers implies a common mechanism of pathogenesis. *Neurology,* 66, S74-78.

Gong, Y., Chang, L., Viola, K.L., Lacor, P.N., Lambert, M.P., Finch, C.E., Krafft, G. A. & Klein, W.L. (2003) Alzheimer's disease-affected brain: presence of oligomeric A beta ligands (ADDLs) suggests a molecular basis for reversible memory loss. *Proc. Natl. Acad. Sci USA*, 100, 10417-10422.

Green, J.D., Kreplak, L., Goldsbury, C., Li Blatter, X., Stolz, M., Cooper, G.S., Seelig, A., Kistler, J. & Aebi, U. (2004) Atomic force microscopy reveals defects within mica supported lipid bilayers induced by the amyloidogenic human amylin peptide. *J. Mol. Biol.*, 342, 877-887.

Hamill, O.P., Marty, A., Neher, E., Sakmann, B. & Sigworth, F.J. (1981) Improved patch-clamp techniques for high-resolution current recording from cells and cell-free membrane patches. *Pflugers. Arch.*, 391, 85-100.

Harmeier, A., Wozny, C., Rost, B.R. Munter, L.M., Hua, H., Georgiev, O., Beyermann, M., Hildebrand, P.W., Weise, C., Schaffner, W., Schmitz, D. & Multhaup, G. (2009) Role of amyloid-beta glycine 33 in oligomerization, toxicity, and neuronal plasticity. J. *Neurosci.,* 29, 7582-7590.

Hartley, D.M., Walsh, D.M., Ye, C.P., Diehl, T., Vasquez, S., Vassilev, P.M., Teplow, D.B. & Selkoe, D.J. (1999) Protofibrillar intermediates of amyloid beta-protein induce acute electrophysiological changes and progressive neurotoxicity in cortical neurons. *J. Neurosci.,* 19, 8876-8884.

Heredia, L., Lin, R., Vigo, F.S., Kedikian, G., Busciglio, J. & Lorenzo, A. (2004) Deposition of amyloid fibrils promotes cell-surface accumulation of amyloid beta precursor protein. *Neurobiol. Dis.*, 16, 617-629.

Holscher, C., Gengler, S., Gault, V.A., Harriott, P. & Mallot, H.A. (2007) Soluble beta-amyloid[25-35] reversibly impairs hippocampal synaptic plasticity and spatial learning. *Eur. J. Pharmacol.*, 561, 85-90.

Hung, L.W., Ciccotosto, G.D., Giannakis, E., Tew, D.J., Perez, K., Masters, C.L., Cappai, R., Wade, J.D. & Barnham, K.J. (2008) Amyloid-beta peptide (A) neurotoxicity is modulated by the rate of peptide aggregation: a dimers and trimers correlate with neurotoxicity. *J. Neurosci.*, 28, 11950-11958.

Hung, Y.H., Bush, A.I. & Cherny, R.A. (2009) Copper in the brain and Alzheimer's disease. JBIC *J. Biol. Inorg. Chem.*, 15, 61-76.

Jang, H., Zheng, J., Lal, R. & Nussinov, R. (2008) New structures help the modeling of toxic amyloidß ion channels. *Trends Biochem. Sci.*, 33, 91-100.

Jang, H., Zheng, J. & Nussinov, R. (2007) Models of beta-amyloid ion channels in the membrane suggest that channel formation in the bilayer is a dynamic process. *Biophys. J.*, 93, 1938-1949.

Ji, S. R., Wu, Y. & Sui, S.F. (2002) Cholesterol is an important factor affecting the membrane insertion of beta-amyloid peptide (A beta 1-40), which may potentially inhibit the fibril formation. *J. Biol. Chem.*, 277, 6273-6279.

Kakio, A., Nishimoto, S., Yanagisawa, K., Kozutsumi, Y. & Matsuzaki, K. (2002) Interactions of amyloid beta-protein with various gangliosides in raft-like membranes: importance of GM1 ganglioside-bound form as an endogenous seed for Alzheimer amyloid. *Biochemistry*, 41, 7385-7390.

Kawahara, M. & Kuroda, Y. (2001) Intracellular calcium changes in neuronal cells induced by Alzheimer's beta-amyloid protein are blocked by estradiol and cholesterol. *Cell. Mol. Neurobiol.*, 21, 1-13.

Kawahara, M., Kuroda, Y., Arispe, N. & Rojas, E. (2000) Alzheimer's beta-amyloid, human islet amylin, and prion protein fragment evoke intracellular free calcium elevations by a common mechanism in a hypothalamic GnRH neuronal cell line. *J. Biol. Chem.*, 275, 14077-14083.

Kawahara, M., Ohtsuka, I., Yokoyama, S., Kato-Negishi, M. & Sadakane, Y. (2011) Membrane incorporation, channel formation, and disruption of calcium homeostasis by Alzheimer's beta-amyloid protein. *Int. J. Alz. Dis.*, 2011, 304583.

Kayed, R., Sokolov, Y., Edmonds, B., McIntire, T.M., Milton, S.C., Hall, J.E. & Glabe, C.G. (2004) Permeabilization of lipid bilayers is a common conformation-dependent activity of soluble amyloid oligomers in protein misfolding diseases. *J. Biol. Chem.*, 279, 46363-46366.

Kedikian, G., Heredia, F., Salvador, V.R., Raimunda, D., Isoardi, N., Heredia, L. & Lorenzo, A. (2010) Secreted amyloid precursor protein and holo-APP bind amyloid beta through distinct domains eliciting different toxic responses on hippocampal neurons. *J. Neurosci. Res.*, 88, 1795-1803.

Kelly, B.L. (2006) beta-amyloid-induced dynamin 1 degradation is mediated by N-Methyl-D-Aspartate receptors in hippocampal neurons. *J. Biol. Chem.*, 281, 28079-28089.

Kelly, B.L., Vassar, R. & Ferreira, A. (2005) Beta-amyloid-induced dynamin 1 depletion in hippocampal neurons. A potential mechanism for early cognitive decline in Alzheimer disease. *J. Biol. Chem.*, 280, 31746-31753.

Kim, S., Jeon, T.J., Oberai, A., Yang, D., Schmidt, J.J. & Bowie, J.U. (2005) Transmembrane glycine zippers: physiological and pathological roles in membrane proteins. *Proc. Natl. Acad. Sci. USA*, 102, 14278-14283.

Kim, S.I., Yi, J.S. & Ko, Y.G. (2006) Amyloid beta oligomerization is induced by brain lipid rafts. *J. Cell. Biochem.*, 99, 878-889.

Kuo, Y.M., Emmerling, M.R., Vigo-Pelfrey, C., Kasunic, T.C., Kirkpatrick, J.B., Murdoch, G.H., Ball, M.J. & Roher, A.E. (1996) Water-soluble Abeta (N-40, N-42) oligomers in normal and Alzheimer disease brains. *J. Biol. Chem.*, 271, 4077-4081.

Lacor, P.N., Buniel, M.C., Chang, L. Fernandez S.J., Gong Y., Viola, K.L., Lambert, M.P., Velasco, P.T., Bigio, E.H., Finch, C.E., Krafft, G.A. & Klein, W.L. (2004) Synaptic targeting by Alzheimer's-related amyloid beta oligomers. *J. Neurosci.*, 24, 10191-10200.

Lacor, P.N., Buniel, M.C., Furlow, P.W., Clemente, A.S., Velasco, P.T., Wood, M., Viola, K.L. & Klein, W.L. (2007) Abeta oligomer-induced aberrations in synapse composition, shape, and density provide a molecular basis for loss of connectivity in Alzheimer's disease. *J. Neurosci.*, 27, 796-807.

Lambert, M.P., Barlow, A.K., Chromy, B.A. Edwards, C., Freed, R., Liosatos, M., Morgan, T.E., Rozovsky ,I., Trommer, B., Viola, K.L., Wals, P., Zhang, C., Finch, C.E., Krafft, G.A. & Klein, W.L. (1998) Diffusible, nonfibrillar ligands derived from Abeta1-42 are potent central nervous system neurotoxins. *Proc. Natl. Acad. Sci, USA,* 95, 6448-6453.

Lashuel, H.A. & Lansbury, P.T., Jr. (2006) Are amyloid diseases caused by protein aggregates that mimic bacterial pore-forming toxins? *Q. Rev. Biophys.,* 39, 167-201.

Lauren, J., Gimbel, D.A., Nygaard, H.B., Gilbert, J.W. & Strittmatter, S.M. (2009) Cellular prion protein mediates impairment of synaptic plasticity by amyloid-beta oligomers. *Nature,* 457, 1128-1132.

Lee, S.J., Liyanage, U., Bickel, P.E., Xia, W., Lansbury, P.T., Jr. & Kosik, K.S. (1998) A detergent-insoluble membrane compartment contains A beta in vivo. *Nat. Med.,* 4, 730-734.

Lorenzo, A., Yuan, M., Zhang, Z. Paganetti, P.A., Sturchler-Pierrat, C., Staufenbiel, M., Mautino, J., Vigo, F.S., Sommer, B. & Yankner, B.A. (2000) Amyloid beta interacts with the amyloid precursor protein: a potential toxic mechanism in Alzheimer's disease. *Nat. Neurosci.*, 3, 460-464.

McLaurin, J., Franklin, T., Fraser, P.E. & Chakrabartty, A. (1998) Structural transitions associated with the interaction of Alzheimer beta-amyloid peptides with gangliosides. *J. Biol. Chem.,* 273, 4506-4515.

Mirzabekov, T.A., Lin, M.C. & Kagan, B.L. (1996) Pore formation by the cytotoxic islet amyloid peptide amylin. *J. Biol. Chem.*, 271, 1988-1992.

Morishima-Kawashima, M. & Ihara, Y. (1998) The presence of amyloid beta-protein in the detergent-insoluble membrane compartment of human neuroblastoma cells. *Biochemistry,* 37, 15247-15253.

Munter, L.M., Voigt, P., Harmeier, A. Kaden, D., Gottschalk, K.E., Weise, C., Pipkorn, R., Schaefer, M., Langosch, D. & Multhaup, G. (2007) GxxxG motifs within the amyloid precursor protein transmembrane sequence are critical for the etiology of Abeta42. *EMBO J.*, 26, 1702-1712.

Nagai, Y. (1995) Functional roles of gangliosides in bio-signaling. *Behav. Brain Res.*, 66, 99-104.

Oddo, S., Caccamo, A., Shepherd, J. D. Murphy, M.P., Golde, T.E., Kayed, R., Metherate, R., Mattson, M.P., Akbari, Y., LaFerla, F.M. (2003) Triple-transgenic model of Alzheimer's disease with plaques and tangles. *Neuron,* 39, 409-421.

Parodi, J., Sepulveda, F.J., Roa, J., Opazo, C., Inestrosa, N.C. & Aguayo, L.G. (2009) beta-amyloid causes depletion of synaptic vesicles leading to neurotransmission failure. *J. Biol. Chem.*, 285, 2506-2514.

Peters, C., Espinoza, M.P., Gallegos, S., Opazo, C. & Aguayo, L.G. (2015) Alzheimer's Abeta interacts with cellular prion protein inducing neuronal membrane damage and synaptotoxicity. *Neurobiol. Aging*, 36, 1369-1377.

Peters, C., Fernandez-Perez, E.J., Burgos, C.F., Espinoza, M.P., Castillo, C., Urrutia, J.C., Streltsov, V.A., Opazo, C. & Aguayo, L.G. (2013) Inhibition of amyloid beta-induced synaptotoxicity by a pentapeptide derived from the glycine zipper region of the neurotoxic peptide. *Neurobiol. Aging*, 34, 2805-2814.

Peters, I., Igbavboa, U., Schütt, T., Haidari, S., Hartig, U., Rosello, X., Böttner, S., Copanaki, E., Deller, T., Kögel, D., Wood, W.G., Müller, W.E., Eckert, G.P. (2009) The interaction of beta-amyloid protein with cellular membranes stimulates its own production. *Biochim. Biophys*. Acta, 1788, 964-972.

Phinney, A.L., Calhoun, M.E., Wolfer, D.P., Lipp, H.P., Zheng, H. & Jucker, M. (1999) No hippocampal neuron or synaptic bouton loss in learning-impaired aged beta-amyloid precursor protein-null mice. *Neuroscience,* 90, 1207-1216.

Prusiner, S.B. (1998) The prion diseases. *Brain Pathol*., 8, 499-513.

Quist, A., Doudevski, I., Lin, H., Azimova, R., Ng, D., Frangione, B., Kagan, B., Ghiso, J. & Lal, R. (2005) Amyloid ion channels: a common structural link for protein-misfolding disease. *Proc. Natl. Acad. Sci. USA*, 102, 10427-10432.

Reddy, P.H., Mani, G., Park, B.S., Jacques, J., Murdoch, G., Whetsell, W., Jr., Kaye, J. & Manczak, M. (2005) Differential loss of synaptic proteins in Alzheimer's disease: implications for synaptic dysfunction. *J. Alz. Dis.,* 7, 103-117; discussion 173-180.

Reitz, C., Brayne, C. & Mayeux, R. (2011) Epidemiology of Alzheimer disease. *Nat. Rev. Neurol*., 7, 137-152.

Richter, L., Munter, L.M., Ness, J. Hildebrand, P.W., Dasari, M., Unterreitmeier, S., Bulic, B., Beyermann, M., Gust, R., Reif, B., Weggen, S., Langosch, D. & Multhaup, G. (2010) Amyloid beta 42 peptide (Abeta42)-lowering compounds directly bind to Abeta and interfere with amyloid precursor protein (APP) transmembrane dimerization. *Proc. Natl. Acad. Sci. USA*, 107, 14597-14602.

Roselli, F., Tirard, M., Lu, J., Hutzler, P., Lamberti, P., Livrea, P., Morabito, M. & Almeida, O.F. (2005) Soluble beta-amyloid1-40 induces NMDA-dependent degradation of postsynaptic density-95 at glutamatergic synapses. *J. Neurosci.,* 25, 11061-11070.

Rovelet-Lecrux, A., Hannequin, D., Raux, G. Le Meur, N., Laquerrière, A., Vital, A., Dumanchin, C., Feuillette, S., Brice, A., Vercelletto, M., Dubas, F., Frebourg, T. & Campion, D. (2006) APP locus duplication causes autosomal dominant early-onset Alzheimer disease with cerebral amyloid angiopathy. *Nat. Genet*., 38, 24-26.

Russ, W.P. & Engelman, D.M. (2000) The GxxxG motif: a framework for transmembrane helix-helix association. *J. Mol. Biol*., 296, 911-919.

Saavedra, L., Mohamed, A., Ma, V., Kar, S. & de Chaves, E.P. (2007) Internalization of beta-amyloid peptide by primary neurons in the absence of apolipoprotein E. *J. Biol. Chem*., 282, 35722-35732.

Seelig, J., Lehrmann, R. & Terzi, E. (1995) Domain formation induced by lipid-ion and lipid-peptide interactions. *Mol. Membr. Biol*., 12, 51-57.

Selkoe, D.J. (2002) Alzheimer's disease is a synaptic failure. *Science,* 298, 789-791.

Selkoe, D.J. (2008) Biochemistry and molecular biology of amyloid beta-protein and the mechanism of Alzheimer's disease. *Handb. Clin. Neurol*., 89, 245-260.

Sepúlveda, F.J., Fierro, H., Fernandez, E., Castillo, C., Peoples, R.W., Opazo, C. & Aguayo, L.G. (2013) Nature of the neurotoxic membrane actions of amyloid-β on hippocampal neurons in Alzheimer's disease. *Neurobiol.* Aging, 35, 472-481.

Sepúlveda, F.J., Fierro, H., Fernandez, E., Castillo, C., Peoples, R.W., Opazo, C. & Aguayo, L.G. (2014) Nature of the neurotoxic membrane actions of amyloid-β on hippocampal neurons in Alzheimer's disease. *Neurobiol.* Aging, 35, 472-481.

Sepulveda, F.J., Parodi, J., Peoples, R.W., Opazo, C. & Aguayo, L.G. (2010) Synaptotoxicity of Alzheimer beta amyloid can be explained by its membrane perforating property. *PLoS One*, 5, e11820.

Shankar, G.M., Bloodgood, B.L., Townsend, M., Walsh, D.M., Selkoe, D.J. & Sabatini, B.L. (2007) Natural oligomers of the Alzheimer amyloid-beta protein induce reversible synapse loss by modulating an NMDA-type glutamate receptor-dependent signaling pathway. *J. Neurosci.,* 27, 2866-2875.

Shankar, G.M., Li, S., Mehta, T.H. Garcia-Munoz, A., Shepardson, N.E., Smith, I., Brett, F.M., Farrell, M.A., Rowan, M.J., Lemere, C.A., Regan, C.M., Walsh, D.M., Sabatini, B.L. & Selkoe, D.J. (2008) Amyloid-β protein dimers isolated directly from Alzheimer's brains impair synaptic plasticity and memory. *Nat. Med.*, 14, 837-842.

Snyder, E.M., Nong, Y., Almeida, C.G. Paul, S., Moran, T., Choi, E.Y., Nairn, A.C., Salter, M.W., Lombroso, P.J., Gouras, G.K. & Greengard, P. (2005) Regulation of NMDA receptor trafficking by amyloid-beta. *Nat. Neurosci.,* 8, 1051-1058.

Sola Vigo, F., Kedikian, G., Heredia, L., Heredia, F., Anel, A.D., Rosa, A.L. & Lorenzo, A. (2009) Amyloid-beta precursor protein mediates neuronal toxicity of amyloid beta through Go protein activation. *Neurobiol. Aging,* 30, 1379-1392.

Stephan, A., Laroche, S. & Davis, S. (2001) Generation of aggregated beta-amyloid in the rat hippocampus impairs synaptic transmission and plasticity and causes memory deficits. *J. Neurosci.,* 21, 5703-5714.

Tanzi, R.E. & Bertram, L. (2005) Twenty years of the Alzheimer's disease amyloid hypothesis: a genetic perspective. *Cell*, 120, 545-555.

Ticku, M.K. (1990) Alcohol and GABA-benzodiazepine receptor function. *Ann. Med.*, 22, 241-246.

Tjernberg, L.O., Naslund, J., Lindqvist, F., Johansson, J., Karlstrom, A.R., Thyberg, J., Terenius, L. & Nordstedt, C. (1996) Arrest of beta-amyloid fibril formation by a pentapeptide ligand. *J. Biol. Chem.*, 271, 8545-8548.

Townsend, M., Shankar, G.M., Mehta, T., Walsh, D.M. & Selkoe, D.J. (2006) Effects of secreted oligomers of amyloid beta-protein on hippocampal synaptic plasticity: a potent role for trimers. *J. Physiol.*, 572, 477-492.

Um, J.W., Kaufman, A.C., Kostylev, M., Heiss, J.K., Stagi, M., Takahashi, H., Kerrisk, M.E., Vortmeyer, A., Wisniewski, T., Koleske, A.J., Gunther, E.C., Nygaard, H.B. & Strittmatter, S.M. (2013) Metabotropic glutamate receptor 5 is a coreceptor for Alzheimer Aβ oligomer bound to cellular prion protein. *Neuron*, 79, 887-902.

van Echten-Deckert, G. & Herget, T. (2006) Sphingolipid metabolism in neural cells. *Biochim. Biophys. Acta*, 1758, 1978-1994.

van Echten-Deckert, G. & Walter, J. (2012) Sphingolipids: critical players in Alzheimer's disease. *Prog. Lipid Res.*, 51, 378-393.

Verdier, Y., Huszar, E., Penke, B. Penke, Z., Woffendin, G., Scigelova, M., Fülöp, L., Szucs, M., Medzihradszky, K., Janáky, T. (2005) Identification of synaptic plasma membrane proteins co-precipitated with fibrillar beta-amyloid peptide. *J. Neurochem.*, 94, 617-628.

Walsh, D.M., Klyubin, I., Fadeeva, J.V., Cullen, W.K., Anwyl, R., Wolfe, M.S., Rowan, M.J. & Selkoe, D.J. (2002) Naturally secreted oligomers of amyloid beta protein potently inhibit hippocampal long-term potentiation in vivo. *Nature,* 416, 535-539.

Wang, H.Y., Lee, D.H., D'Andrea, M.R., Peterson, P.A., Shank, R.P. & Reitz, A.B. (2000) beta-Amyloid(1-42) binds to alpha7 nicotinic acetylcholine receptor with high affinity. Implications for Alzheimer's disease pathology. *J. Biol. Chem.*, 275, 5626-5632.

Wang, Z., Song, D. & Berger, T.W. (2002) Contribution of NMDA receptor channels to the expression of LTP in the hippocampal dentate gyrus. *Hippocampus,* 12, 680-688.

Yan, S.D., Chen, X., Fu, J., Chen, M., Zhu, H., Roher, A., Slattery, T., Zhao, L., Nagashima, M., Morser, J., Migheli, A., Nawroth, P., Stern, D. & Schmidt, A.M. (1996) RAGE and amyloid-beta peptide neurotoxicity in Alzheimer's disease. *Nature*, 382, 685-691.

Yanagisawa, K., McLaurin, J., Michikawa, M., Chakrabartty, A. & Ihara, Y. (1997) Amyloid beta-protein (A beta) associated with lipid molecules: immunoreactivity distinct from that of soluble A beta. *FEBS Lett.*, 420, 43-46.

Yanagisawa, K., Odaka, A., Suzuki, N. & Ihara, Y. (1995) GM1 ganglioside-bound amyloid beta-protein (A beta): a possible form of preamyloid in Alzheimer's disease. *Nat. Med.*, 1, 1062-1066.

Yip, C.M., Elton, E.A., Darabie, A.A., Morrison, M.R. & McLaurin, J. (2001) Cholesterol, a modulator of membrane-associated Abeta-fibrillogenesis and neurotoxicity. *J. Mol. Biol.*, 311, 723-734.

Zampagni, M., Evangelisti, E., Cascella, R. Liguri, G., Becatti, M., Pensalfini, A., Uberti, D., Cenini, G., Memo, M., Bagnoli, S., Nacmias, B., Sorbi, S. & Cecchi, C. (2010) Lipid rafts are primary mediators of amyloid oxidative attack on plasma membrane. *J. Mol. Med.* (Berl), 88, 597-608.

Zhao, G., Cui, M.Z., Mao, G., Dong, Y., Tan, J., Sun, L. & Xu, X. (2005) gamma-Cleavage is dependent on zeta-cleavage during the proteolytic processing of amyloid precursor protein within its transmembrane domain. *J. Biol. Chem.*, 280, 37689-37697.

Zheng, H. & Koo, E.H. (2006) The amyloid precursor protein: beyond amyloid. *Mol. Neurodegener.*, 1, 5.

Zou, W.Q., Xiao, X., Yuan, J., Puoti, G., Fujioka, H., Wang, X., Richardson, S., Zhou, X., Zou, R., Li, S., Zhu, X., McGeer, P.L., McGeehan, J., Kneale, G., Rincon-Limas, D.E., Fernandez-Funez, P., Lee, H.G., Smith, M.A., Petersen, R.B. & Guo, J.P. (2011) Amyloid-beta42 interacts mainly with insoluble prion protein in the Alzheimer brain. *J. Biol. Chem.*, 286, 15095-15105.

In: Synaptic Fundamentals of Memory Performance
Editor: Ignacio González-Burgos

ISBN: 978-1-63483-279-3

Chapter 9

CELLULAR AND MOLECULAR TARGETS AS STARTING POINTS TO ATTENUATE THE SYNAPTIC FAILURE IN ALZHEIMER BETA AMYLOID TOXICITY: THE PURINERGIC TRANSMISSION

Jorge Fuentealba*[1,*]*, Pamela Godoy*[1]*, Tiare Silva-Grecchi*[1]*,
***Francisco Saez-Orellana*[1] *and Luis G. Aguayo*[2]**

[1] Neuroactive Compound Screening Unit,
Department of Physiology, University of Concepcion, Chile
[2]Laboratory of Neurophysiology, Department of Physiology,
Faculty of Biological Sciences, University of Concepcion, Chile

ABSTRACT

Memory, emotional and behavioral disorders that are characteristic of early and advanced Alzheimer´s disease (AD) are currently associated to synaptic failure as a consequence of the effects of amyloid beta peptide (Aβ) on neuronal networks. Unfortunately, many years of research in this area have not been able to provide an effective treatment to this devastating disease. The advances in combinatorial or synthetic chemistry and bioinformatics have systematically failed to elicit this aim. The identification of new anti-AD drugs to attack specific targets has been slow due to adverse drug reactions (ADRs). Therefore, the main challenge is to identify innovative strategies in order to discover new drugs and treatments for an ever-increasing number of AD patients. Although the finding of new molecules that efficiently modulate some classical targets in AD models (i.e. nAChR) has been turned into a global health priority, a more interesting option for the development of new therapeutic strategies would be to discover and propose a novel target that is effectively proven to interfere with Aβ toxicity. Purinergic transmission has been classically associated to glial inflammatory responses, but recent work has found that modulation of neuronal ionotropic purinergic

* Send correspondence to: Jorge Fuentealba, PhD, Neuroactive Compound Screening Unit, Department of Physiology, Faculty of Biological Sciences, University of Concepcion, Barrio Universitario s/n, Concepcion, Chile. P. O. Box 160-C. Phone: 56-41-2661082. Email: jorgefuentealba@udec.cl

P2X receptors (P2XR) is a key element in the potentiation of Aβ toxicity. For example, use of P2XR antagonists have shown promising results in *in vitro* studies by demonstrating an important recovery in neuronal network activity through the modulation of crosstalk between P2XR and other neuronal receptors, intracellular key proteins and mitochondria. These results provide us with a novel opportunity to develop new drug therapies for AD that could potentiate or replace the current treatment. However, these therapies must be associated to the development of biomarkers that could identify the disease in the earliest stages so that pharmacological treatment could begin as soon as possible. In this chapter, we will discuss the main advances in this field and provide different rational approaches.

Keywords: Alzheimer´s disease, Synaptic failure, amyloid beta, purinergic receptors, neurodegeneration

1. Introduction

1.1. Population Ageing as a Consequence of Technology Development and Biomedical Advances

Ageing can be defined as a process that involves a physiological wear and tear of the normal function of the body, mainly related with a decrease on the dynamic range of physical capacities and the sensorial and cognitive abilities that people require to maintain communication with the environment and especially with their social network. In the 90s there were 4 million Americans aged 85 and older, and the projections estimate that in 2040, there will be 40 million people considered old; which is based on the capacity of people to live over 65 years (Bowling & Dieppe, 2005). In fact, every country has a growing ageing population, especially low and middle income countries. The factors involved in this phenomenon are related to changes in epidemiology indicators associated with the increase in life expectancies, declining fertility and mortality rates (United-Nations 2014), health advances and better life conditions (United-Nations, 2013); all of which are correlated with technological development and the access of the population to these advances. Most developed countries have many decades in this process; however, developing countries are recently experiencing a rise in ageing. Therefore, the most aged population is in developed countries, while the majority of older people are from developing countries (United-Nations, 2013). The percentage of elderly people (over 60 years old) in the world was 9% of the population in 1994, 12% in 2014 and it is expected to reach 21% in 2050, while the "oldest elder" (over 80 years old) was 14% in 2014 and is projected to be 19% in 2050 (United-Nations, 2014). For example, Chile is a developing country, and the life expectancy at birth will increase about 10 years by 2020 (from 1980). This gain in life expectancy is twice the world average, suggesting that the Chilean population has aged faster than the world average (INE, 2006). All these changes induce a strong economic impact on the health and social security systems determining whether people will have the opportunity to age successfully.

Successful ageing can be defined from several points of view, but mainly this concept is related with objective and subjective indicators such as: individual perception of oneself, subjective well-being, absence of disease, physical and functional capacities to develop daily tasks with independence and proper cognitive functioning. All of these indicators provide the subjects with a perception of their quality of life and life satisfaction. Two groups of factors have been associated as predictors of physiological ageing and cognitive functions: 1) intrauterine environment, that determines birth size, brain tissue volume and age-related cognitive function at birth; and 2) the access and quality of education, since a lower educational level is important for cognitive function decline rate in later life, particularly in subjects with poor intrauterine environment (Muller, et al., 2014). Taken together, it appears that the strongest impact on population ageing would be in countries that have a developing economy, where the access and resources to obtain available biomedical advances are restricted, and where social benefits are lower.

When physiological ageing is altered, affecting the cognitive function, the ageing process is transformed into a complex scenario that requires special health and social policies to support the needs of those people suffering from this condition.

2. Dementias and Alzheimer's Disease: Unsuccessful Ageing of Key Areas in the Central Nervous System

Dementias are multifactorial syndromes that have common symptoms like memory deficit, defective thinking, behavioral changes, motor dysfunctions, cognitive deficit, etc (Burns, 2009). One important characteristic is their progressive condition that generates dependence, disability and loss in the quality of life of elderly people. Moreover, the prevalence of these syndromes can double each 5 years (Prince, 2014). Dementias are a big problem to all public health and social systems since the treatment and care of demented people and the family group have a high economic cost and a deep social impact. This becomes relevant when indicators show an exponential increase in people with dementia, especially in low and middle income countries, which is a logical consequence of the epidemiological indicators previously discussed.

Dementias can be classified in 4 main groups sorted by prevalence: Frontotemporal dementia (5-10%), Dementia with Lewy bodies (<5%), Vascular Dementia (20-30%) and Alzheimer´s Disease (AD, 50-70%). AD represents the most important type of dementia (Burns, 2009; Prince 2014) and is characterized as a slow, neurodegenerative process that does not have a fully determined etiology (Burns, 2009, Castellani et al., 2010). AD has had the most potent increase among selected causes of deaths such as stroke, prostate cancer, breast cancer, heart disease and HIV; showing an increase of 68%. Recent reports from the Alzheimer's Association indicate that the American population over 65 years old that have AD is almost 5 million people, making AD the fifth leading cause of death in this age group (Hebert et al., 2013). Furthermore, in 2005 the number of people affected by AD around the world was close to 24 million (Ferri et al., 2006), and according to the projections made in 2011, this number will increase to 80 million in 2040 (Thies, 2011). From an economical point of view, the cost of care for AD patients was 604 billion dollars in 2010 (Wimo & Prince 2010; Thies & Bleiler, 2011), in addition to the indirect costs associated to the stress and related diseases in caregivers (Wimo & Prince, 2010).

With regards to brain structure and morphology, a reduction in brain mass and an increase in ventricular volume that reflects the associated neuronal death has been described (Ballard, 2011). This process is histologically recognized by the presence of two markers:

senile plaques (ultracondensed amyloid beta peptide aggregates) and neurofibrillary tangles (hyperphosphorylated Tau protein fibrils (Ballard, 2011). There exists a scientific consensus about the key role of amyloid beta peptide (Aβ) in the pathophysiology and toxic effects seen in AD (Glenner et al., 1984; Selkoe, 1991; Hardy & Mullan, 1992; Sokolov et al., 2006). The abnormal processing of amyloid precursor protein (APP) (Tomiyama et al., 2008) generates two principal toxic species: Aβ 1-40, the more predominant species which contains 40 amino acids, and Aβ 1-42/43, the more toxic species having 42-43 amino acids (Selkoe, 1994; Suh & Checler, 2002). Considering that AD is a complex disease, several hypotheses have been proposed to explain its mechanism such as APP mutation (E693Δ) (Thinakaran & Koo, 2008), and other mutations described as important in the presenilin 1 gene (chromosome 14), presenilin 2 gene (chromosome 1) and APP gene (chromosome 21) (Cruts & van Broeckhoven, 1998; Suh & Checler 2002; Bertram et al., 2010; Cruts et al., 2012). All of these are focused on the abnormal processing of APP that enhances the amyloidogenic pathway and generates an increase in the Aβ concentrations (Bertram et al., 2010); a process that has been directly associated with the early onset of the toxic effects (Selkoe, 2008). Several years ago, senile plaques were considered the responsible cause for the neuronal toxic effects (neuronal death and synaptic connection loss) and symptoms (learning and memory deficits) associated with AD (Glenner et al., 1984; Palop & Mucke 2010; Ballard, 2011). However, as previously mentioned, wide scientific evidence has re-focused the attention on small Aβ aggregates that have been suggested as central toxic elements in the pathology, and have been described to interact with different membrane proteins such as NMDA receptors (Decker et al., 2010), lipoprotein receptor-related protein 6 (LRP6) (De Ferrari et al., 2007) and α-7 nicotinic acetylcholine receptor (α-7 AChR) (Wang et al., 2000). However, stronger evidence points to a direct interaction of Aβ with the plasma membrane and the subsequent changes induced in its properties (dielectric and permeability) (Sokolov et al., 2006; Valincius et al., 2008; Kawahara et al., 2011). On the other hand, elements such as Zn^{2+} have been suggested to be a promoter or accelerating agent of Aβ aggregation (Tõugu et al., 2008); while the pH (Wong et al., 2009) or cholesterol depletion have been considered as modulating factors in the process (D'Errico et al., 2008; Jones et al., 2010), and high concentrations of Cu^{2+} and Fe^{2+} have been associated with Aβ deposits in AD brains (Barnham & Bush 2008; Bush & Tanzi 2008; Strozyk et al., 2009). All of these factors could potentiate or modulate Aβ toxicity.

All the cytotoxic changes induced by the interaction of Aβ peptide with the plasma membrane have been associated to initial disruption of neuronal ionic homeostasis (Bezprozvanny & Mattson 2008; Camandola & Mattson, 2011), and supported mainly by post mortem observations related with the presence of plaques in intact areas and neurodegenerated areas without the presence of plaques (Lesné et al., 2008; Carlo, 2010), suggesting that the presence of "soluble oligomeric" aggregates (SO-Aβ, 17 to 55 kDa) must be the key and central element in the onset of neurotoxicity (a more earlier event than plaque formation) (Haass & Selkoe 2007; DaRocha-Souto et al., 2011; Prangkio et al., 2012). These SO-Aβ show a potent and fast neurotoxicity in the micromolar range (Lesné et al., 2006), leading to several alterations such as structural and functional changes of the synapse (for review see (Haass & Selkoe, 2007, Carlo, 2010, Palop & Mucke 2010), overexpression of Arc (a synaptic immediate-early gene related with dysfunctional learning) (Lacor et al., 2004), inhibition of hippocampal long term potentiation (LTP) (Walsh et al., 2002; Wang et al., 2002; Selkoe, 2008; Palop & Mucke, 2010) and finally induction of cell death (Wang et al., 2002; Lacor et al., 2004; Wong et al., 2009; Carlo, 2010; DaRocha-Souto et al., 2011). All together, these data suggest that SO-Aβ are the initial responsible agents for the neurodegenerative effects of the disease, based on early ionic dyshomeostasis, permeability alterations and adaptive changes in the expression levels of proteins and signaling pathway activation. Therefore, any modulator that could alter the toxic events related with Aβ physiopathology must be considered as a target to be studied and developed.

3. The Cholinergic Hypothesis and Therapies: Nicotinic Responses As Classical Targets

The cholinergic hypothesis was one of the first theories to explain AD and was based on the loss of cholinergic activity commonly observed in the brain of patients with this form of dementia (Craig et al., 2011). The cholinergic system is the most characterized in the physiopathology of AD. Therefore, a role for acetylcholine (ACh) in learning and memory, two of the principal functions impaired in AD, has been extensively described (Craig et al., 2011). The cholinergic hypothesis asserts that in the brains of patients with AD there is a reduced synthesis of ACh, a decrease in the number of nicotinic and muscarinic receptors, and an increase in acetylcholinesterase activity (Perry et al., 1990; Sakurada et al., 1990). Seventeen subunits of neuronal nicotinic acetylcholine receptors (nAChRs) have been found that are denominated as α1-α10, β1-β4, γ, δ and ε (Millar & Gotti 2009), and it has been suggested that there are receptors with only α and β subunits in neurons (Role, 1992; Drisdel & Green, 2000). These receptors are permeable to Na^+ and K^+, but some are also permeable to Ca^{2+}, especially the homomeric isoform such as α7 (Itier & Bertrand, 2001). The nAChRs have been associated with different neurological disorders as Alzheimer's Disease, Parkinson's Disease, Schizophrenia and epilepsy (Nordberg, 2001; Posadas et al., 2013).

The nAChRs are expressed in the pre-synaptic membranes where they modulate the release of ACh and other neurotransmitters and in the post-synaptic membranes where they regulate cell excitability (Wonnacott, 1997; Dajas-Bailador & Wonnacott, 2004; Gotti & Clementi, 2004; Sher et al., 2004; Jensen et al., 2005). These receptors are in cholinergic neurons that are involved in important processes like memory, motor control, reward, arousal, anxiety and pain; and therefore they are extensively studied and are possible therapeutic targets (Wonnacott, 1997; Gotti & Clementi, 2004; Jensen et al., 2005). The most common nAChRs in the CNS are α4β2 and α7 subtypes, which have their highest expression in cortex and hippocampus, areas with cholinergic degeneration in AD. Moreover, the activation of α7 nAChRs may promote neuronal survival (Orr-Urtreger et al., 1997; Shinotoh et al., 2000; Picciotto et al., 2001). It has been demonstrated that a perturbation in α7 nAChRs provokes dysfunction and neurodegeneration, while stimulation protects neurons from Aβ. These findings converted α7 nAChR in a central target for the first drugs that tried to fight AD deterioration (D'Andrea & Nagele 2006; Buckingham et al., 2009). Then, scientific efforts were focused on the search and development of new drugs with safer profiles to treat the cholinergic deficit and reverse the cognitive dysfunction. This led to the use of acetylcholinesterase (AChE) inhibitors, Donepezil, Galantamine and Rivastigmine to treat AD with partial results. Donepezil showed improvement in cognitive function in mild, moderate and severe dementia for AD patients (Birks & Harvey, 2003) by stimulation of the

$\alpha 7$ receptor in addition to its inhibiting function (Shen et al., 2010). Galantamine, besides inhibiting AChE, acts as an allosteric modulator ligand for nAChRs to increase ACh release (Woodruff-Pak et al., 2001), and it showed a partial beneficial effect on cognitive functions, behavior and daily activities (Corey-Bloom, 2003). Rivastigmine is classified as a pseudo-irreversible inhibitor because its effects on AChE lasts up to 10 hours (long as compared to other inhibitors) and it has CNS selectivity (Jann, 2000). Also, this drug has been shown to slow the progression of AD symptoms (Rösler et al., 1999). The partial benefit of the above mentioned drugs is the reason why new pharmaceutics to modulate nAChRs have not been approved in recent years. However, growing scientific evidence has shown that neuronal nicotinic receptors are still a key target for the development of new drugs having beneficial properties for AD. For example, Huperzine A, another inhibitor of AChE, was shown to be a well-tolerated drug that improved cognitive performance in patients, had a longer effect and higher therapeutic index than tacrine and donepezil, and the peripherical cholinergic side effects were minimal (Bai et al., 2000; Wang et al., 2009).

The importance of nAChRs in the physiopathology of AD is reinforced by evidence that suggests that nicotine prevents amyloid formation, and in primary neuronal cultures, it prevented the toxicity of Aβ and other toxic agents (Salomon et al., 1996; Liu & Zhao, 2004; Yu et al., 2011; Posadas et al., 2013). The mechanism for this effect seems to require activation of the PI3K/AKT pathway and the enhancement of anti-apoptotic proteins Bcl-2 and Bcl-x (Kihara et al., 2001; Buckingham et al., 2009; Yu et al., 2011; Posadas et al., 2013), as has been recently shown with the use of new alkaloids isolated from plants (Araya et al., 2014). All of these findings allow to re-validate nAChRs and cholinergic transmission as important targets for modulating the toxicity in AD (Figure 1), and this leads to the challenge of finding novel molecules to become the leaders in the development of new drugs with better selectivity and potency (Fuentealba et al., 2004; Posadas et al., 2013).

4. Calcium Channels and Other Calcium Sources As Potential Targets to Treat AD

Calcium is the main intracellular messenger that mediates responses to neurotransmitter release at the synapses and activation of postsynaptic receptors, controls key intracellular processes, modulates mitochondrial function and pro- and anti-apoptotic pathways, and mainly controls neurotransmission and synaptic functions such as vesicle transport and release (Green & LaFerla, 2008).

Several neurodegenerative diseases, such as Parkinson's disease and Alzheimer's disease, have been related to the dysregulation of intracellular calcium homeostasis (Bezprozvanny & Mattson, 2008; Bezprozvanny, 2009). Therefore, modulation of the main extracellular Ca+2 source, calcium channels, have been widely studied to determine their role in the neuroprotective effect on neurons under pathophysiological conditions (Demuro et al., 2010; Camandola & Mattson, 2011).

Intracellular Ca^{+2} is mainly regulated by the endoplasmic reticulum, mitochondria, and cytosolic proteins; then, intracellular dyshomeostasis suggests also an organelles dysfunction. It has been found that the pores formed by Aβ oligomers lead to calcium influx in a concentration gradient manner (Valincius et al., 2008; Diaz et al., 2009).

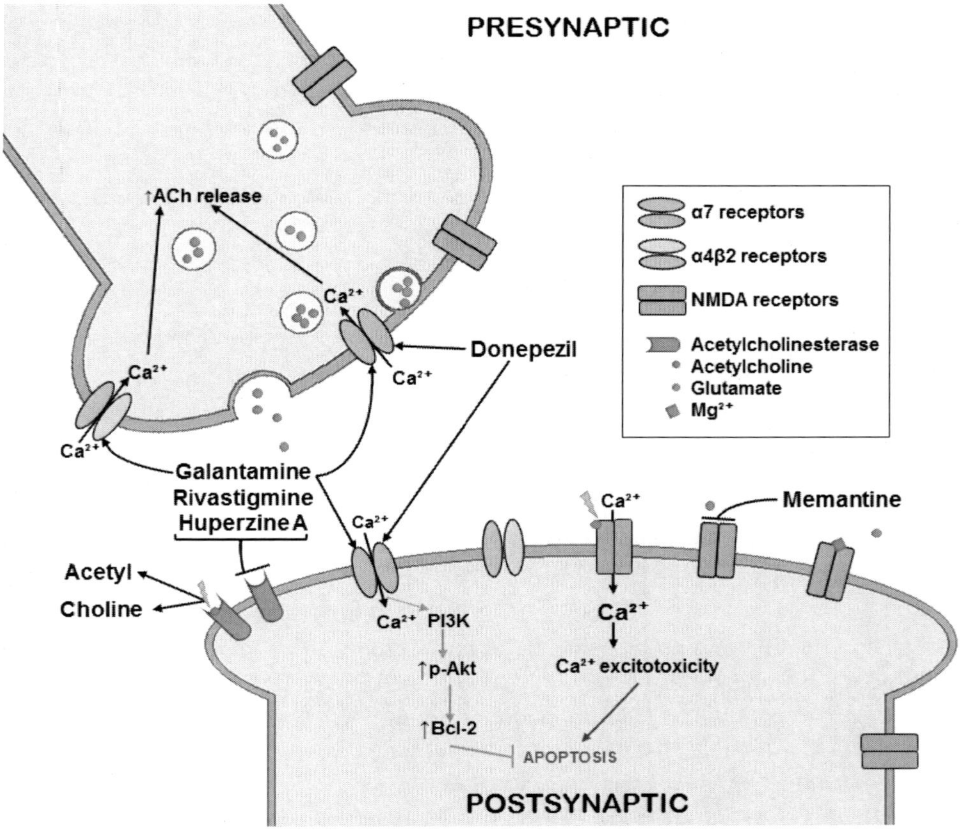

Figure 1. Schematic representation of a neuronal synapse and pharmacological modulation sites. Neuronal synapses have several susceptible areas to be modulated. The inhibition of Acetylcholinesterase (1) by galantamine, rivastigmine and huperizine A. The modulation of nicotinic Acetylcholine receptors α7 by donepezil (2), with the additional activation of the survival pathways (PI3K/Akt, (3)). Finally, the modulation of NMDAR by memantine (4).

It has also been demonstrated that Aβ induces a sustained mitochondrial Ca^{+2} overload (Sanz-Blasco et al., 2008), promoting the opening of mitochondrial transition pores, which induces a loss of mitochondrial membrane potential, inhibition of ATP production, release of cytochrome C and activation of apoptotic pathways (Celsi et al., 2009; Du et al., 2010; Camandola & Mattson, 2011; Rao et al., 2014). Therefore, modulation of Ca^{+2} influx into the cytosol seems to be important. For example, the effect of bexarotene, an anticancer drug, which possesses the same binding domain with Aβ 1-42 and Aβ 25-35 oligomers as cholesterol and inhibits the binding of Aβ to cell membranes was found to decrease the Ca^{+2} influx (Cramer et al., 2012). Estradiol, cholesterol and other substances have also been shown to decrease the concentration of intracellular calcium induced by Aβ (Green & LaFerla, 2008; Demuro et al., 2010). The previous examples are just some of the several studies that have been done to block the massive influx of calcium and the toxic consequences to the cell.

In parallel, a classical blocker of voltage dependent calcium channels (VDCC), dihydropyridine, commonly used in hypertension, angina and arrhythmia, decreases the risk of suffering Parkinson´s disease by 26-30% (Lee et al., 2014). Furthermore, it has been described that blockade of type L voltage-dependent channels using nimodipine, for instance, attenuates Aβ toxicity, but this drug does not decrease the concentration of radicals produced by Aβ. Also dihydropyridines, like israpidine, have been used in AD models as calcium channel modulators, and was found to render neuroprotection (Pasternak et al., 2012). No promissory advances in the development of new calcium modulators as approved drugs have been observed in the last years, suggesting that calcium dysregulation in AD could be a late event that is unable to reverse the condition, despite the interesting in vitro results reported in the literature.

5. NMDA Receptors and Neurodegenerative Disorders

The N-methyl-D-aspartate receptors (NMDARs) are glutamate gated ion channels that constitute a major class of receptors in the mammalian brain (Paoletti & Neyton 2007). They are localized in the postsynaptic membrane of excitatory synapses, and underlie a variety of functions in the CNS, including neuronal differentiation and synapse consolidation, activity dependent forms of synaptic plasticity, and long-term potentiation (Hynd et al., 2004). These receptors are heterotetramers consisting of two obligatory GluN1 subunits and two of four possible GluN2 subunits: GluN2A, GluN2B, GluN2C, and GluN2D; or a GluN2 and GluN3A or GluN3B. The GluN2 subunits present in the adult hippocampus and cortex are usually GluN2A and GluN2B, and the ratio of GluN2B to GluN2A decreases with age in diverse animal species (including humans), starting from or before the onset of sexual maturity (Li & Tsien 2009). NMDAR subunits share a common membrane topology characterized by a large extracellular N-terminus, a membrane region comprising three transmembrane segments (TM1, 3 and 4) plus a re-entrant pore loop (M2), an extracellular loop between TM3 and TM4, and a cytoplasmic C-terminus, which varies in size depending upon the subunit and provides multiple sites of interaction with numerous intracellular proteins (Paoletti & Neyton 2007).

This ion channel is subject to a voltage-dependent blockade by Mg^{+2} whose liberation by depolarizing potentials gives the receptor the capacity to act as a molecular "coincidence" detector, allowing ion flow only when pre and postsynaptic cells are excited in unison (Paoletti et al., 2013). In addition, the initial activation of NMDARs requires the presence not only of glutamate, but also of the co-agonists glycine or d-serine (Cull-Candy & Leszkiewicz 2004). The Mg^{2+} blockade and the high Ca^{2+} permeability of these channels are all influenced by their subunit composition. For example, di-heteromeric GluN2A or GluN2B containing receptors generate 'high-conductance' channel openings (main conductance of ~50 pS) with high sensitivity to Mg^{+2} blockade (half-maximal inhibitory concentration (IC50) of ~15 μM at –70 mV) and Ca^{+2} permeability (pCa/pCs of ~7.5). By contrast, GluN2C or GluN2D containing di-heteromeric receptors have lower conductances (37 pS), sensitivity to Mg^{+2} (IC50 of 80 μM) and Ca^{+2} permeability (pCa/pCs of 4.5) (Paoletti et al., 2013).

Under chronic and pathological conditions, persistent depolarization of the neuronal cell membrane releases the Mg^{+2} blockade on NMDARs leading to increased amounts of intracellular $Ca^{+2.}$ This excessive activation can lead to the excitotoxic necrosis of both cortical and subcortical neurons, a phenomenon commonly known as "excitotoxicity" (Hynd et al., 2004). NMDAR dysfunction, which may cause hyperactivity or hypofunction, is expressed either as altered subunit expression, trafficking, localization or activity, and it can contribute to numerous neurological and psychiatric conditions (Paoletti et al., 2013). This excitotoxic damage occurs in neurodegenerative disorders like Alzheimer's disease (in which glutamate excitotoxicity is one of the contributing factors for neuronal death), cerebral ischemia (dying neurons at the core release glutamate to overstimulate the neurons nearby), Parkinson's and Huntington's disease (in which compromised neurons are sensitized to glutamate excitotoxicity, though excess of glutamate is not seen) (Sonkusare et al., 2005), and probably epilepsy (Cuevas et al., 2011), among others.

6. The Role of NMDA and NMDAR's in AD: Synaptic Function and Neuronal Plasticity

Neuropathological and neurochemical studies of the AD brain have shown that degeneration of glutamate mediated pathways occurs early in the disease and in a pattern that corresponds with the distribution of plaques and tangles (Hynd et al., 2004). Additionally, activation of GluN2B containing NMDARs mediates the alterations induced by Aβ in synaptic plasticity and synapse loss (Paoletti et al., 2013). The activation of extrasynaptic NMDARs enhances the production of Aβ and thus the aberrant activation of extrasynaptic GluN2B-containing NMDARs is probably mediated by an Aβ-induced deficit in glutamate uptake by excitatory amino acid transporters (EAATs), which also leads to impaired long-term potentiation (LTP) and facilitated induction of long-term depression (LTD) (Paoletti et al., 2013). All neurons in the CNS carry the NMDA subtype of ionotropic-glutamate receptors, which are able to mediate post-synaptic Ca^{+2} influx. The excitotoxicity resulting from excessive activation of NMDA receptors may enhance the vulnerability of neurons in a manner consistent with AD neuropathology, which may be a consequence of an altered regional distribution of NMDA receptor subtypes (Hynd et al., 2004).

7. NMDAR's as Potential Therapeutic Targets

NMDARs have always triggered an intense interest as potential therapeutic drug targets because they are involved in many brain disorders (Paoletti & Neyton 2007). So far, there is one approved drug currently in use that affects NMDARs, Memantine, which acts as a non–competitive inhibitor of NMDARs and affects the pathological but not the physiological functions of these receptors, and in addition, it has antioxidant action and enhances the production of brain-derived neurotrophic factor (BDNF). However, Memantine has side effects (hallucinations, confusion, dizziness, gastrointestinal problems, among others) that have led to restrictions on the use of this drug in AD patients (Sonkusare et al., 2005). Another drug that is currently under study is dizolcipine (MK801), which is a strong non-competitive antagonist that prevents neurodegeneration in various pathological conditions. Nevertheless, the use of MK801 has been limited to animal and tissue experiments since it exhibited psychotropic effects in pre-clinical trials (Hynd et al., 2004).

Previous to these studies, there were many other searches for NMDAR antagonists, but these first generation compounds failed because they were unable to discriminate between the different subunits. Nowadays, there are compounds that selectively inhibit NMDARs that contain GluN2B subunits which have shown high neuroprotective potential and have been used as pain killers in various animal models. Furthermore, they have a higher tolerance because they do not inhibit NMDARs that do not contain GluN2B subunits (Paoletti & Neyton 2007). Taken together, NMDARs are still an important target for the development of new molecules with higher selectivity that could avoid ADRs and contribute to the recovery of neuronal function.

8. P2X Receptors As Possible Drug Targets in AD

A novel therapeutic target for AD and other neurodegenerative diseases could be the P2X receptors (P2XRs). These receptors are activated by ATP and form trimeric ion channels that mediate cation flux (Manago et al., 2005) and are made up of 7 different subunits (P2X1-7) that can form homo or heterotrimers (Khakh & North 2012). These receptors are expressed in neuron and glial cells and have different roles such as neurotransmission and trophic actions (Volonté, Amadio et al. 2003). Recently they have been related to injury, metabolism impairment, excitotoxicity and neurodegeneration (Apolloni et al., 2009), mostly because ATP may leave cells through their plasma membranes damaged by mechanical injury and inflammation (Lazarowski et al., 2000; Franke et al., 2006).

P2XRs are expressed in glial cells, and in presynaptic and postsynaptic neuron membranes where they have been shown to modulate the synapsis (North, 2002). Particularly, the P2X2 receptor is widely expressed in different regions of the CNS like cortex, cerebellum, hypothalamus, striatum and hippocampus; and it has a wide range of functions in the regulation of neuronal processes such as memory and learning (Apolloni et al., 2009), both impaired in AD.

ATP acts as a neurotransmitter and neuromodulator. For example, presynaptic P2XRs facilitate the release of GABA (Vavra et al., 2011), glutamate (Cho et al., 2010), and dopamine (Choi et al., 2009) in several brain areas including the hippocampus.

At the postsynaptic level, P2XRs can modulate the insertion of AMPARs in the hippocampus (Sim et al., 2006; Baxter et al., 2011; Pougnet et al., 2014), and they can also directly inhibit GABARs promoting excitability of neuronal networks (Boué-Grabot et al., 2003; Boué-Grabot et al., 2004; Boué-Grabot et al., 2004), as well as participate in the integration with astrocytes and modulate the function of the synapse as a whole (Gordon et al., 2005; Gordon et al., 2009; Poskanzer & Yuste 2011; Khakh & North, 2012) (see Figure 2 for more detail).

Therefore, this type of receptor can modify or amplify the pathophysiological effects (Apolloni et al., 2009) of certain conditions such as AD. The release of ATP from injury or deregulation can transform P2XRs into important actors in neuropathological conditions; therefore, it is important to identify the correct tools for effective pharmacological approaches (Burnstock, 2008).

On the other hand, it has been described that hyperactive microglia are crucial for the pathogenesis of several neurodegenerative disorders like AD, and activated glia is one of the major sources for extracellular ATP that acts as a cell death mediator (Nakajima & Kohsaka, 1993; Amadio et al., 2002; Koles et al., 2005).

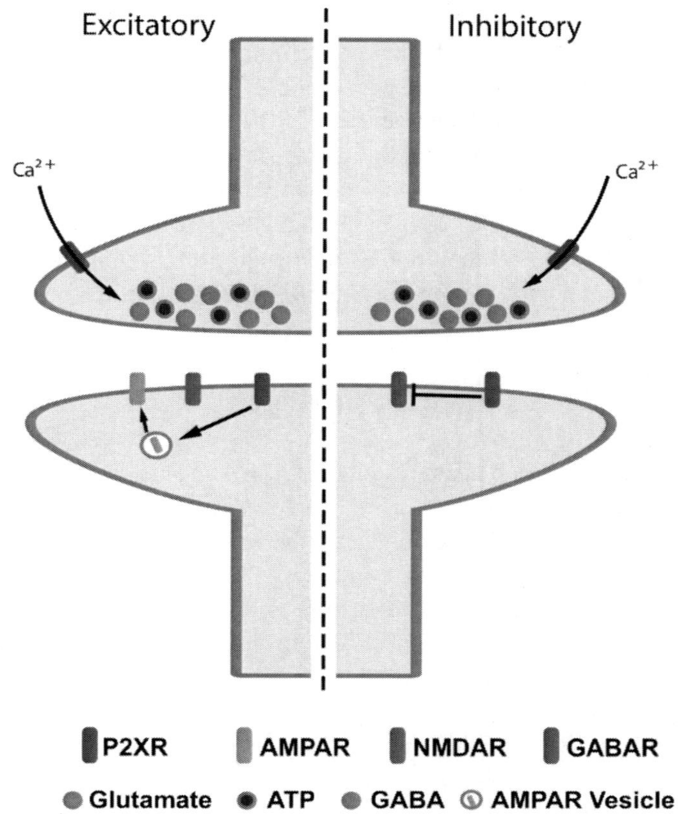

Figure 2. Pathophysiological roles of P2XR in AD. Due to their normal physiological role as neuromodulators, P2XRs can participate in neurodegenerative processes such as AD. At excitatory and inhibitory presynapses, P2XR activation increases Ca^{2+} concentration facilitating neurotransmitter release; and in the case of glutamatergic synapses this provokes a positive feedback loop in excitotoxicity increasing this effect. Also, P2XR activation can modulate the insertion of AMPAR at excitatory postsynapses promoting an increase in the release of neurotransmitters in postsynaptic neurons. In parallel, P2XR can directly inhibit GABAR at inhibitory postsynaptic neurons increasing the excitability of these neurons.

Several studies suggest that P2X7 receptors contribute to neurodegenerative processes observed in the CNS, including multiple sclerosis, Huntington's disease, PD and AD. Importantly, an up-regulation of these receptors has been reported in animal models and patients with neurodegenerative diseases (Kaczmarek-Hájek et al., 2012). It has been demonstrated that P2X7Rs enhance their expression in microglia around Aβ plaques in a mouse model of AD, in microglia from brains of patients with this disease, in cultured fetal human microglia treated with Aβ and in rat hippocampus injected with the peptide (Parvathenani et al., 2003; McLarnon et al., 2006). The expression of P2X7R in microglia can be induced by Aβ very early in the onset of AD which may induce excessive production of ROS (Lee et al., 2010), and it has been demonstrated that P2X7R participates in the activation of microglia and other effects induced by the Aβ peptide (Sanz et al., 2009) such as the stimulation of the release of ATP that activates NADPH oxidase and the subsequent ROS production from microglia, and the modulation of cytokine secretion from macrophages and microglia (Parvathenani et al., 2003; Rampe et al., 2004; Apolloni et al., 2009). Moreover, a specific P2X7R antagonist, brilliant blue G, confers a significant degree of neuroprotection in an animal model of AD, probably by reducing the inflammation mediated by the microglia that indirectly protects the neurons (Ryu & McLarnon, 2008).

All this evidence leads to the conclusion that P2X7Rs play a key role in the inflammatory response by microglia in AD brains, and antagonists for this receptor could be a possible treatment to reduce the inflammatory processes that occur in AD, and consequently, protect neurons. Therefore, it is important to advance in the study of these receptors, and with new and more effective tools that are continuously created, achieve an understanding of the underlying mechanism and potential drugs to treat this disease.

Conclusion

The etiology of Alzheimer's disease is still unknown and represents the most important barrier to finding an adequate therapy. The lack of specific predictors like an efficient biomarker raises the difficulty in establishing early therapy and treatment. Therefore, the most important tools for discovering efficient therapies appear to be drug development to modulate these new targets, which could be used safely and with a low incidence of ADRs. Accordingly, recent evidence shows that P2XRs, which have been related to several neurodegenerative diseases and have been the focus of a great amount of research, show promissory results in animal models providing an additional paradigm to attack the pathology. Hence, new purinergic drugs with high selectivity, efficacy and potency will be required to define the ideal purinergic modulator.

References

Amadio, S., D'Ambrosi, N., Cavaliere, F., Murra, B., Sancesario, G., Bernardi, G., Burnstock, G. & Volonté, C. (2002) P2 receptor modulation and cytotoxic function in cultured CNS neurons. *Neuropharmacology*, 42, 489-501.

Apolloni, S., Montilli, C., Finocchi, P. & Amadio, S. (2009) Membrane compartments and purinergic signalling: P2X receptors in neurodegenerative and neuroinflammatory events. *FEBS J.*, 276, 354-364.

Araya, J.A., Ramírez, AE., Figueroa-Araca, D., Sotes, G.J., Pérez, C., Becerra, J., Sáez-Orellana, F., Guzmán, L., Aguayo, L.G. & Fuentealba, J. (2014) Modulation of neuronal nicotinic receptor by quinolizidine alkaloids causes neuroprotection on a cellular Alzheimer model. *J. Alz. Dis.*, 42, 143-155.

Bai, D., Tang, X.C. & Él, X.C. (2000) Huperzine A, a potential therapeutic agent for treatment of Alzheimer's disease. Curr. Med. Chem., 7, 355-374.

Ballard, C. Gauthiers, S., Corbett, A., Brayne, C., Aarsland, D & Jones, E. (2011) Alzheimer's disease. *Lancet,* 377, 9770.

Barnham, K.J. & Bush, A.I. (2008) Metals in Alzheimer's and Parkinson's diseases. *Curr. Op. Chem. Biol.*, 12, 222-228.

Baxter, A.W., Choi, S.J., Sim, J.A. & Norte, R.A. (2011) Role of P2X4 receptors in synaptic strengthening in mouse CA1 hippocampal neurons. *Eur. J. Neurosci.*, 34, 213-220.

Bertram, L., Lill, C.M. & Tanzi, R.E. (2010) The genetics of Alzheimer disease: back to the future. *Neuron*, 68, 270-281.

Bezprozvanny, I. (2009) Calcium signaling and neurodegenerative diseases. *Trends Mol. Med.*, 15, 89-100.

Bezprozvanny, I. & Mattson, M.P. (2008) Neuronal calcium mishandling and the pathogenesis of Alzheimer's disease. *TINS,* 31, 454-463.

Birks, J. & Harvey R. (2003) Donepezil for dementia due to Alzheimer's disease. The Cochrane Library.

Boué-Grabot, É., Barajas- López, C., Chakfe, Y., Blais, D., Bélanger, D., Emerit, M. B. & Séquéla, P. (2003) Intracellular cross talk and physical interaction between two classes of neurotransmitter-gated channels. *J. Neurosci.,* 23, 1246-1253.

Boué-Grabot, É., Emerit, M.B., Toulme, E., Séquéla, P. & Garret, M. (2004) Cross-talk and co-trafficking between ρ1/GABA receptors and ATP-gated channels. *J. Biol. Chem.*, 279, 6967-6975.

Boué-Grabot, É., Toulme, E. Emerit, M.B. & Garret, M. (2004) Subunit-specific coupling between γ-aminobutyric acid type A and P2X2 receptor channels. *J. Biol. Chem.*, 279, 52517-52525.

Bowling, A. & Dieppe, P. (2005) What is successful ageing and who should define it?. BMJ, 331, 1548-1551.

Buckingham, S.D., Jones, A.K., Marrón, L.A. & Sattelle, D.B. (2009) Nicotinic acetylcholine receptor signalling: roles in Alzheimer's disease and amyloid neuroprotection. *Pharmacol. Rev.*, 61, 39-61.

Burns, A. & Iliffe, S. (2009) Dementia. BMJ, 338, b75.

Burnstock, G. (2008) Purinergic signalling and disorders of the central nervous system. *Nat. Rev. Drug Disc.*, 7, 575-590.

Bush, A.I. & Tanzi, R.E. (2008) Therapeutics for Alzheimer's disease based on the metal hypothesis. *Neurotherapeutics,* 5, 421-432.

Camandola, S. & Mattson, M.P. (2011) Aberrant subcellular neuronal calcium regulation in aging and Alzheimer's disease. *Biochim. Bioph. Acta Mol.* Cell Res., 1813, 965-973.

Carlo, M.D. (2010) b amyloid peptide: from different aggregation forms to the activation of different biochemical pathways. *Eur. Bioph. J.,* 39, 877-888.

Castellani, R.J., Roston, R.K. & Smith, M.A. (2010) Alzheimer disease. Disease-a-month: DM, 56, 484.

Celsi, F., Pizzo, P., Brini, M., Leo, S., Fotino, C., Pinton, P. & Rizzuto, R. (2009) Mitochondria, calcium and cell death: A deadly triad in neurodegeneration. *Biochim. Bioph. Acta Bioenergetics*, 1787, 335-344.

Corey-Bloom, J. (2003) Galantamine: a review of its use in Alzheimer's disease and vascular dementia. *Int. J. Clin. Prac.,* 57, 219-223.

Craig, L.A., Hong, N.S. & McDonald, R.J. (2011) Revisiting the cholinergic hypothesis in the development of Alzheimer's disease. Neuroscience *Biobeh. Rev.,* 35, 1397-1409.

Cramer, P.E., Cirrito, J.R., Wesson, D.W., Lee, C.Y., Karlo, J.C., Zinn, A.E., Casali, B.T., Restivo, J.L., Goebel, W.D., James, M.J., Brunder, K.R., Wilson, D.A. & Landreth, G.E. (2012) ApoE-directed therapeutics rapidly clear β-amyloid and reverse deficits in AD mouse models. *Science,* 335, 1503-1506.

Cruts, M., Theuns, J. & Van Broeckhoven, C. (2012) Locus-specific mutation databases for neurodegenerative brain diseases. *Hum. Mut.*, 33, 1340-1344.

Cruts, M. & Van Broeckhoven, C. (1998) Molecular genetics of Alzheimer's disease. *Ann. Med.*, 30, 560-565.

Cuevas, M.E., Haensger, H., Sepúlveda, F.J., Zegers, G., Roa, J., Opazo, C. & Aguayo, L.G. (2011) Soluble Abeta(1-40) peptide increases excitatory neurotransmission and induces epileptiform activity in hippocampal neurons. *J. Alz. Dis.*, 23, 673-687.

Cull-Candy, S.G. & Leszkiewicz, D.N. (2004) Role of distinct NMDA receptor subtypes at central synapses. *Sci STKE*, 2004, re16.

Cho, J.H., Choi, E.S. & Jang, E.S. (2010) P2X7 receptors enhance glutamate release in hippocampal hilar neurons. *Neuroreport,* 21, 865-870.

Choi, Y. M., Jang, J.Y., Jang, M., Kim, S.H., Kang, Y.K., Cho, H., Chung, S. & Parque, M.K. (2009) Modulation of firing activity by ATP in dopamine neurons of the rat *substantia nigra pars compacta*. *Neuroscience,* 160, 587-595.

D'Andrea, M.R. & Nagele, R.G. (2006) Targeting the alpha 7 nicotinic acetylcholine receptor to reduce amyloid accumulation in Alzheimer's disease pyramidal neurons. *Curr. Pharm. Des.*, 12, 677-684.

D'Errico, G., Vitiello, G., Ortona, O., Tedeschi, A., Ramunno, A. & D´Ursi, A.M. (2008) Interaction between Alzheimer's Ab_{25-35} peptide and phospholipid bilayers: The role of cholesterol. *Biochim. Bioph. Acta Biomembranes,* 1778, 2710-2716.

Dajas-Bailador, F. & Wonnacott, S. (2004) Nicotinic acetylcholine receptors and the regulation of neuronal signalling. *Trends Pharm. Sci.*, 25, 317-324.

DaRocha-Souto, B., Scotton, T.C., Coma, M., Serrano-Pozo, A., Hashimoto, T., Serenó, L., Rodríguez, M., Sánchez, B., Hyman, B.T. & Gómez-Isla, T. (2011) Brain oligomeric β-amyloid but not total amyloid plaque burden correlates with neuronal loss and astrocyte inflammatory response in amyloid precursor protein/tau transgenic mice. *J. Neuropathol. Exp. Neurol.,* 70, 360-376.

De Ferrari, G.V., Papassotiropoulos, A., Biechele, T., Wavrant De-Vrieze, F., Ávila, M.E., Major, M.B., Myers, A., Sáez, K., Henríquez, J.P., Zhao, A., Wollmer, M.A., Nitsch, R.M., Morris, C.M., Hardy, J. & Luna, R.T. (2007) Common genetic variation within the low-density lipoprotein receptor-related protein 6 and late-onset Alzheimer's disease. *Proc. Nat. Acad. Sci.,* 104, 9434-9439.

Decker, H., Jürgensen, S., Adrover, M.F., Brito-Moreira, J., Bomfim, T.R., Klein, W.L., Epstein, A.L., De Felice, F.G., Jerusalinsky, D. & Ferreira, S.T. (2010) N-Methyl-D-aspartate receptors are required for synaptic targeting of Alzheimer's toxic amyloid-β peptide oligomers. *J. Neurochem.,* 115, 1520-1529.

Demuro, A., Parker, I. & Stutzmann, G.E. (2010) Calcium Signaling and Amyloid Toxicity in Alzheimer Disease. *J. Biol. Chem.,* 285, 12463-12468.

Diaz, J. C., Simakova, O., Jacobson, K.A., Arispe, N. & Pollard, H.B. (2009) Small molecule blockers of the Alzheimer Ab calcium channel potently protect neurons from Ab cytotoxicity. *Proc. Nat. Acad. Sci.*, 106, 3348-3353.

Drisdel, R.C. & Green, W.N. (2000) Neuronal α-bungarotoxin receptors are α7 subunit homomers. *J. Neurosci.,* 20, 133-139.

Du, H., Guo, L., Yan, S., Sosunov, A.A., McKhann, G.M. & Yan, S.S. (2010) Early deficits in synaptic mitochondria in an Alzheimer's disease mouse model. *Proc. Nat. Acad. Sci.,* 107, 18670-18675.

Ferri, C.P., Prince, M., Brayne, C., Brodaty, H., Fratiglioni, L., Ganguli, M., Hall, K., Hasegawa, K., Hendrie, H., Huang, Y., Jorm, A., Mathers, C., Menezes, P.R., Rimmer, E.

& Scazufca, M. (2005) Global prevalence of dementia: a Delphi consensus study. *Lancet*, 366, 2112-2117.

Franke, H., Krügel, U. & Illes, P. (2006) P2 receptors and neuronal injury. *Pflügers Arch.*, 452, 622-644.

Fuentealba, J., Olivares, R., Alés, E., Tapia, L., Rojo, J., Arroyo, G., Aldea, M., Criado, M., Gandía, L. & García, A.G. (2004) A choline-evoked [Ca2+] c signal causes catecholamine release and hyperpolarization of chromaffin cells. *FASEB J.*, 18, 1468-1470.

Glenner, G.G., Wong, C.W., Quaranta, V., Eanes, E.D. (1984) The amyloid deposits in Alzheimer's disease: their nature and pathogenesis. *Appl. Pathol.*, 2, 357-369.

Gordon, G.R., Baimoukhametova, D.V., Hewitt, S.A., Rajapaksha, W.R., Fisher, T.E. & Bains, J.S. (2005) Norepinephrine triggers release of glial ATP to increase postsynaptic efficacy. *Nat. Neurosci.*, 8, 1078-1086.

Gordon, G.R., Iremonger, K.J., Kantevari, S., Ellis-Davies, G.C., MacVicar, B.A. & Bains, J.S. (2009) Astrocyte-Mediated Distributed Plasticity at Hypothalamic Glutamate Synapses. *Neuron*, 64, 391-403.

Gotti, C. & Clementi, F. (2004) Neuronal nicotinic receptors: from structure to pathology. *Prog. Neurobiol.*, 74, 363-396.

Green, K.N. & LaFerla, F.M. (2008) Linking calcium to Ab and Alzheimer's disease. *Neuron,* 59, 190-194.

Haass, C. & Selkoe, D.J. (2007) Soluble protein oligomers in neurodegeneration: lessons from the Alzheimer's amyloid β-peptide. *Nat. Rev. Mol. Cell Biol.*, 8, 101-112.

Hardy, J. & Mullan, M. (1992) Alzheimer's disease. In search of the soluble. *Nature,* 359, 268-269.

Hebert, L.E., Weuve, J., Scherr, P.A. & Evans, D.A. (2013) Alzheimer disease in the United States (2010–2050) estimated using the 2010 census. *Neurology*, 80, 1778-1783.

Hynd, M.R., Scott, H.L. & Dodd, P.R. (2004) Glutamate-mediated excitotoxicity and neurodegeneration in Alzheimer's disease. *Neurochem.* Int., 45, 583-595.

INE (2006). Demografía, Ganancia en años de vida y riesgo de muerte. Chile. Enfoque estadístico, Instituto Nacional de Estadisticas de Chile.

Itier, V. & Bertrand, D. (2001) Neuronal nicotinic receptors: from protein structure to function. *FEBS Letters*, 504, 118-125.

Jann, M.W. (2000) Rivastigmine, a new-generation cholinesterase inhibitor for the treatment of Alzheimer's disease. *J. Hum. Pharmacol. Drug Ther.*, 20, 1-12.

Jensen, A.A., Frølund, B., Liljefors, T., Krogsgaard-Larsen, P. (2005) Neuronal nicotinic acetylcholine receptors: structural revelations, target identifications, and therapeutic inspirations. *J. Med. Chem.*, 48(15), 4705-4745.

Jones, L., Holmans, P.A., Hamshere, M.L., Harold, D., Moskvina, V., Ivanov, D., Pocklington, A., et. al. (2010) Genetic evidence implicates the immune system and cholesterol metabolism in the aetiology of Alzheimer's disease. *PLOS one*, 5, e13950.

Kaczmarek-Hájek, K., Lörinczi, E., Hausmann, R. & Nicke, A. (2012) Molecular and functional properties of P2X receptors—recent progress and persisting challenges. *Purinergic signall.*, 8, 375-417.

Kawahara, M., Ohtsuka, I., Yokoyama, S., Kato-Negishi, M. & Sadakane, Y. (2011) Membrane incorporation, channel formation, and disruption of calcium homeostasis by Alzheimer-b-amyloid protein. *Int. J. Alz. Dis.,* 2011.

Khakh, B. S. & North, R.A. (2012) Neuromodulation by extracellular ATP and P2X receptors in the CNS. *Neuron*, 76, 51-69.

Kihara, T., Shimohama, S., Sawada, H., Honda, K., Nakamizo, T., Shibasaki, H., Kume, T. & Akaike, A. (2001) α7 nicotinic receptor transduces signals to phosphatidylinositol 3-kinase to block A β-amyloid-induced neurotoxicity. *J. Biol. Chem.,* 276, 13541-13546.

Koles, L., Furst, S. & Illes, P. (2005) P2X and P2Y receptors as possible targets of therapeutic manipulations in CNS illnesses. *Drug News* Perspect., 18, 85.

Lacor, P. N., Buniel, M.C., Chang, L., Fernandez, S.J., Gong, Y., Viola, K.L., Lambert, M.P., Velasco, P.T., Bigio, E.H., Finch, C.E., Krafft, G.A. & Klein, W.L. (2004) Synaptic targeting by Alzheimer's-related amyloid β oligomers. *J. Neurosci.,* 24, 10191-10200.

Lazarowski, E.R., Boucher, R.C. & Harden, T.K. (2000) Constitutive release of ATP and evidence for major contribution of ecto-nucleotide pyrophosphatase and nucleoside diphosphokinase to extracellular nucleotide concentrations. *J. Biol. Chem.*, 275, 31061-31068.

Lee, H.G., Won, S.M., Gwag, B.J. & Lee, Y.B. (2010) Microglial P2X7 receptor expression is accompanied by neuronal damage in the cerebral cortex of the APPswe/PS1dE9 mouse model of Alzheimer's disease. *Exp. Mol. Med.*, 43, 7-14.

Lee, Y.C., Lin, C.H., Wu, R.M., Lin, J.W., Chang, C.H. & Lai, M.S. (2014) Antihypertensive agents and risk of Parkinson's disease: A nationwide cohort study. *PLOS one*, 9, e98961.

Lesné, S., Kotilinek, L. & Ashe, K.H. (2008) Plaque-bearing mice with reduced levels of oligomeric amyloid-β assemblies have intact memory function. *Neuroscience,* 151, 745-749.

Lesné, S., Koh, M.T., Kotilinek, L., Kayed, R., Glabe, C.G., Yang, A., Gallagher, M. & Ashe, K.H. (2006) A specific amyloid-b protein assembly in the brain impairs memory. *Nat. Lett.*, 440, 352-357.

Li, F. & Tsien, J.Z. (2009) Memory and the NMDA receptors. *N. Engl. J.* Med., 361, 302-303.

Liu, Q. & Zhao, B. (2004) Nicotine attenuates β-amyloid peptide-induced neurotoxicity, free radical and calcium accumulation in hippocampal neuronal cultures. *Brit. J. Pharmacol.*, 141, 746-754.

Manago, Y., Kanahori, Y., Shimada, A., Sato, A., Amano, T., Sato-Sano, Y., Setsuie, R., Sakurai, M., Aoki, S., Wang, Y.L., Osaka, H., Wada, K. & Noda, M. (2005) Potentiation of ATP-induced currents due to the activation of P2X receptors by ubiquitin carboxy-terminal hydrolase L1. *J. Neurochem.*, 92, 1061-1072.

McLarnon, J. G., Ryu, J.K., Walker, D.G. & Choi, H.B. (2006) Upregulated expression of purinergic p2x7 receptor in Alzheimer disease and amyloid-β peptide-treated microglia and in peptide-injected rat hippocampus. J. Neuropathol. *Exper. Neurol.*, 65, 1090-1097

Millar, N.S. & Gotti, C. (2009) Diversity of vertebrate nicotinic acetylcholine receptors. *Neuropharmacology,* 56, 237-246.

Muller, M., Sigurdsson, S., Kjartansson, O., Jonsson, P.V., Garcia, M., Von Bonsdorff, M.B., Gunnarsdottir, I., Thorsdottir, I., Harris, T.B., Van Buchem, M., Gudnason, V. & Launer, L.J. (2014) Birth size and brain function 75 years later. *Pediatrics,* 134, 761-770.

Nakajima, K. & Kohsaka, S. (1993) Functional roles of microglia in the brain. *Neurosci. Res.,* 17, 187-203.

Nordberg, A. (2001) Nicotinic receptor abnormalities of Alzheimer's disease: therapeutic implications. *Biol. Psych.*, 49, 200-210.

North, R.A. (2002) Molecular physiology of P2X receptors. *Physiol. Rev.*, 82, 1013-1067.

Orr-Urtreger, A., Göldner, F.M., Saeki, M., Lorenzo, I., Goldberg, L., De Biasi, M., Dani, J.A., Patrick, J.W. & Beaudet, A.L. (1997) Mice deficient in the α7 neuronal nicotinic acetylcholine receptor lack α-bungarotoxin binding sites and hippocampal fast nicotinic currents. *J. Neurosci.*, 17, 9165-9171.

Palop, J.J. & Mucke, L. (2010) Amyloid-b-induced neuronal dysfunction in Alzheimer's disease: from synapses toward neural networks. *Nat. Neurosci.,* 13, 812-818.

Paoletti, P., Bellone, C. & Zhou, Q. (2013) NMDA receptor subunit diversity: impact on receptor properties, synaptic plasticity and disease. *Nat. Rev. Neurosci.,* 14, 383-400.

Paoletti, P. & Neyton, J. (2007) NMDA receptor subunits: function and pharmacology. *Curr. Op. Pharmacol.*, 7, 39-47.

Parvathenani, L.K., Tertyshnikova, S., Greco, C.R., Roberts, S.B., Robertson, B. & Posmantur, R. (2003) P2X7 mediates superoxide production in primary microglia and is up-regulated in a transgenic mouse model of Alzheimer's disease. *J. Biol. Chem.*, 278, 13309-13317.

Pasternak, B., Svanström, H., Nielsen, N.M., Fugger, L., Melbye, M. & Hviid, A. (2012) Use of calcium channel blockers and Parkinson's disease. *Am. J. Epidemiol.*, 175, 627-635.

Perry, E., Smith, C.J., Court, J.A. & Perry, R.H. (1990) Cholinergic nicotinic and muscarinic receptors in dementia of Alzheimer, Parkinson and Lewy body types. *J. Neural Trans. Parkinson's Dis. Dem. Section*, 2, 149-158.

Picciotto, M. R., Caldarone, B.J., Brunzell, D.H., Zachariou, V., Stevens, T.R. & King, S.L. (2001) Neuronal nicotinic acetylcholine receptor subunit knockout mice: physiological and behavioral phenotypes and possible clinical implications. *Pharmacol. Ther.*, 92, 89-108.

Posadas, I., López-Hernández, B. & Ceña, V. (2013) Nicotinic receptors in neurodegeneration. *Curr. Neuropharmacol.*, 11, 298.

Poskanzer, K.E. & Yuste, R. (2011) Astrocytic regulation of cortical UP states. *Proc. Nat. Acad. Sci.*, 108, 18453-18458.

Pougnet, J.T., Toulme, E., Martinez, A., Choquet, D., Hosy, E. & Boué-Grabot, E. (2014) ATP P2X receptors downregulate AMPA receptor trafficking and postsynaptic efficacy in hippocampal neurons. *Neuron,* 83, 417-430.

Prangkio, P., Yusko, E.C., Sept, D., Yang, J. & Mayer, M. (2012) Multivariate analyses of amyloid-b oligomer populations indicate a connection between pore formation and cytotoxicity. *PLOS one*, 7, e47261.

Prince, M.A. (2014) World Alzheimer report 2014 dementia and risk reduction: an analysis of protective and modificable factors. *Lon. Alz. Dis.* Int., 104.

Rampe, D., Wang, L. & Ringheim, G.E. (2004) P2X7 receptor modulation of β-amyloid-and LPS-induced cytokine secretion from human macrophages and microglia. *J. Neuroimmunol.*, 147, 56-61.

Rao, V. K., Carlson, E.A. & Yan, S.S. (2014) Mitochondrial permeability transition pore is a potential drug target for neurodegeneration. Biochim. *Biophys. Acta Mol. Basis Dis.*, 1842, 1267-1272.

Role, L.W. (1992) Diversity in primary structure and function of neuronal nicotinic acetylcholine receptor channels. *Curr. Op. Neurobiol.*, 2, 254-262.

Rösler, M., Retz, W., Retz-Junginger, P. & Dennler, H.J. (1999) Effects of two-year treatment with the cholinesterase inhibitor rivastigmine on behavioural symptoms in Alzheimer's disease. *Behav. Neurol.*, 11, 211-216.

Ryu, J. K. & McLarnon, J.G. (2008) Block of purinergic P2X7 receptor is neuroprotective in an animal model of Alzheimer's disease. *Neuroreport,* 19, 1715-1719.

Sakurada, T., Alufuzoff, I., Winblad, B. & Nordberg, A. (1990) Substance P-like immunoreactivity, choline acetyltransferase activity and cholinergic muscarinic receptors in Alzheimer's disease and multi-infarct dementia. *Brain Res.*, 521, 329-332.

Salomon, A. R., Marcinowski, K.J., Friedland, R.P. & Zagorski, M.G. (1996) Nicotine inhibits amyloid formation by the β-peptide. *Biochemistry,* 35, 13568-13578.

Sanz-Blasco, S., Valero, R.A., Rodríguez-Crespo, I., Villalobos, C. & Núñez, L. (2008) Mitochondrial Ca^{2+} Overload underlies ab oligomers neurotoxicity providing an unexpected mechanism of neuroprotection by NSAID's. *PLOS one,* 3, 1-16.

Sanz, J. M., Chiozzi, P., Ferrari, D., Colaianna, M., Idzko, M., Falzoni, S., Fellin, R., Trabace, L. & Di Virgilio, F. (2009) Activation of microglia by amyloid β requires P2X7 receptor expression. *J. Immunol.*, 182, 4378-4385.

Selkoe, D.J. (1991) The molecular pathology of Alzheimer's disease. Neuron, 6, 487-498.

Selkoe, D.J. (1994) Alzheimer's disease: a central role for amyloid. *J. Neuropathol. Exp. Neurol*, 53, 438-447.

Selkoe, D.J. (2008) Soluble oligomers of the amyloid b-protein impair synaptic plasticity and behavior. *Behav. Brain Res.*, 192, 106-113.

Shen, H., Kihara, T., Hongo, H., Wu, X., Kem, W.R., Shimohama, S., Akaike, A., Niidome, T. & Sugimoto, H. (2010) Neuroprotection by donepezil against glutamate excitotoxicity involves stimulation of α7 nicotinic receptors and internalization of NMDA receptors. *Br. J. Pharmacol.*, 161,127-139.

Sher, E., Chen, Y., Sharples, T.J., Broad, L.M., Benedetti, G., Zwart, R., McPhie, G.I., Pearson, K.H., Baldwinson, T. & De Filippi, G. (2004) Physiological roles of neuronal nicotinic receptors subtypes: new insights on the nicotinic modulation of neurotransmitter release, synaptic transmission and plasticity. *Curr. Topics Med. Chem.*, 4, 283-297.

Shinotoh, H., Namba, H., Fukushi, K., Nagatsuka, S., Tanaka, N., Aotsuka, A., Ota, T., Tanada, S. & Irie, T. (2000) Progressive loss of cortical acetylcholinesterase activity in association with cognitive decline in Alzheimer's disease: a positron emission tomography study. *Ann. Neurol.*, 48, 194-200.

Sim, J. A., Chaumont, S., Jo, J., Ulmann, L., Young, M.T., Cho, K., Buell, G., North, R.A. & Rassendren, F. (2006) Altered hippocampal synaptic potentiation in P2X4 knock-out mice. *J. Neurosci.*, 26, 9006-9009.

Sokolov, Y., Kozak, J.A., Kayed, R., Chanturiya, A., Glabe, C. & Hall, J.E. (2006) Soluble amyloid oligomers increase bilayer conductance by altering dielectric structure. *J. Gen. Physiol.*, 128(6), 637-647.

Sonkusare, S.K., Kaul, C.L. & Ramarao, P. (2005) Dementia of Alzheimer's disease and other neurodegenerative disorders--memantine, a new hope. *Pharmacol. Res.,* 51(1), 1-17.

Strozyk, D., Launer, L.J., Adlard, P.A., Cherny, R.A., Tsatsanis, A., Volitakis, I., Blennow, K., Petrovitch, H., White, L.R. & Bush, A.I. (2009) Zinc and copper modulate Alzheimer Ab levels in human cerebrospinal fluid. *Neurobiol. Aging,* 30, 1069-1077.

Suh, Y.H. & Checler, F. (2002) Amyloid precursor protein, presenilins, and alpha-synuclein: molecular pathogenesis and pharmacological applications in Alzheimer's disease. *Pharmacol. Rev.,* 54, 469-525.

Thies, W. (2011) Stopping a thief and killer: Alzheimer's disease crisis demands greater commitment to research. *Alz. Dem.*, 7, 175-176.

Thies, W. & Bleiler, L. (2011) 2011 Alzheimer's disease facts and figures. *Alz. Dem.*, 7, 208-244.

Thinakaran, G. & Koo, E.H. (2008) Amyloid precursor protein trafficking, processing, and function. *J. Biol. Chem.*, 283, 29615–29619.

Tomiyama, T., Nagata, T., Shimada, H., Teraoka, R., Fukushima, A., Kanemitsu, H., Takuma, H., Kuwano, R., Imagawa, M., Ataka, S., Wada, Y., Yoshioka, E., Nishizaki, T.,Watanabe, Y. & Mori, H. (2008) A new amyloid beta variant favoring oligomerization in Alzheimer's-type dementia. *Ann. Neurol.*, 63, 377-387.

Töugu, V., Karafin, A. & Palumaa, P. (2008) Binding of zinc(II) and copper(II) to the full-length Alzheimer's amyloid-b peptide. *J. Neurochem.*, 104, 1249-1259.

United-Nations. (2013) World Population Ageing 2013. New York, Department of Economic and Social Affairs Population Division, United Nations, 114.

United-Nations. (2014) Concise Report on the World Population Situation in 2014. New York, Department of Economic and Social Affairs, Population Division United Nations, 35.

Valincius, G., Heinrich, F., Budvytyte, R., Vanderah, D.J., McGillivray, D.J., Sokolov, Y., Hall, J.E. & Lösche, M. (2008) Soluble amyloid b-oligomers affect dielectric membrane properties by bilayer insertion and domain formation: implications for cell toxicity. *Biophys. J.,* 95, 4845-4861.

Vavra, V., Bhattacharya, A. & Zemkova, H. (2011) Facilitation of glutamate and GABA release by P2X receptor activation in supraoptic neurons from freshly isolated rat brain slices. *Neuroscience,* 188, 1-12.

Volonté, C., Apolloni, S., Skaper, S.D. & Burnstock, G. (2003) Extracellular ATP and neurodegeneration. *Curr. Drug Tar. CNS Neurol. Dis*., 2, 403-412.

Walsh, D. M., Klyubin, I., Fadeeva, J.V., Cullen, W.K., Anwyl, R., Wolfe, M.S., Rowan, M.J. & Selkoe, D.J. (2002) Naturally secreted oligomers of amyloid [beta] protein potently inhibit hippocampal long-term potentiation in vivo. *Nature*, 416, 535-539.

Wang, B.S., Wang, H., Wei, Z.H., Song, Y.Y., Zhang, L. & Chen, H.Z. (2009) Efficacy and safety of natural acetylcholinesterase inhibitor huperzine A in the treatment of Alzheimer's disease: an updated meta-analysis. *J. Neural Transm.,* 116, 457-465.

Wang, H.W., Pasternak, J.F., Kuo, H., Ristic, H., Lambert, M.P., Chromy, B., Viola, K.L., Klein, W.L., Stine, W.B., Krafft, G.A. & Trommer, B.L. (2002) Soluble oligomers of β amyloid (1-42) inhibit long-term potentiation but not long-term depression in rat dentate gyrus. *Brain Res.,* 924, 133-140.

Wang, H.Y., Lee, D.H., D'Andrea, M.R., Peterson, P.A., Shank, R.P. & Reitz, A.B. (2000) β-Amyloid1–42 binds to α7 nicotinic acetylcholine receptor with high affinity: implications for alzheimer's disease pathology. *J. Biol. Chem.,* 275, 5626-5632.

Wimo, A. & Prince, M.J. (2010) World Alzheimer Report 2010: the global economic impact of dementia, Alzheimer's Disease International.

Wong, P.T., Schauerte, J.A., Wisser, K.C., Ding, H., Lee, E.L., Steel, D.G. & Gafni, A. (2009) Amyloid-b Membrane binding and permeabilization are distinct processes influenced separately by membrane charge and fluidity. *J. Mol. Biol.,* 386, 81-96.

Wonnacott, S. (1997) Presynaptic nicotinic ACh receptors. TINS, 20, 92-98.

Woodruff-Pak, D. S., Vogel, R.W. 3rd, & Wenk, G.L. (2001) Galantamine: effect on nicotinic receptor binding, acetylcholinesterase inhibition, and learning. *Proc. Nat. Acad. Sci.*, 98, 2089-2094.

Yu, W., Mechawar, N., Krantic. S. & Quirion, R. (2011) α7 Nicotinic receptor activation reduces β-amyloid-induced apoptosis by inhibiting caspase-independent death through phosphatidylinositol 3-kinase signaling. *J. Neurochem.*, 119, 848-858.

INDEX

#

A

B

C

D

E

F

G

H

I

K

L

M

N

O

P

R

S

T

U

V

W

Z

A

B

Γ

Δ